Applied and Economic Zoology

A Textbook of Zoological Science

THE AUTHORS

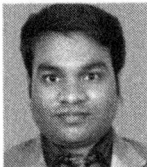

Dr. Ashok K. Rathoure shares his knowledge and experience in the field of Environment Impact Assessment with a doctoral degree in Bioremediation for M/s En-vision Group Surat. Previously he was associated with En-vision Enviro Engineers Pvt. Ltd. for EIA studies; Himachal Institute of Life Sciences Paonta and Beehive College of Ad. Studies Dehradun for teaching to Biotechnology, Microbiology, Biochemistry and other biosciences subjects. He is also associated as Editor-in-Chief for Octa Journal of Environmental Research, Managing Editor for Octa Journal of Biosciences and Executive Editor for Scientific India Magazine. His area of research is environmental biotechnology and publication includes 58 full length research papers in international and national journals of repute, 8 Course books from reputed publishers in India, 4 Research books and 6 Book chapters in Springer-verlag USA, CRC press Tayer & Francis Florida, I.K. Publishers Mumbai and Daya Publishers New Delhi, respectively. He had reviewed more than 70 research manuscript for many international journals. He is member of APCBEES (Hong Kong), IACSIT (Singapore), EFB (Spain), Society for Conservation Biology (Washington) and founder member of Scientific Planet Society (Dehradun). He has supervised 24 research scholars (UG, PG and Diploma). Dr. Rathoure was born in 1983 in village Hariharpur (UP) and completed his basic education in Hariharpur, Tandiyawan and Hardoi. He came to Kanpur for M.Sc. and was moved to Pauri for M.Tech. (G.B. Pant Engineering College) and has travelled extensively in the major cities of Northern and Western India for his education and as a teacher, trainer and taught to widen the horizon of knowledge and to sharpen his intellect. Moreover, He has also received PG Diploma in Human Resource Management (HRM) from Algappa University Karaikudi Tamilnadu.

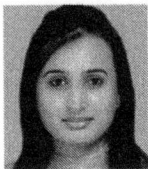

Dr. Nazneen Z. Deshmukh is working as an Assistant Professor in Department of Zoology, H.P.T. Arts and R.Y.K. Science College, Nasik (MS). She has about 5 years of teaching experience at undergraduate and postgraduate level. She is a gold medalist and topper of M.Sc. Zoology (2007) and she was awarded Ph.D. in Protozoology (2011) from Dr. B.A.M. University, Aurangabad. Dr. Deshmukh has intense experience of laboratory techniques including DNA Barcoding of Marine Fishes of India. She is member of editorial board of Trends in Biotechnology Research. She has presented many research papers in national and international conferences, seminars and symposia. She has published various research papers in national and international journals and received Young Scientist Award from the Society of Life Science in 2010.

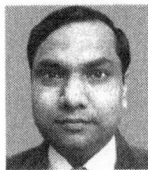

Dinesh Kumar has received his master degree in Biochemistry from Patna University in 2007, followed by M.Phil.in Biochemistry from Vinayaka Mission University in 2009. He is pursuing Ph.D. in Biochemistry in UTU, Dehradun since Feb 2010. He has also received MBA in HR from Sikkim Manipal University. His area of research is Isolation of bioactive compound and antimicrobial properties. His publication includes 10 full length research papers in international and national journals of repute. He has attained many conferences, workshops and seminars. He has undergone various pathological training and having industrial exposure. Presently, he is working as Senior Lecturer in Uttaranchal Dental and Medical Research Institute, Dehradun. He has more than 7 years of teaching experience.

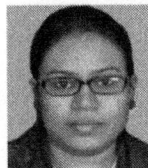

Rachna Goswami is working as Assistant Professor in Department of Zoology, Baba Ram Das Degree College, Bareilly, Uttar Pradesh. After completion of M.Sc. in Biotechnology from HNB Garhwal University, she joined C.C.S. University Meerut for B.Ed. She learnt extensively about Techniques used in Pharmaceutical, Composting of Bioremediation solid and liquid waste using Biotic sets and tissue culture techniques for *Ageratum houstonianum* etc. She has also undergone training from N.B.R.I. Lucknow, I.V.R.I. Bareilly, IPCA Laboratory. Her area of interest is Environmental Biotechnology, Microbial Biotechnology in the field of Environment. She is very active in research and development with her creative mind.

Applied and Economic Zoology

A Textbook of Zoological Science

– *Authors* –

Dr. Ashok K. Rathoure

Dr. Nazneen Z. Deshmukh

Dinesh Kumar

Rachna Goswami

2015

Daya Publishing House®

A Division of

Astral International Pvt. Ltd

New Delhi-110002

Cataloging in Publication Data—DK
Courtesy: D.K. Agencies (P) Ltd. <docinfo@dkagencies.com>

Rathoure, Ashok K., author.
  Applied and economic zoology : a textbook of zoological science / authors, Dr. Ashok K. Rathoure, Dr. Nazneen Z. Deshmukh, Dinesh Kumar, Rachna Goswami.
    pages   cm
  Includes bibliographical references (pages   ).
  ISBN 978-93-5130-687-0 (International Edition)

  1. Zoology, Economic—India. 2. Zoology, Economic. 3. Zoology, Medical—India. 4. Zoology, Medical. 5. Animals—India.   I. Deshmukh, Nazneen Z., author. II. Kumar, Dinesh (Senior lecturer in biochemistry), author. III. Goswami, Rachna, author. IV. Title.

DDC 591.60954   23

Published by   :   **Daya Publishing House®**
A Division of
Astral International Pvt. Ltd.
– ISO 9001:2008 Certified Company –
4760-61/23, Ansari Road, Darya Ganj
New Delhi-110 002
Ph. 011-43549197, 23278134
E-mail: info@astralint.com
Website: www.astralint.com

Laser Typesetting: **SSMG Computer Graphics,** Delhi - 110 084

Printed at   :   **Replika Press Pvt Ltd**

PRINTED IN INDIA

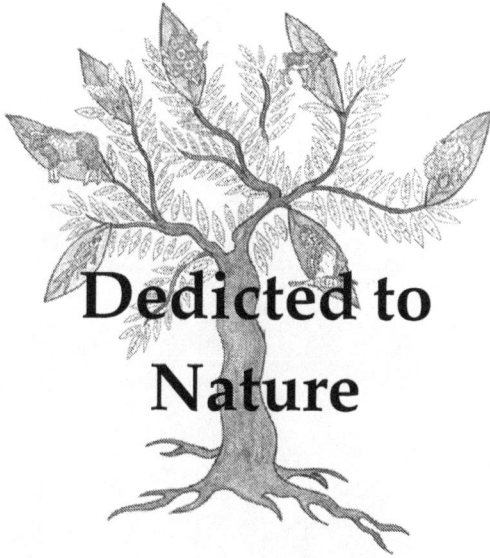
Dedicted to
Nature

Preface

Recently Applied and Economic Zoology has been included in national syllabus by UGC in unified syllabus for undergraduates. All these applied fields are very vast and it is hard to cover up all aspects of each field. The book examines insect pests, animal pests, natural enemies, beneficial insects, beneficial animals, agricultural chemicals and more. A foundation for learning various subjects had already been provided in the lower classes. The current book is blueprint for undergraduate students to aware about our natural wild life and its economic importance. The book contains four chapters with illustrations and boxed materials.

In the chapter 1, we have covered parasitology, in which we have deliberately discussed about parasites of domestic animals and human, structures, life cycles, pathogenicity, diseases, symptoms and it control. In chapter 2, we consciously talk about vectors and pests. Here, we covered life cycles and control of pest and vectors such as Gundhi bug, Sugarcane leafhopper, Rodents, Termites and Mosquitoes. Chapter 3 is about animal breeding and animal cultures. In this, we stared with basic introduction about breeding and culture, difference between them and then detailed discussion about Animals and Human Society, Animal Breeding, Genetic engineering applications in Animal Breeding, Breeding and Variation, Aquaculture, Pisciculture, Poultry farming, Sericulture, Apiculture, Lac-culture. The last chapter has wild life of India. In this chapter we provided detail for Wild Life Protection and Acts, Documentation of Wild Life, Rare, Endangered and Endemic species, Protected Area Network, Conservation of Wild Life, *In-situ* and *Ex-situ* conservation. Additional feature of this book includes boxed materials which enclose in depth explanation of some pertinent topics to extent the scope and coverage area beyond the main text.

This book will extensively assist students, teachers and academicians to further extend their knowledge beyond the course work and related subject. We did not claim perfection but if we get co-operation from the readers in the form of constructive suggestions, we hope, we would be able to improve it further in the next edition.

Authors

Acknowledgements

"By the grace of almighty, we have reached this opportunity to thank all those who have been instrumental in bringing this book to completion."

Book writing whether original or compilation is a tedious job requiring academic labor. The present book is purely a research compilation of literature from authorized publication/readings/excerpts/notes/reviews/researches/literature, authored by eminent scholars and distinguished writers. During research and compilation, the authors have also taken assistance/reference/literature from various websites through internet.

The authors, therefore humble acknowledge the contribution of all those eminent writers/scholars along with their respective publishers and websites from those learned writings/displays/references/literature have been taken while preparing the work.

Authors are also thankful to Dr. Meena Srivastava, Professor and Head Dept. of Zoology, MP Govt. PG College, Hardoi (UP), Prof. Akhilesh Kumar, Principal, M.P. Govt. (PG) College Hardoi (UP) India, Prof. B.S. Bisht, Dept. of Zoology, HNBGU (A Central University), SRT Campus Badshahithaul Tehri (Uttarakhand), India, Prof. N. Singh Dept. of Biotechnology and Zoology, Prof. S.C. Tiwari and Prof. J.P. Mehta, Dept. of Microbiology and Botany HNBGU (A Central University), Srinagar-Garhwal (Uttarakhand), Dr. D. K. Srivastava, Principal, Govt PG College, Rajajipuram, Lucknow (India), Dr. I.D. Singh, Ex Head, Dept. of Botany, M. P. Govt (PG) College Hardoi (UP), India, Dr. V.D. Joshi, Principal, Govt. PG College Purola, Uttarkashi (Uttarakhand) India, Dr. Manoj Bhatt, Dept. of Biotechnology, G.B. Pant Engineering College, Pauri-Garhwal, Dr. Arun Kumar, Director Research, Dolphin Institute of Biomedical and Natural Sciences, Dr. A. K. Chopra, Dr. P.C. Joshi, Dept. of Zoology, Gurukul Kangari University, Haridwar, Dr. Sanjay Gupta, Dept. of Biotech, SBS College Dehradun, Dr.Mrs. Susheel V. Nikam, Professor, Protozoology Laboratory, Department of Zoology, Dr. Babasaheb Ambedkar Marathwada University,

Aurangabad for discussions and valuable comments which have helped to improve the matter.

Our sincere thanks to all other friends and colleagues whose names we have not mentioned here for want of space.

Thank you all forever!!!

Authors

Contents

Chapter 1

Parasitology

1.1 Introduction

Parasitology is the study of parasites and their relationships to their hosts. While it is entirely proper to classify many bacteria and fungi and all viruses as parasites, parasitology has traditionally been limited to parasitic protozoa, helminthes and arthropod, as well as those species of arthropods that serve as vector for parasites. It follows that parasitology encompasses elements of protozoology, helminthology and medical arthropodology. Human parasitology, an important part of parasitology, studies the medical parasites including their morphology, life cycle, the relationship with host and environment. According to the very broad definition of parasitology, parasites should include the viruses, bacteria, fungi, protozoa and metazoa (multicelled organisms) which infect their host species. Parasites are living things which harm udders by becoming metabolically dependent on them. It is an old animal relationship based on the concept of dependence for nutrition and support. Parasitology is studied in a wide variety of headings and it is a dynamic aspect of zoology with links to other fields of sciences and social sciences. No biological association is of greater medical importance than parasitism. Parasites plague humanity and are at the root cause of many diseases especially in the tropics, the need for a dedicated branch of zoology to study these exciting but disturbing polyphyletic animal groups. Parasitology is an applied field of biology dedicated to the study of the biology, ecology and relationships which parasites are involved in with other organisms known as the host.

Depending on the specific bias, there are different fields of parasitology and some of these include medical parsitology, veterinary parasitology, structural parasitology, quantitative parasitology, parasite ecology, conservation of parasites, malariology, helminthology, parasite immunology etc. The term parasitism may be defined as a two species association in which one species *i.e.* parasite lives on or in a second species *i.e.* host for a significant period of its life and obtains nourishment from it. This is a commonly accepted working definition of parasitism and using it we can emphasize several important features of the host parasite relationship. The following are important features of parasitism:

a. Parasitism always involves two species *i.e.* parasite and host.

b. Many of these parasitic associations produce pathological changes in hosts that may result in disease.

c. Successful treatment and control of parasitic diseases requires not only comprehensive information about the parasite itself but also a good understanding of the nature of parasites' interactions with their hosts.

d. The parasite is always the beneficiary and the host is always the provider in any host parasite relationship.

This definition of parasitism is a general one but it tells us nothing about parasites themselves. It does not address which particular infectious organisms of domestic animals we might include in the realm of parasitology. The protozoa, arthropods and helminths are traditionally defined as parasites. However, there are members of the scientific community who designate all infectious agents of animals as parasites including viruses, bacteria and fungi. This broader definition of parasites includes viruses, bacteria and fungi as well as the arthropods, helminths and protozoa. Within this broad definition, parasites are further divided into microparasites and macroparasites. From the table 1.1, we can differentiate between micro and macro parasites.

Table 1.1: Microparasites and Macroparasites

S.No.	Micro-parasites	Macro-parasites
1.	Unicellular or acellular organisms.	Multicellular organisms.
2.	Usually multiply in the host so that a few infecting organisms may give rise to many in a non-immune host.	Rarely multiply in a host.
3.	Short generation time, hours or days.	Long generation time, usually weeks or months.
4.	Acute infections most commonly seen. Infected animals may succumb, may recover and show significant protective immunity or the infection may, in some cases revert to a chronic state.	Chronic infections are most commonly seen but acute infections may be seen in young, susceptible animals. Recovery from acute infections does not necessarily confer immune protection on the host.
5.	Bacteria, Viruses, Fungi, Protozoa.	Arthropods, Helminths.

Parasites are an extremely varied group. They range from flies, such as the blood sucking mosquitoes, nematodes such as the heartworm of dogs, liver flukes of cattle and sheep, fleas commonly found on dogs and cats, lice and ticks found on almost all domestic animals and protozoa such as Giardia which are found in most domestic animals but are of particular significance in cattle and dogs. An important feature to note about parasites is that they are not equally parasitic. Parasitism is seen as a spectrum. It includes organisms at one of the spectrum that spend most or all of their lives as independent free living creatures, seeking a host only to feed. The other end of the spectrum includes parasites that spend their entire lives in or on a host and cannot survive at any stage of their life cycles without a host. Between these two extremes we see a whole host of parasitic configurations with differing degrees of host dependency.

(i) Protozoa (Greek words: protos = first and zoon = animal)

The protozoan parasites are fall into the following groups:

- Protozoa transmitted by resistant cysts.
- Protozoa transmitted through coitus.
- Protozoa transmitted by insects.
- Protozoa transmitted by ticks.

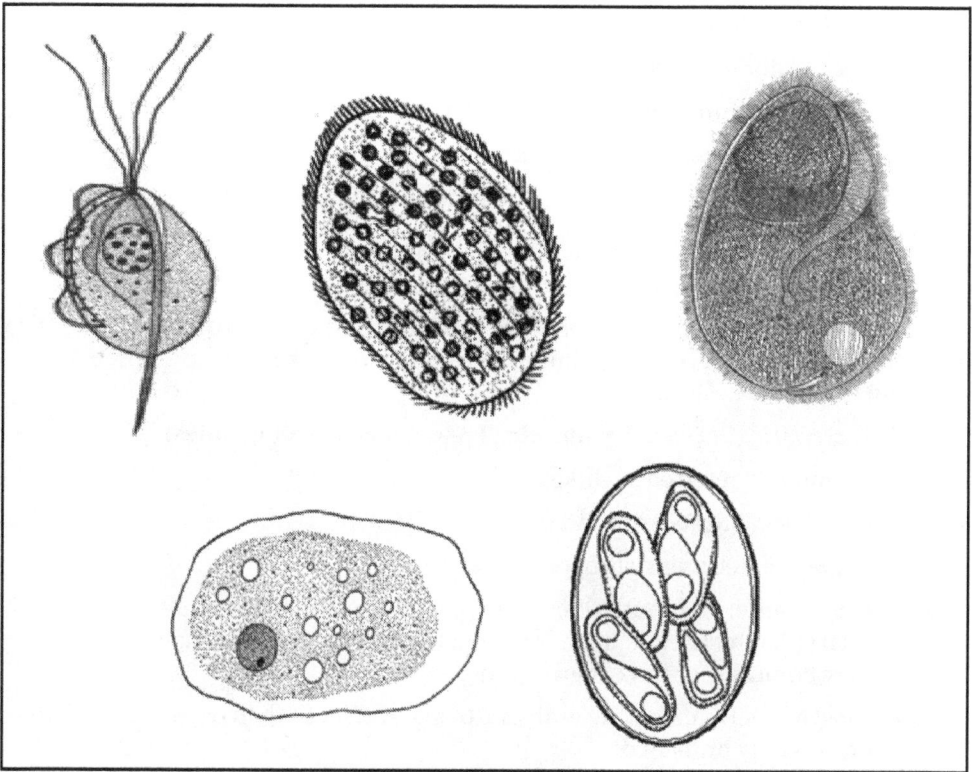

Mastigophora- *Trichomonas*

Sarcodina- *Entamoeba*

Apicomplexa - *Eimeria*

Ciliophora - *Opalina* and *Nyctotherus*

Figure 1.1: Protozoa

(ii) Helminths (Greek word helminth or helminthos = worm)

The helminth parasites fall into three groups:

- Trematodes (Flukes).
- Cestodes (Tapeworms).
- Nematodes (Roundworms).

The helminths of medical and veterinary importance belong to:

(a) Phylum Platyhelminthes.

(b) Phylum Nematoda (Roundworms).

(c) Phylum Acanthocephala (Sting headed worms).

(a) Phylum Playhelminthes

- Body is dorsoventrally flattened.
- Bialateral symmetry.
- No definite anus, no body cavity.
- Organ embedded in specialized connective tissue.
- Usually hermaphrodite.
- Respiratory and circulatory systems absent.

There are four classes in the phylum Platyhelminthes. Two of these Tubellaria and Monogenea are of no medical importance. The two classes of medical importance are Trematoda and Cestoda.

Characteristics of Class Trematoda (Trematodes = having holes)

- Commonly referred as flukes.
- Parasitic, with suckers and sometimes hooks.
- Unsegmented; consists of only one piece.
- Has an anterior mouth often with oral sucker and a muscular pharynx which leads to an intestine which is usually bifurcated but may be simple or have many branches.
- Most are hermaphrodite with one ovary and more than one testis. T h e s e organs may branched.
- Eggs are encapsulated (operculated at one pole).

Of the three orders within Class Trematoda only the order Digenea is of medical importance. The order Monogena is mostly ectoparasites of cold blooded aquatic vertebrates while the order Aspidogastrea is mostly endoparasites of aquatic hosts.

Digenic Trematodes: These constitute the flukes which parasitize the domestic animals and man. Fish can be the primary or intermediate host depending on the digenean species. They are found externally or internally, in any organ. For the majority of digenean trematodes, pathogenicity to the host is limited. The characteristics of digenic trematodes include:

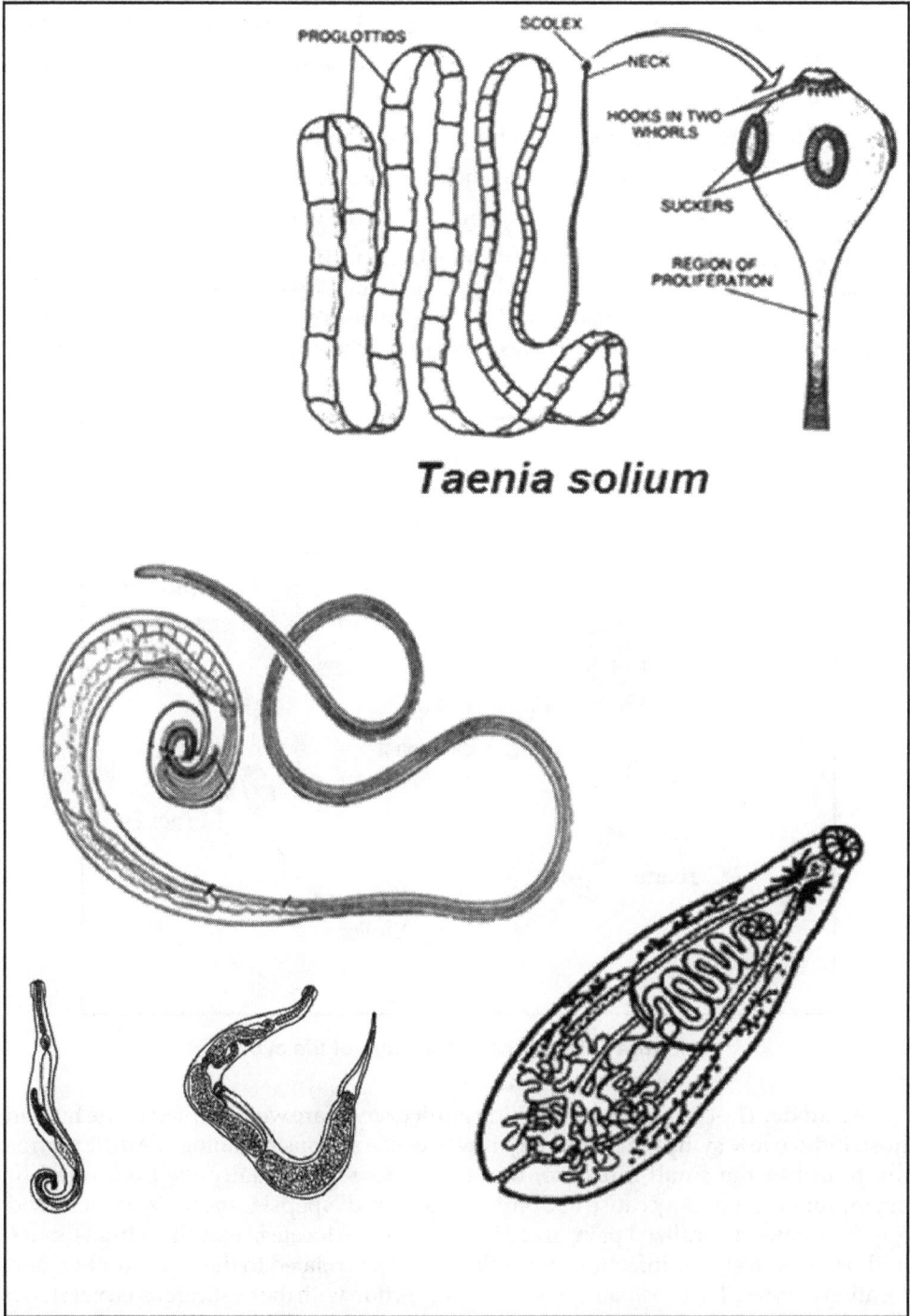

Taenia solium

Figure 1.2: Adult Heminth Parasites

- Most are dorsoventrally flattened but some may be rounded. Majority are long and narrow, some are leaf shaped while some have thick fleshy bodies.
- The tegument (body covering) is usually smooth, although it can be spiny in a few trematodes.
- There are two organs of attachment. These are:
  - Anterior sucker = oral sucker (surrounds mouth at the anterior end).
  - Ventral sucker = Acetabulum (on the ventral surface).

In a group of trematodes (holostomes), an additional large adhesive organ call holdfast occurs behind the acetabulum. Another fluke is Clinostonum, often called yellow grub. It is a large trematode and although it does not cause any major problems for fish, it is readily seen and will make fish unmarketable for aesthetic reasons.

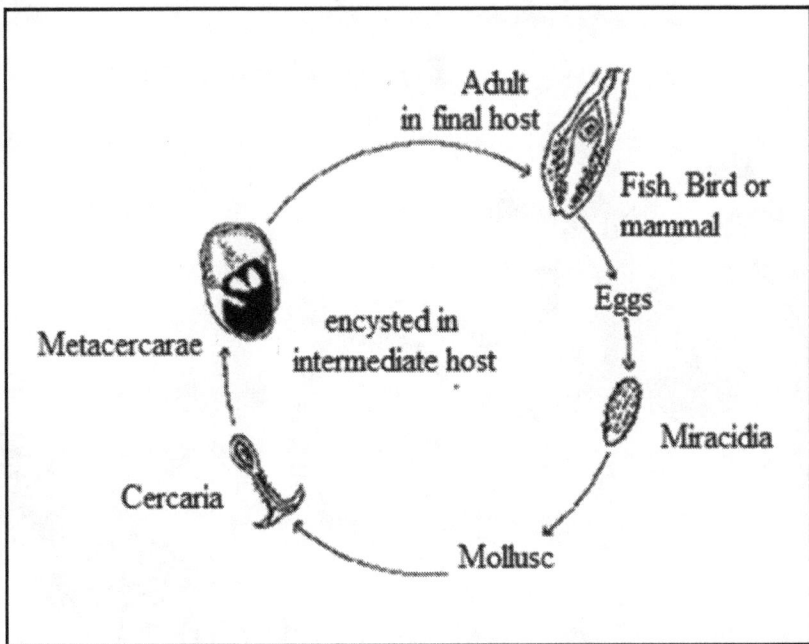

Figure 1.3: Metacercaria stage of life cycle

Cestode: The common gut-dwelling adult _cestodes_ are well adapted to the human host, induce few symptoms and only rarely cause serious pathology. Adult worms are found in the small intestine; these infections are usually well tolerated or asymptomatic, but may cause abdominal distress, dyspepsia, anorexia or increased appetite, nausea, localized pain, and diarrhea. Larvae locate in extraintestinal tissues and produce systemic infections with clinical effects related to the size, number, and location of cysts. _Taenia solium_ cysticercosis (infection with the cysticercus larval stage) is often asymptomatic and chronic; neurocysticercosis, ophthalmic cysticercosis, and subcutaneous and muscular cysticercosis are, however, frequently and other organs,

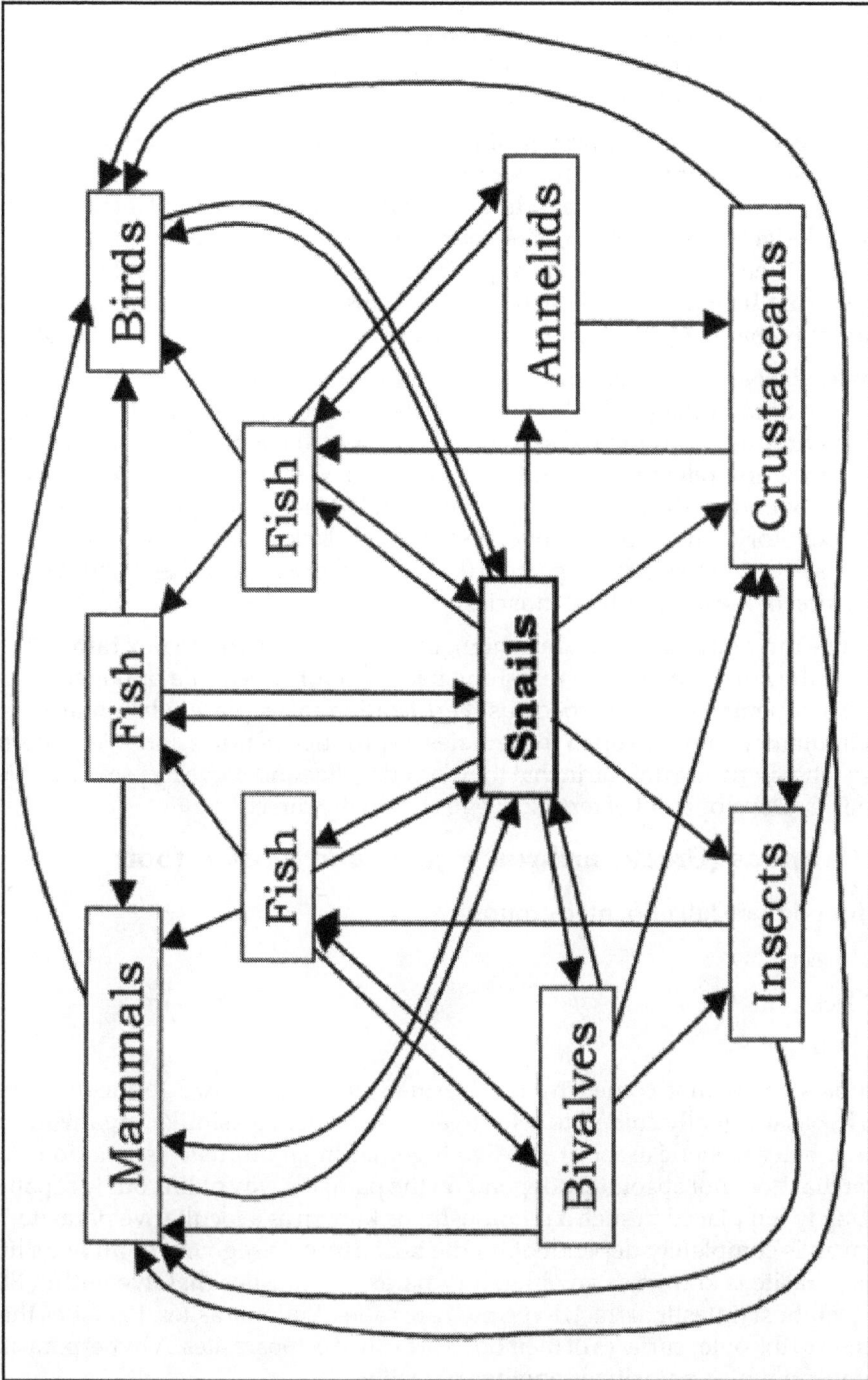

Figure 1.4: Transmission of Digenic Trematodes

including long bones and the central nervous system. Adults, which mature sexually in the definitive or final host, are ribbon-shaped, multisegmented, hermaphroditic flatworms; each segment has a complete male and female reproductive system. An anterior holdfast organ (the scolex) is followed by a germinative portion (neck) and segments at successively later stages of development.

Larvae encyst in various tissues of the intermediate host; larval cysts contain one or many scoleces of future adult worms. Tapeworms are ribbon-shaped multi-segmented flatworms that dwell as adults entirely in the human small intestine. The larval forms lodge in skin, liver, muscles, the central nervous system, or any of various other organs. Their life cycles involve a specialized pattern of survival and transfer to specific intermediate hosts, by which they are transferred to another human host. Each pattern is characteristic of a given tapeworm species.

Nematode: Nematodes are structurally simple organisms. Adult nematodes are comprised of approximately 1,000 somatic cells, and potentially hundreds of cells associated with the reproductive system. Nematodes have been characterized as a tube within a tube; referring to the alimentary canal which extends from the mouth on the anterior end, to the anus located near the tail. Nematodes possess digestive, nervous, excretory, and reproductive systems, but lack a discrete circulatory or respiratory system. In size they range from 0.3 mm to over 8 meters. Nematodes move by contraction of the longitudinal muscles.

Because their internal pressure is high, this causes the body to flex rather than flatten, and the animal moves by thrashing back and forth. No cilia or flagellae are present. Most nematodes are dioecious. Fertilization takes place when males use special copulatory spines to open the females' reproductive tracts and inject sperm into them. The sperm are unique in that they lack flagellae and move by pseudopodia, like amoebas. Development of fertilized eggs is usually direct.

(iii) Arthropods (Greek: arthron = joint and pous = foot)

The Arthropods are fall into three groups:

- Insects,
- Ticks,
- Mites.

Symbiosis was first coined by the German de Bary in 1879 to mean living togetherIt was originally coined to refer to all cases where dissimilar organisms or species *e.g.* heterogenetic associations live together in an intimate association. An organism that does not absolutely depend on the parasitic way of life, but is capable of adapting to it if placed in such a relationship is known as a facultative parasite. If an organism is completely dependent on the host during a segment or all of its life cycle the parasite is known as an obligatory parasite. Parasites that live within the body of their host (intestinal tract, liver, etc.) are called Endoparasites. Parasites that are attached to the outer surfaces of their hosts are called ectoparasites. A hyperparasite is an organism which parasitizes another parasite.

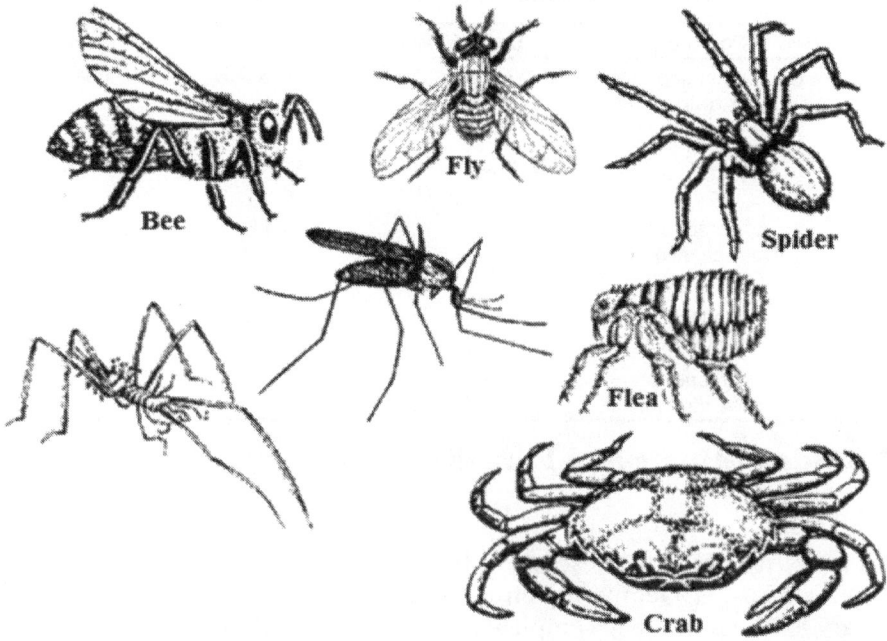

Figure 1.5a: Arthropods

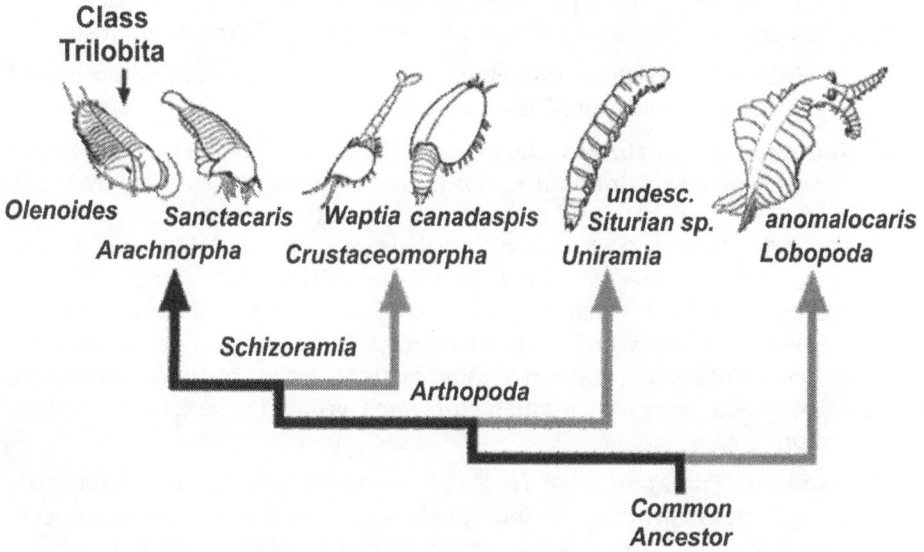

Figure 1.5b: Primitive Arthropods

Table 1.2: Taxonomic classification of Protozoa

Sub-kingdom	Phylum	Sub-phylum	Genus	Species
Protozoa	Sarcomastigophora (Further divided into 2 sub-	Sarcodina(Move by pseudopodia)	Entamoeba	*E. histolytica*
		Mastigophora(Move by flagella)	Giardia	*G. lamblia*
	Apicomplexa (No organelle of locomotion)	-	Plasmodium	*P. falciparum, P. vivax, P. malariae,P. ovale*
	Ciliophora (Move by cilia)		Balantidium	*B. coli*
	Microspora (Spore forming)	-	Enterocytozoa	*E. bienusi*

1.2 Kinds of Hosts and Parasites

1.2.1 Host

A definitive host is the host in which the parasite becomes sexually mature. An intermediate host is a temporary environment for the parasite, but is nonetheless necessary for the parasite to complete its life cycle. Parasites do not reach sexually maturity in an intermediate host; they can undergo asexual reproduction in this type of host. A paramedic (transfer host) is one in which the parasite does not undergo development, but one in which it remains alive and infective to another host. Any organisms (typically arthropods) that serve as intermediate hosts as well as carriers for protozoans and other small parasites are called vectors. Animals that harbor an infection that can be transmitted to humans are referred to as reservoir hosts.

- **Definitive host or Primary host:** Harbors the adult or sexually mature stage of the parasite (Mosquito-Plasmodium).

- **Intermediate host/Secondary host:** This is the host which harbors the developing larval, immature, and juvenile young stages of a parasite. The intermediate host may harbor many immature stages of a parasite *e.g.* Cercaria, Redia and Sporocysts which are all immature stages of Fasciola in the snail intermediate host. Some parasites require more than one intermediate host which is designated as first, second intermediate, etc. The parasitic disease which require intermediate hosts for transmission are restricted to the distribution of those hosts. The distribution of intermediate hosts is determined by many factors such as climate, vegetation, historical factors, etc.

- **Paratenic/Transport host:** This is a host in which the immature stage of the parasite does not normally undergo development but only remains encysted until the paratenic host is consumed by the final host *e.g.* second stage larva of Toxocara in chickens, lambs, rodent, invertebrates, etc.

- **Reservoir host:** This is a vertebrate host in which a parasite or disease occurs naturally and which is a source of infection for man or domestic animals.

The parasite usually exists in massive numbers in a reservoir host and man or domestic animal may become infected when they enter the locality where the parasites or diseases exist. Such a locality is known as ridus and is used primarily in connection with vector borne diseases.

- **Tangenital/Incidental host:** This is a host which is only infected with a parasite circumstantially.

- **Carrier:** A carrier is an animal or man which has a light infection with a parasite but is not harmed by it, usually due to immunity resulting from previous infection, but which serves as a source of infection for susceptible animals or men. For example:

  (a) Adult sheep and cattle may be lightly infected with gastrointestinal nematodes without noticeable effect, but their lambs and calves may become heavily parasitized from grazing with them. The condition in the adults is called parasitiasis and in the young, parasitosis.

  (b) Chickens rarely suffer from coccidiosis because they have recovered from a clinical or subclinical attack when they were young. However, they still harbor a light infection and continue to shed fee oocysts (coccidiasis) which is a source of infection to the young chicks.

  (c) Cattle previously exposed to anaplasmosis become pre-immune to the infection (few parasites in the blood) but continue to be a source of infection to the ticks.

- **Vector:** This is an organism usually an arthropod which transfers infective forms of a parasite from one host to the other. We differentiate between a mechanical and a biological vector. In a mechanical vector, the parasite does not undergo development before the transfer to another host is affected. Biological vector is characterized by the development of the parasite before its transfer to another host.

1.2.2 Parasites

The parasite is an organism which lives in or on another organism (its host) and benefits by deriving nutrients at the other's expense. In mid 16th century: via Latin from Greek *parasitos* (person) eating at another's table from *para-* alongside + *sitos* food. There are different types of parasites:

(a) **Ectoparasites:** Parasites which live on body surfaces of the host *e.g.* lice, fleas, ticks, etc.

(b) **Endoparasites:** Parasites which live inside the host body in tissues or organs such as blood, peritoneal cavity, brain, etc. *e.g.* liver fluke, Ascaris, malaria parasites, etc.

(c) **Facultative parasite:** An organism which is able to live either a free living or parasitic existence *e.g.* Strongyloids Stercoralis of man.

(d) **Obligatory parasite:** Organism which has become completely dependent upon its host for existence.

(e)   **Aberrant parasite:** Found in locations in the host where they normally do not occur *e.g.* Ascaris larvae may migrate to the brain.

(f)   **Insidental parasite:** Occurs in hosts where it does not normally occur *e.g.* Fasciola normally does not occur in man but is incidental if found in man's liver.

(g)   **Periodic parasite:** Feeds on host but does not live on host *e.g.* blood sucking flies.

(h)   **Hyperparasite:** Parasitizes another parasite *e.g. Histomonas meleagridis* (a protozoan) is hyperprsitic on the nematode worm *Heterakis gallinae.*

(i)   **Monoxenous parasites:** Those with direct life cycles *i.e.* within one host.

(j)   **Heteroxenous parasites:** Those with indirect life cycles requiring an intermediate host *i.e.* involves 2 or more hosts.

(k)   **Heterogenetic Parasites:** One with alteration of generations *e.g.* Coccidial parasites and Strongyloides.

(l)   **Euryxenous parasites:** Those with a broad host range.

(m)   **Stenoxenous parasites:** Those with a narrow host range *e.g.* host specific coccidia.

1.3 Branches of Parasitology

There are many branches of parasitology. Some of them are described here.

*   **Medical parasitology:** This is the science that deals with organisms living in the human body (host) and the medical significance of host parasite relationship. It's also concerned with the various methods of their diagnosis, treatment and finally their prevention and control.

*   **Veterinary parasitology:** The study of parasites that cause economic losses in agriculture or aquaculture operations or which infect companion animals. This is becoming particularly important as emerging diseases threatens global food security.

*   **Structural parsitology:** This is the study of structures of proteins from parasites. Determination of parasitic protein structures may help to better understand how these proteins function differently from homologous proteins in humans. In addition, protein structures may inform the process of drug discovery.

*   **Quantitative parasitology:** Parasites exhibit an aggregated distribution among host individuals, thus the majority of parasites live in the minority of hosts. This feature forces parasitologists to use advanced biostatistical methodologies.

*   **Parasite ecology:** Parasites can provide information about host population ecology. In fisheries biology, parasite communities can be used to distinguish distinct populations of the same fish species co-inhabiting a region. Additionally, parasites possess a variety of specialized traits and life history

strategies that enable them to colonize hosts. Understanding these aspects of parasite ecology can illuminate parasite avoidance strategies employed by host.

- **Malariology:** This is an aspect of parasitology which focuses mainly on the study of Protozon parasite, *Plasmodium,* its species, their biology, pathogenicity, epidemiology and management of the parasitic infection.

- **Helminthology:** Helminth means worms. Hence as the name implies it is the study of vermiform parasites ranging from trematodes to Cestodans, Nematodans and leeches.

- **Parasite immunology:** This is an aspect which deals with parasite survival in host as well as host susceptibility. This aspect is particularly important when formulating concentrations of chemotherapeutic agents and vaccines.

1.4 Parasites of Domestic Animals and Humans

Parasites are dynamic in their distribution; some are endemic while many are ubiquitous. The environment plays a key role in their survival and transmission. Generally, they rely of vectors mostly arthropods, for their transmission. By virtue of their nature, parasites reside in their hosts, depend on their hosts for physiological and nutritional ends and hence result in adverse effects on their host. The parasite-host interaction does not occur in isolation; rather it is affected by conditions known as risk factors.

A risk factor which must occur for a disease situation to arise is known as the necessary risk while the organism/parasite which causes the disease is called an agent. The causal web is a simple triangle which shows the inevitable link between the agent (parasite), the host and the environment. Organisms live within various habitats ranging from air, water and soil; interacting with each other in the environment. These associations are characterized by diverse benefits such as provision of food, transport, protection, etc. Within the environment, living organisms exhibit diverse forms of associations which may be broadly divided to two categories namely:

- Homospecific/Intraspecific/ Homogenetic,
- Heterospecific/Interspecific/Heterogametic.

Phoresis (Transport commensalism) is a form of loose association in which an organism provides shelter, support or transport for the other organism, usually a sedentary animal of a different species. The passenger can survive without its usually motile substratum or attachment surface. There is no conflict of interest in this association. Examples are barnacles on limpet mollusks, dung beetle, *Aphodius fimentarius* carrying dauver lavae of *Pledora coactatata* (free living nematode which feeds on bacteria) etc.

Commensalism (Co= together, Mensa= table) is an association between two organisms in which one benefits, but the host is not hurt nor injured. It usually occurs between species that are either vulnerable to predation, danger or with an inefficient means of locomotion, feeding or defense. It is the most indefinite and least obligatory inter specific relationship. The host neither benefits nor looses in the relationship.

Mutualism: This is a non-competitive, physiologically interdependent association between organisms of two different species. It is considered as the most advanced form of symbiosis because it involves reciprocal benefits. They always live together and mutualism is recognized as a special case of parasitism, in which metabolic by-products of the associates are of value to the partners *e.g. Trichonympha campanula* (intestinal flagellates) feeds on the wood chips in the gut of termites and wood roaches. They by-products of cellulose digestion and cellulose of the flagellated protozoan are useful to the insect. The sexual reproduction of the protozoa is stimulated and regulated by the insect molting hormone, ecdysome. The anaerobic environment of the insect's gut is integral to the survival of the flagellate. The two organisms depend on each other for survival. Physiological dependence is an essential component of mutualistic relationships.

Nematode Parasites of Animals

Of the eighteen Orders in the phylum Nematoda, seven contain nematodes that are parasites or associates of invertebrates and six include species that are parasites of vertebrate animals. Nematodes are reported as parasites and associates of many invertebrate animals, especially in the Annelida, Mollusca and Arthropoda. In some cases, the invertebrate functions as the intermediate host in a life cycle that includes parasitism of a vertebrate. In other cases, the invertebrate, usually an insect, functions as a vector between vertebrate hosts or the nematode is passively transported by the insect. Several interesting plant-parasitic nematodes fall into this latter group and, significantly, they are closely related to nematode species that are parasites of insects. A considerable research effort has been applied toward using nematode parasites of insects as biological control agents *e.g.* mosquitos and black flies. Some of the nematode associates of insects are important because they vector bacteria that kill the insect. The nematode invades or is consumed by the insect and bacteria are released into the insect hemolymph. When the insect is dead or near death, growth and subsequent development of nematodes occur as they utilize essential steroids supplied by the insect. These nematodes are also used extensively in the biological control of insects and are particularly effective against those insects that pass through at least one life stage in the soil. Some 5,000 species of nematodes are estimated to be parasites of vertebrate animals and humans. These species are characterized in a larger group of worm parasites as helminths. Nematode parasites of domestic vertebrate animals are managed by strategies that include control of secondary hosts or vectors and the use of chemical anthelminthics. Helminth infections of wild animals are not managed, except by attrition of infected individuals. As human demography patterns change throughout the world, the interface between the ranges and habitats of wild and domestic animals change and overlap. Consequently, the pattern of exposure of domestic animals to helminth infections is also changing and new associations continue to be reported; the incidence of heartworm (*Dirofilaria immitis*) infection in dogs is currently increasing. Both freshwater and marine fish are subject to nematode infections. The impact of the infections on the health and longevity of fish in nature is generally unknown. Frequently, nematodes are observed in the tissues of fish purchased by consumers. The nematodes are usually killed during cooking, but certainly the transfer of live fish parasites to humans can occur during consumption of sashimi and other raw fish products. Generally, these nematodes will not establish a permanent infection in humans, but they may cause intestinal disorders in attempting to do so.

Humans

There are other well known examples of the transfer of nematodes to humans. In most cases, the incidence of infection is relatively low due to regulatory inspection of food products, public educationand cooking of food. An example is trichinosis caused by the nematode *Trichinella spiralis*. Humans become infected by *Trichinella* by eating raw or undercooked pork. The nematode parasites of humans cause a variety of disease conditions and symptoms, ranging from lack of energy and vigor to blindness and malformations. Pinworms, hookwormsand roundworms are extremely common intestinal helminth infections of humans; worldwide, roundworms are probably the most common. Pinworm transmittal generally occurs through ingestion of fecal contaminated material and infection occurs commonly in children. Other helminth infections are vectored as filarial worms by insects such as mosquitosor the filaria may penetrate directly through the skin from water or soil. Filarial worms cause such diseases as river blindness (*Onchocerca volvulus*) and elephantiasis which are major health problems in some third world countries. Most helminth infections of humans can be controlled by public health programmes, public education, vector control, intermediate host control and anthelminthic drugs.

Helminth Parasites

The word helminth is a general term meaning worm, but there are many different types of worms. Prefixes are therefore used to designate types such as platyhelminths for flat-worms and nematohelminths for round-worms. All helminths are multicellular eukaryotic invertebrates with tube like or flattened bodies exhibiting bilateral symmetry. They are triploblastic (with endo, meso and ecto-dermal tissues) but the flatworms are acoelomate (do not have body cavities) while the roundworms are pseudocoelomate with body cavities not enclosed by mesoderm. In contrast, segmented annelids such as earthworms are coelomate with body cavities enclosed by mesoderm. Many helminths are free living organisms in aquatic and terrestrial environments whereas others occur as parasites in most animals and some plants. Parasitic helminths are an almost universal feature of vertebrate animals; most species have worms in them somewhere. Three major assemblages of parasitic helminths are recognized; Nemathelminthes (nematodes) and Platyhelminthes (flatworms), the latter being subdivided into Cestoda (tapeworms) and the Trematoda (flukes). Nematodes (roundworms) have long thin un-segmented tube like bodies with anterior mouths and longitudinal digestive tracts. They have a fluid filled internal body cavity (pseudocoelum) which acts as a hydrostatic skeleton providing rigidity, so called tubes under pressure. Worms use longitudinal muscles to produce a sideways thrashing motion. Adult worms form separate sexes with well developed reproductive systems.

Cestodes (tapeworms) have long flat ribbon like bodies with a single anterior holdfast organ (scolex) and numerous segments. They do not have a gut and all nutrients are taken up through the tegument.

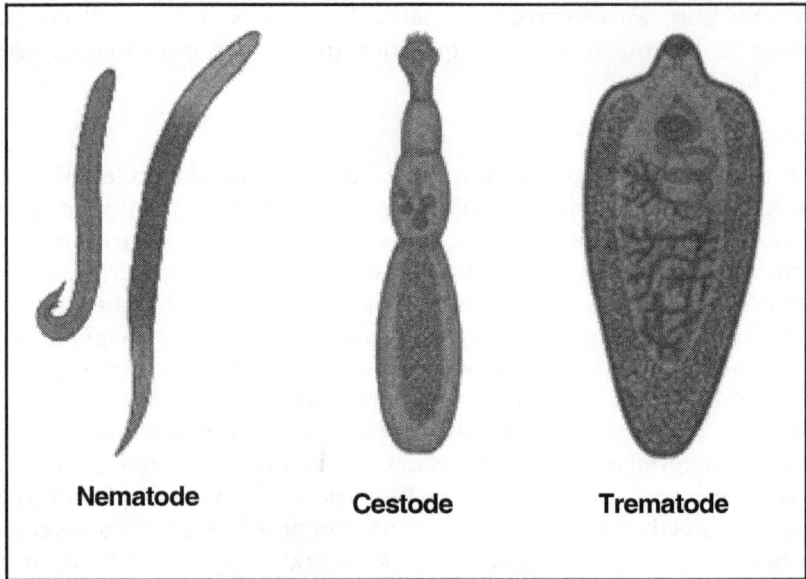

Figure 1.6: Helminths

They do not have a body cavity (acoelomate) and are flattened to facilitate perfusion to all tissues. Segments exhibit slow body flexion produced by longitudinal and transverse muscles. All tapeworms are hermaphroditic and each segment contains both male and female organs. Trematodes (flukes) have small flat leaf like bodies with oral and ventral suckers and a blind sac like gut. They do not have a body cavity (acoelomate) and are dorsoventrally flattened with bilateral symmetry. They exhibit elaborate gliding or creeping motion over substrates using compact 3D arrays of muscles. Most species are hermaphroditic (individuals with male and female reproductive systems) although some blood flukes form separate male and female adults.

Unlike other pathogens such as viruses, bacteria, protozoa and fungi, helminths do not proliferate within their hosts. Worms grow, moult, mature and then produce offspring which are voided from the host to infect new hosts. Worm burdens in individual hosts and the severity of infection are therefore dependent on intake, number of infective stages taken up. Worms develop slowly compared to other infectious pathogens so any resultant diseases are slow in onset and chronic in nature. Although, most helminth infections are well tolerated by their hosts and are often asymptomatic, subclinical infections have been associated with significant loss of condition in infected hosts. Other helminths cause serious clinical diseases characterized by high morbidity and mortality. Clinical signs of infection vary considerably depending on the site and duration of infection. Larval and adult nematodes lodge, migrate or encyst within tissues resulting in obstruction, inflammation, oedema, anaemia, lesions and granuloma formation. Infections by adult cestodes are generally benign as they are not invasive, but the larval stages penetrate and encyst within tissues leading to inflammation, space occupying lesions and organ malfunction. Adult flukes usually cause obstruction, inflammation and fibrosis in tubular organs, but the eggs of blood flukes can lodge in tissues causing extensive granulomatous reactions and hypertension.

Taxonomy of Helminth

Two classes of nematodes are recognized on the basis of the presence or absence of special chemoreceptors known as phasmids; Secernentea (Phasmidea) and Adenophorea (Aphasmidea). While many different orders are recognized within these classes, the main parasitic assemblages infecting humans and domestic animals include one aphasmid order (Trichocephalida) and 6 phasmid orders (Oxyurida, Ascaridida, Strongylida, Rhabditida, Camallanida and Spirurida). The trichocephalid whipworms have long thin anterior ends which they embed in the intestinal mucosa of their hosts. They have simple life cycles where infections are acquired by the ingestion of eggs and emergent larvae moult and mature to adults in the gut. *Trichuris* infections in humans may cause inflammation, tenesmus, straining and rectal prolapse. Oxyurid pin worms have small thin bodies with blunt anterior ends. They have simple life cycles, but with an unusual modification. Female worms emerge from the anus of their hosts at night and attach eggs to the skin. This causes peri-anal itching and eggs are transferred by hand to mouth. Infections by *Enterobius* cause irritability and sleeplessness in humans, especially children.

i.   **Ascarid roundworms:** They have large bodies with 3 prominent anterior lips. Their life cycles involve a stage of pulmonary migration where larvae released from ingested eggs invade the tissues and migrate through the lungs before returning to the gut to mature as adults. *Ascaris* infections in humans cause gastroenteritis, protein depletion and malnutrition and heavy infections can cause gut obstruction.

ii. **Strongyle hookworms:** They have dorsally curved mouths armed with ventral cutting plates or teeth which they embed in host tissues to feed on blood. They have complex life cycles where larvae develop in the external environment (as geo-helminths) before infecting hosts by penetrating the skin. Once inside, they undergo pulmonary migration before settling in the gut to feed. Heavy infections by *Ancylostoma* and *Necator* cause severe iron deficient anaemia in humans, especially children.

iii. **Rhabditid threadworms:** They have tiny bodies which become embedded in the host mucosa. Their life cycle includes parasitic parthenogenetic females producing eggs which may hatch internally leading to auto infection or externally leading to transmission of infection or formation of free living male and female adults. Super infections by *Strongyloides* may cause severe haemorrhagic enteritis in humans.

iv. **Camallanid guinea worms:** They infect host tissues where the large females cause painful blisters on the feet and legs. When hosts seek relief by immersion in water, the blisters rupture releasing live larvae which infect copepods that are subsequently ingested with contaminated drinking water. The fiery serpents mentioned in historical texts are thought to refer to *Dracunculus* infections. The spirurid filarial worms occur as long thread like adults in blood vessels or connective tissues of their hosts. The large female worms release live larvae (microfilariae) into the blood or tissues which are taken up by blood sucking mosquitoes or pool feeding flies and transmitted to new hosts. *Onchocerca* infections cause nodules, skin lesions and blindness in humans, while those of *Wuchereria* cause elephantitis.

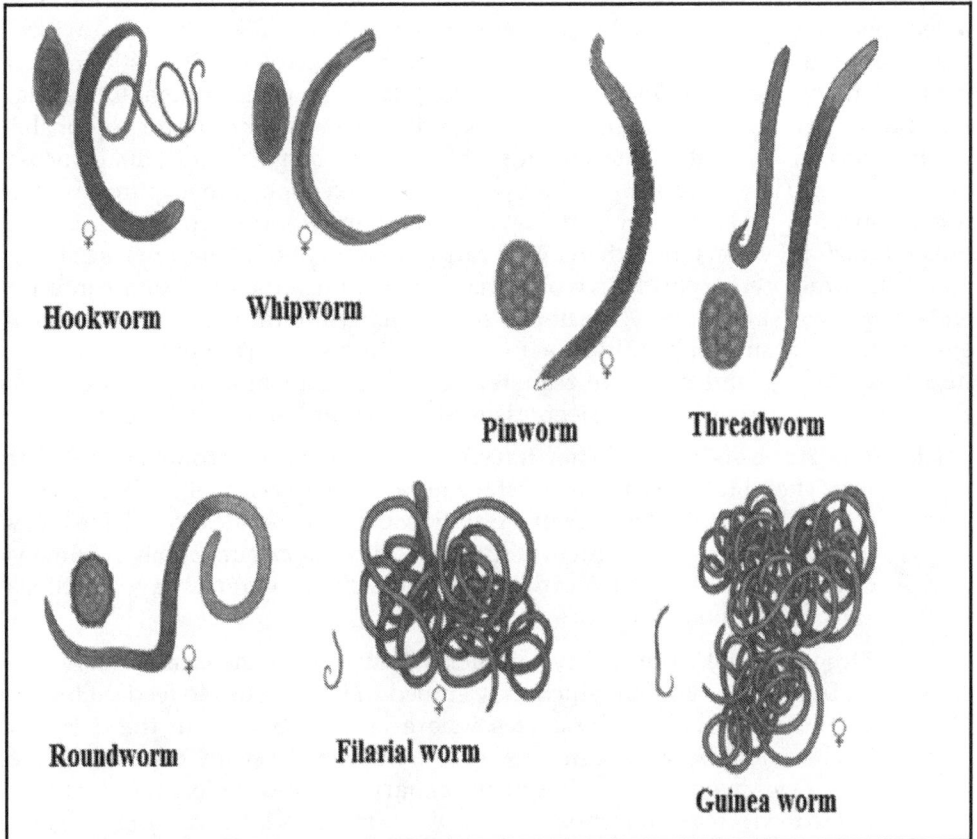

Figure 1.7: Different types of Helminths parasite

Two subclasses of cestodes are differentiated on the basis of the numbers of larval hooks, the Cestodaria being decacanth (10 hooks) and Eucestoda being hexacanth (6 hooks). Collectively, 14 orders of cestodes have been identified according to differences in parasite morphology and developmental cycles. Two orders have particular significance as parasites of medical and veterinary importance.

   a. **Cyclophyllidean cestodes:** They have terrestrial 2 host life cycles where adult tapeworms develop in carnivores (scolex with 4 suckers and sometimes hooks) while larval metacestodes form bladder like cysts in the tissues of herbivores. The larvae of *Taenia* spp. cause cysticercosis in cattle, pigs and humans, while those of *Echinococcus* cause hydatid disease in humans, domestic and wild animals.

b. **Pseudophyllidean cestodes:** They have aquatic 3 host life cycles, involving the sequential formation of adult tapeworms in fish eating animals (scolex with 2 longitudinal bothria), procercoid larval stages in aquatic invertebrates (copepods) and then plerocercoid (spargana) stages in fish *e.g. Diphyllobothrium* in humans, dogs and cats being transmitted through copepods and fish.

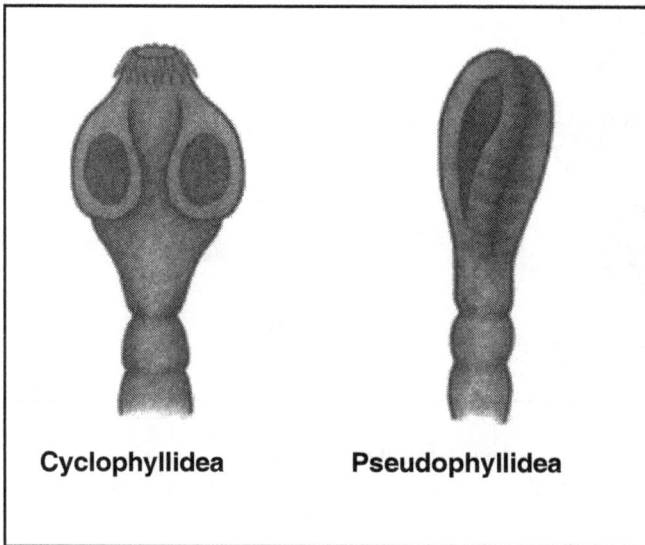

Cyclophyllidea **Pseudophyllidea**

Figure 1.8: Cyclophyllidea and Pseudophyllidea

Two major groups of trematodes are recognized on the basis of their structure and development; monogenean trematodes with complex posterior adhesive organs and direct life cycles involving larvae called oncomiracidia; and digenean trematodes with oral and posterior suckers and heteroxenous life cycles where adult worms infect vertebrates and larval miracidia infect molluscs to proliferate and produce free swimming cercariae. Monogenea are almost exclusively ectoparasites of fishes while Digenea are endoparasites in many vertebrate hosts and have snails as vectors. Some 10 digenean orders are recognized on the basis of morphologic and biologic differences, two orders of particular medical and veterinary significance.

a. **Echinostomatid fasciolids** (*liver flukes*): They live as adults in hepatic bile ducts of mammals where they cause fibrotic pipestem disease. The parasites proliferate in freshwater snails and mammals become infected by ingesting metacercariae attached to aquatic vegetation. Several *Fasciola* sp. cause hepatic disease in domestic ruminants and occasionally in humans.

b. **Strigeatid schistosomes** (*blood flukes*): They are unusual in that the adults are not hermaphroditic but form separate sexes which live conjoined in mesenteric veins in mammals. Female worms lay eggs which actively penetrate tissues to be excreted in urine/faeces or they become trapped in organs where they cause granuloma formation. Miracidia released from eggs infect aquatic snails and produce fork tailed cerceriae which actively penetrate the skin of their hosts. Several *Schistosoma* sp. cause schistosomiasis/bilharzia in humans.

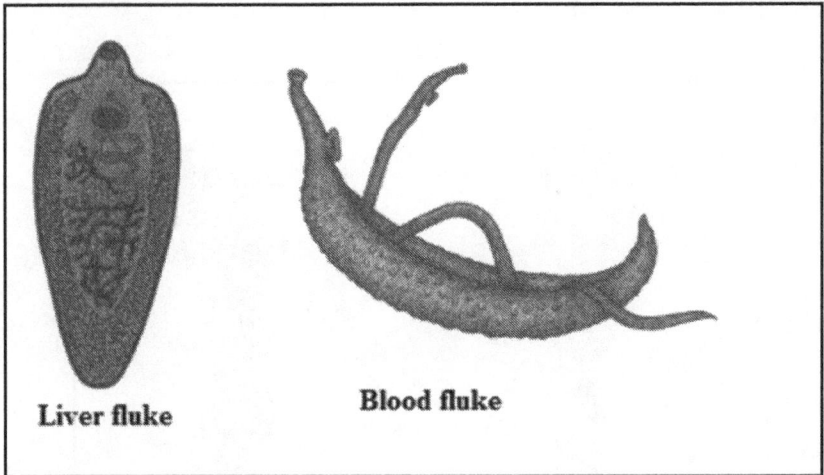

Liver fluke   **Blood fluke**

Figure 1.9: Flukes

Life cycle of Helminths

Helminths form three main life cycle stages; eggs, larvae and adults. Adult worms infect definitive hosts (those in which sexual development occurs) whereas larval stages may be free living or parasitize invertebrate vectors, intermediate or paratenic hosts. Nematodes produce eggs that embryonate in utero or outside the host. The emergent larvae undergo 4 metamorphoses (moults) before they mature as adult male or female worms. Cestode eggs released from gravid segments embryonate to produce 6 hooked embryos (hexacanth oncospheres) which are ingested by intermediate hosts. The oncospheres penetrate host tissues and become metacestodes (encysted larvae). When eaten by definitive hosts, they excyst and form adult tapeworms. Trematodes have more complex life cycles where larval stages undergo asexual amplification in snail intermediate hosts. Eggs hatch to release free swimming miracidia which actively infect snails and multiply in sac like sporocysts to produce numerous rediae. These stages mature to cercariae which are released from the snails and either actively infect new definitive hosts or form encysted metacercariae on aquatic vegetation which is eaten by definitive hosts.

Helminth eggs have tough resistant walls to protect the embryo while it develops. Mature eggs hatch to release larvae either within a host or into the external environment. The four main modes of transmission by which the larvae infect new hosts are faecal-oral, transdermal, vector borne and predator-prey transmission.

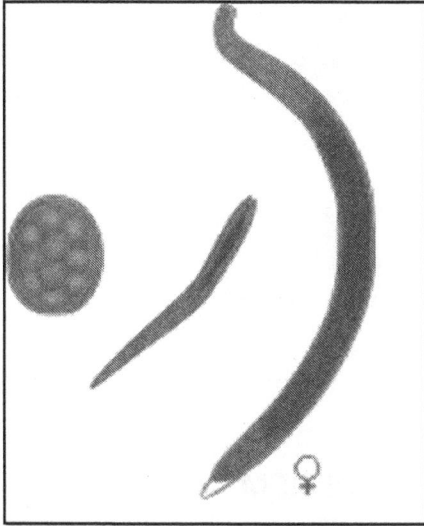

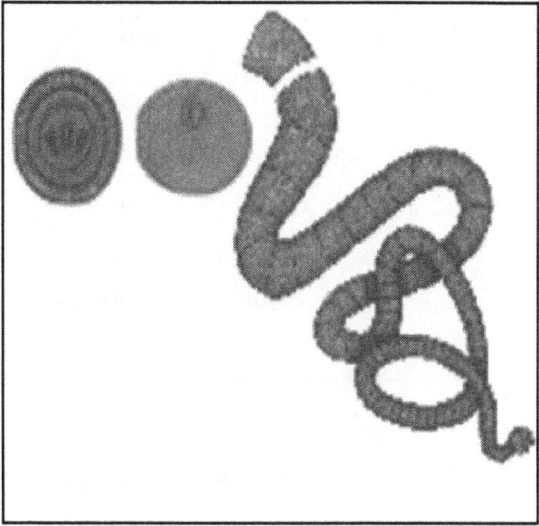

Nematode cycle (Egg→ Larvae →Adult)

Cestode cycle (Egg→Metacestode→Adult)

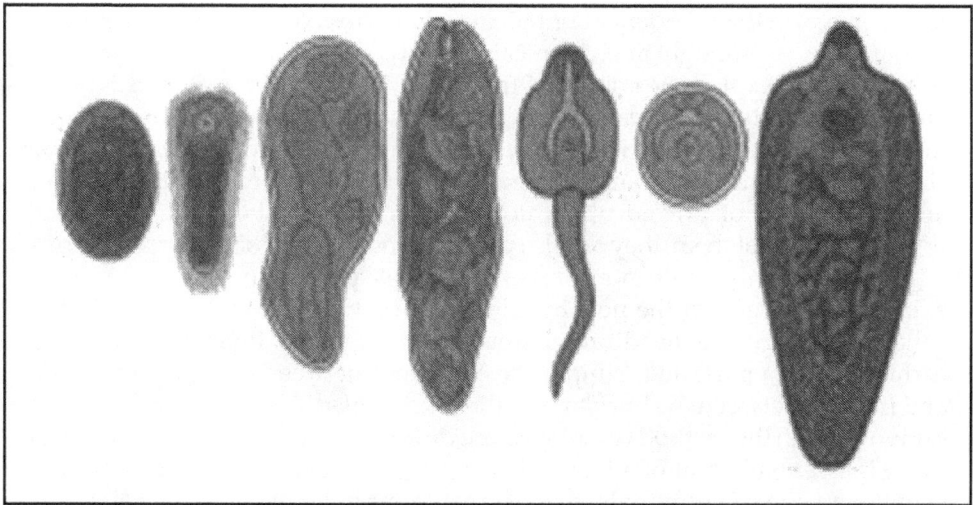

Trematode cycle (Egg→Miracidium→Sporocyst→Redia→ Cercaria→Metacercaria→Adult)

Figure 1.10: Lify cycle of Nematode, Cestode and Teamatode

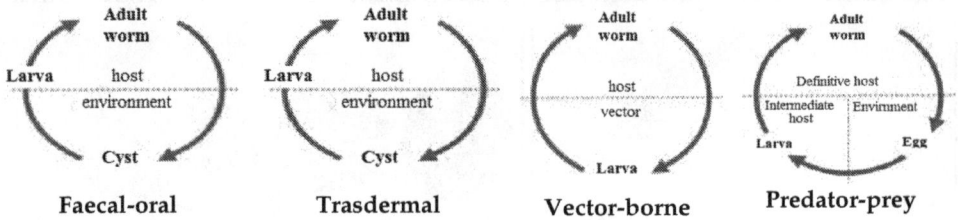

Figure 1.11: Transmission of Larvae to Host

BOX 1.1

PARASITES AND PARASITISM

Nature of Parasitism: The world of animal life consists of communities of organisms which live by eating each other. In a broad sense all animals are parasites, in that they are helpless without other organisms to produce food for them, on which they are dependent. Plants alone are able to build up their body substance out of sunlight and chemicals. Herbivorous animals, when they feed on vegetation, exploit the energy of the plants for their own use. Carnivorous animals exploit the energies of the herbivorous ones, larger carnivores exploit the smaller ones, etc. thus whole series constituting what ecologists call a food chain; many such chains can be traced in any animal community. But animals and plants are not preyed upon alone by successively larger forms which overpower and eat them; they are also preyed upon by successively smaller forms which destroy only small, more or less replaceable portions or even more subtly exploit the energies of the host by subsisting on the food which the host has collected with great expenditure of time and energy. The difference between a carnivore and a parasite is simply the difference between living upon capital and income, between the burglar and the blackmailer. The general result is the same although the methods employed are different. A man's relation to his beef cattle is essentially that of a tiger to its prey; his relation to his milk cattle and sugar maple trees is essentially that of tapeworms or hookworms to their hosts. There is every gradation between parasites and carnivores *e.g.* hookworms, leeches, horseflies, bloodsucking bats and tigers; there are also all gradations between parasites and saprophytes or organisms which live on the wastes or leftovers *e.g.* *Endam (Bba histolytica,* feeding on the tissue of the host; *Trichomonas hominis,* feeding on digested foods which would otherwise be converted into tissues; *Endamaeba coli,* feeding on still undigested particles and bacteria and the coprozoic amoebae, feeding on the waste fecal matter of the host.

General Relations to Hosts: The parasites are more oblique in their habits than other animals, as they were taking some unfair and mean advantage of their hosts. Carnivores and herbivores have no interest in the welfare of their prey and ruthlessly destroy them; parasites cannot be so inconsiderate, for their welfare is intimately bound up with the welfare of the host. A dead host is seldom of any use to a parasite in its adult state, though it may capitalize the death of an intermediate host as a means of attaining its destination in the definitive host. Food of the right kind and in sufficient quantity is the burning question in all animal society, for parasites this resolves itself into the question of what to do when the host dies; most internal parasites, as adults, are so specialized for a protected life in the body of the host that they are unable to take any steps to deal with this situation. The result is that they make no attempt to do so and resign themselves to dying with their hosts, leaving it to their offspring to find their way to another host in order to continue the race and since the offspring have to run enormous risks in order to succeed, they have to be produced in correspondingly enormous numbers, running into millions.

Parasites and Food Habits: Since food is the hub of the wheel of animal life, it is natural to find that many parasites have taken advantage of the food habits of their hosts in order to propagate themselves from host to host. Intestinal Protozoa such as amoebae and flagellates, usually solve the problem by entering into a resistant cystic stage in which they can survive outside the body until they can re-enter a host with its food or water; blood Protozoa such as trypanosomes and malaria parasites are adapted to live temporarily in bloodsucking insects which feed on the host and subsequently re-inject them into another host. Most flukes and tapeworms lay eggs which develop in the bodies of animals which the host habitually eats or which are eaten by a third animal which is then eaten by the definitive host. Some intestinal nematodes, such as the spiruroids, do likewise such as ascaris, follow the tactics of intestinal Protozoa; and still others, such as hookworms, produce self reliant embryos which actively burrow into the skin of their hosts; most parasitic arthropods are able to migrate from host to host when these come in contact with each other, directly or indirectly; but the bloodsucking flies, which anticipated airplane transportation, have no worries about this matter and can go at will from host to host. The result of the dependence of parasites to such a large extent on the food habits of animals is that the food habits largely determine Protozoa, etc., are abundant where unsanitary conditions favor fecal contamination of food or water; may fluke infections of man are abundant in localities in the Far East where fish is habitually eaten raw and spiruroid infections occur only accidentally in man because the human animal is nowhere habitually insectivorous in habit.

Origin of Parasitism: Parasitism, in the restricted sense of a small organism living on or in and at the expense of, a larger one, probably rose soon after life began to differentiate in the world. It would be difficult to explain step by step the details of the process of evolution by which some of the highly specialized parasites reached their present condition. Parasitism at times has probably grown out of a harmless association of different kinds of organisms, one of the members of the association, by virtue, perhaps, of characteristics already possessed, developing the power of living at the expense of the other and ultimately becoming more and more dependent upon it. It is easy to understand the general mechanism by which parasites of the alimentary canal were evolved from free living organisms which were accidentally or purposely swallowed and which were able to survive in the environment in which they found themselves and to adapt themselves to it. It is also easy to see how some of these parasites might eventually have developed further territorial ambitions and have extended their operations beyond the confines of the alimentary canal. The development of some of the blood Protozoa of vertebrates, on the other hand, seems clearly to have taken place in two steps: first, adaptation to life in the gut of insects and second, adaptation to life in vertebrates' blood or tissues when inoculated by hosts with skin piercing and blood sucking habits.

Kinds of Parasites: Parasitism is of all kinds and degrees. There are facultative parasites which may be parasitic or free living at will and obligatory parasites which must live on or in sopie other organism during all or part of their lives and which perish if prevented from doing so. There are intermittent parasites which visit and leave their hosts at intervals. Some, as mosquitoes, visit their hosts only long enough to get a meal; others, as certain lice, leave their hosts only for the purpose of moulting and laying eggs and still others, as the cattle tick, *Boophilus annulatus,* never leave except to lay eggs. Some parasites pass only part of their life cycles as parasites such as botflies are parasitic only as larva, hookworms only as adults. Some organ different species, in the course of their life histories. There are permanent parasites which live their whole lives, from the time of hatching to death, in a single host, hut in which the eggs or the corresponding cysts in the case of Protozoa must be transferred to a new host before a second generation can develop. Such are many intestinal protozoan and roundworms. The final degree of parasitism is reached, perhaps, in those parasites which live not only their whole lives, but also generation after generation on a single host becoming transferred from host to host only by direct contact. Such are the scab mites and many species of lice. Every gradation is found among all the types of parasites and a complete classification of parasites according to mode of life would contain almost as many types as kinds of parasites. It is sometimes convenient to classify parasites according to whether they are external or internal. External parasites or ecto parasites, living on the surface of the body of their hosts, suck blood or feed upon hair, feathers, skin or secretions of the skin. Internal parasites, living inside the body, occupy the digestive tract or other cavities of the body or live in various organs, blood, tissues or even within cells. No sharp line of demarcation can be drawn between external and internal parasites since inhabitants of the mouth and nasal cavities and such worms and mites as burrow just under the surface of the skin, might be placed in either category.

Effects of Parasitism on Parasites: Aside from the toning down of their effects on the host, parasites are often very highly modified in structure to meet the demands of their particular environment. As a group, parasites have little need for sense organs and seldom have them as highly developed as do related free living animals. Fixed parasites do not need and do not have, well developed organs of locomotion, if they possess any. Intestinal parasites do not need highly organized digestive tracts and the tapeworms and spiny headed worms have lost this portion of their anatomy completely. On the other hand, parasites must be specialized, often to .a very high degree, to adhere to or to make their way about in their particular host or the particular part of the host in which they find suitable conditions for existence. Every structure, every function, every instinct of many of these parasites is modified, to a certain extent, for the sole purpose of reproduction. A fluke does not eat to live, it eats only to reproduce. The inevitable death of the host is the parasite's doomsday, against which it must prepare by producing all the offspring possible, in the hope that enough will survive to keep the race from extinction. The complexity to which the development of the reproductive systems may go is almost incredible. In some adult tapeworms not only does every segment bear complete male and female reproductive systems, but it also bears two sets of each. The number of eggs produced by many parasitic worms may run well into the millions. The complexity of the life history is no less remarkable. Not only are free living stages interposed and intermediate hosts made to serve as transmitting agents, but also often asexual multiplications are passed through during the course of these remarkable experiences.

Mutual Tolerance of Hosts and Parasites: The effect of parasitism is felt by both parasite and host. A sort of mutual adaptation between the two is developed in proportion to the time that the relationship of host and parasite has existed. It is obviously to the disadvantage of internal parasites to cause the death of their host, for in so doing they destroy themselves. It is likewise to the disadvantage of external parasites, not so much to cause the death of their host, as to produce such pain or irritation as to lead to their own destruction at the hands of the irritated host. In well established host-parasite relations the host succeeds in protecting itself against the injurious effects of the parasites, partly by developing antibodies which neutralize poisonous or injurious products of the parasites, partly by placing its blood forming or tissue repairing mechanisms on a plane of higher efficiency and partly by less well understood immune mechanisms, enforcing birth control or at least family quotas upon the parasites. The efficient parasite is one which is able to survive under these conditions, content to live in a restricted manner in a host which is in consequence not sufficiently aroused to put forth the effort necessary to eliminate it entirely. An African native living in a highly malarial district in apparently good health, in spite of having harbored malaria parasites approximately from birth, affords a good example. It is a well established fact that a disease introduced into a place where it is not endemic *i.e.* does not normally exist, is more destructive than in places where it has long been present. In an abnormal host the delicate adjustment between host and parasite is missing and usually either the parasite fails to survivor else the host is severely injured or destroyed; a high degree of pathogenicity of a parasite may be considered *prima facie* evidence of a recent and still imperfect development of the host-parasite relation. An organism and the parasites which are particularly adapted to live with it may be looked upon as a sort of compound organism.

Modes of Infection and Transmission: The portals of entry and means of transmission of parasites are of the most vital importance from the standpoint of preventive medicine. In the past few decades wonderful strides in our knowledge along these lines have been made, but much is yet to be found out. Many parasites may be spread by direct or indirect contact with infected parts *e.g.* spirochetes of syphilis and yaws, the mouth amoebae, itch mites and free moving ecto-parasites. The parasites of the digestive system and of other internal organs gain entrance in one of two ways. They may bore directly through the skin as larvae *e.g.* hookworms. More commonly they enter the mouth as cysts or eggs *e.g.* dysentery amoebae and ascaris as larvae *e.g.* tapeworms; or as adults *e.g.* leeches. Access to the mouth is gained in many different ways, but chiefly with impure water, with unwashed vegetables fertilized with night soil, with food contaminated by dust, flies or unclean hands or with the flesh of an animal which has served as an intermediate host. The parasites of the blood or lymphatic systems usually rely on biting arthropods (insects, ticks and mites) to transmit them from host to.

Geographic Distribution: The distribution of parasites over the surface of the earth is dependent on the presence of suitable hosts on habits and environmental conditions which make possible the transfer from host to host. A human parasite which does not utilize an intermediate host is likely to be found in every inhabited region of the world, providing its particular requirements with respect to habits and environmental conditions are met and if it can also live as a parasite in other animals it may occur even beyond the limits of human habitation. Parasites such as amoebae, intestinal flagellates, pinworms and itch mites, which require only slight carelessness and also depend on habits for their transfer and are largely independent of external conditions, are practically cosmopolitan, but vary in abundance with the extent of the carelessness on which their propagation depends. Ascaris and Trichuris are only slightly more limited since they require some time outside the body to reach the infective stage and are susceptible to heat and dryness. Hookworms are more limited, since they have to brave the dangers of the outside world as free living organisms, unprotected by resistant egg shells. Therefore, not only heat and dryness but also such factors as cold and nature of the soil come into play. When an intermediate host is involved, distribution is more limited, for not only must both hosts be present together, but the relations between them must be such as to favor the transfer of the parasites from one to the other. Sleeping sickness never occurs outside the range of certain species of tsetse flies, malaria beyond the range of certain species of Anopheles, nor kala-azar outside the range of certain species of Phlebotomus. Usually the distribution of the parasites is not as great as the distribution of their necessary intermediate hosts. A guinea worm not only requires both man and certain species of Cyclops, but it also requires conditions under which the Cyclops can be reached by the embryos and under which the infected Cyclops can be ingested by man. Even in the presence of both man and mosquitoes, filaria may not thrive, since it must have atmospheric conditions which give it time to penetrate human skin, after a mosquito has landed it there, before it dries up and it has little chance in a place where houses and porches have mosquito-proof screens. Clonorchis requires not only the simultaneous presence of man, certain snails and certain fish, but it also requires unsanitary conditions making possible the access of eggs to the snails, a free association of infected snails and fish and an established habit of eating raw fish. Sometimes ability to infect other hosts than man may keep alive an infection even when human habits prevent the possibility of more than occasional or rare access to the human body.

1.5 *Trypanosoma*

Trypanosoma is a group of unicellular parasitic flagellate heteroxenous protozoan, requiring more than one obligate host to complete life cycle and are transmitted via vector. These infect a variety of hosts and cause various diseases, including the fatal human diseases sleeping sickness caused by *Trypanosoma brucei* and Chagas disease caused by *Trypanosoma cruzi*. *Trypanosoma gambiense* is digenetic and polymorphic (trypanosome or adult form in human; crithidial, leptomonal and leishmania forms are developmental forms in Tse-Tse fly) infective stage is called metacyclic stage. Although trypanosomes were first discovered in 1841, which is very ancient history in parasitology, the first connection with disease was the discovery in 1880 that they were the cause of surra in horses and other animals in India. In 1895, Bruce showed that nagana of domestic animals in Africa was caused by a trypanosome which now bears his name. In 1902, Forde and Dutton discovered the presence of trypanosomes in human blood in a case of Gambia fever, the preliminary stage of sleeping sickness. In 1903, Castellani found trypanosomes in the cerebrospinal fluid of cases of sleeping sickness in Uganda. Trypanosomes live as parasites in all sorts of vertebrates, fish, amphibians, reptiles, birds and mammals living in the blood, lymph or tissues of their hosts. A great number of different species have been named; usually any trypanosome found in a new host is named after the host as a tentative label, until more is found out about it. Though this procedure is not in accordance with rules of naming animals, it is better than the alternatives of having numerous nameless trypanosomes to deal with or of identifying them with species from which they may subsequently be found to differ. In form most trypanosomes are active wriggling little creatures somewhat suggesting diminutive delphins or eels, according to their slenderness.

They swim in the direction of the pointed end of the body, being propelled by the wave motions of the undulating membrane. Some of them dart in and about among the blood corpuscles with great rapidity, but others swim in a more leisurely manner. The body is shaped like a curved, flattened blade, tapering to a fine point anteriorly, from which a free flagellum often continues forward. This flagellum continues to near the posterior end of the body and is connected with the body by an undulating membrane, like a long fin or crest; whereas in some species it is thrown into numerous graceful ripples, in certain others *e.g. Trypanosoma cruzi, it* is only slightly rippled. The body contains a nucleus which varies in its position in different species and under different circumstances.

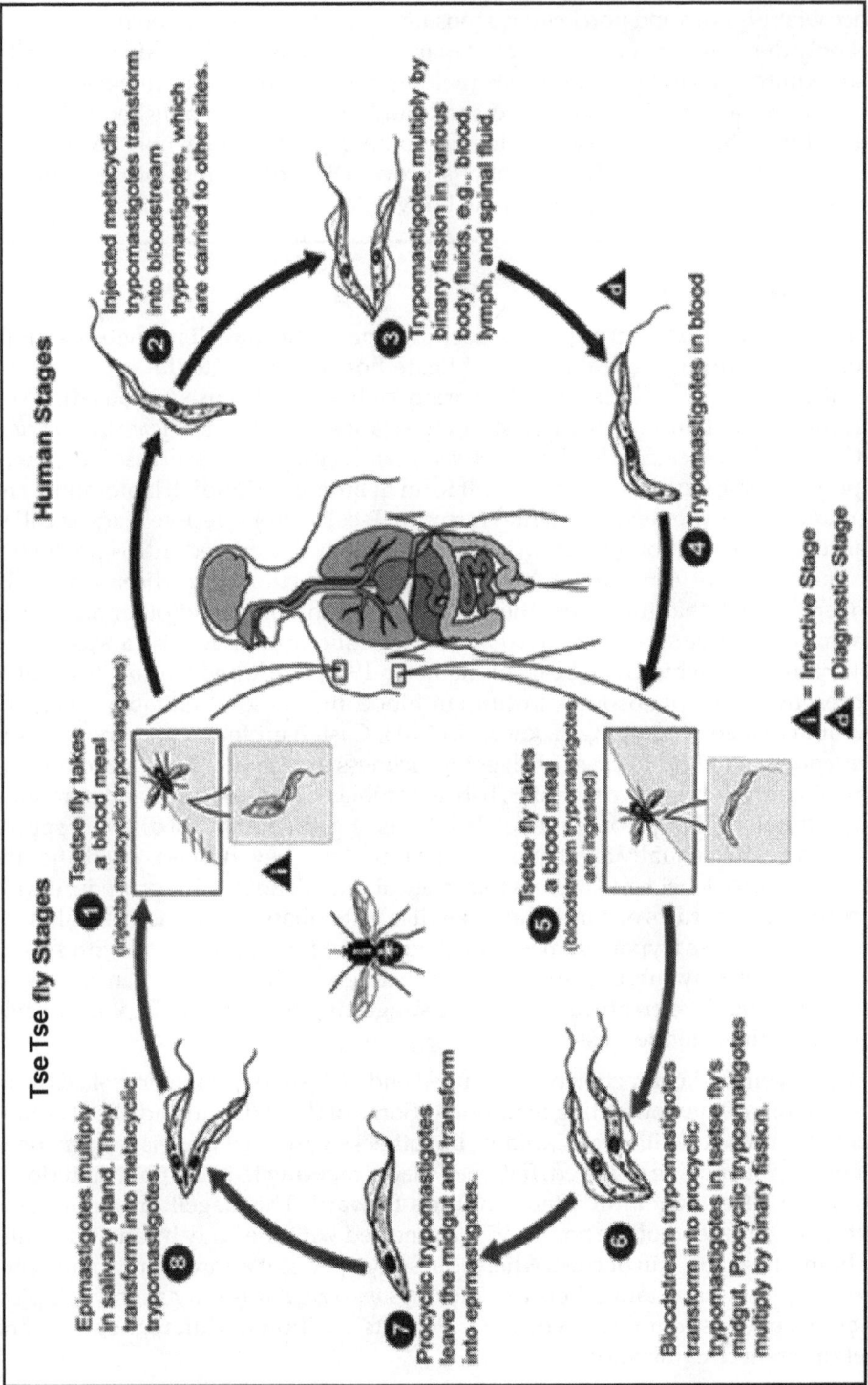

Figure 1.12: Life cycle of Trypanosome (Adopted from CDC)

Human Stages

② Injected metacyclic trypomastigotes transform into bloodstream trypomastigotes, which are carried to other sites.

③ Trypomastigotes multiply by binary fission in various body fluids, e.g., blood, lymph, and spinal fluid.

④ Trypomastigotes in blood

Tse Tse fly Stages

① Tsetse fly takes a blood meal (injects metacyclic trypomastigotes)

⑤ Tsetse fly takes a blood meal (bloodstream trypomastigotes are ingested)

⑥ Bloodstream trypomastigotes transform into procyclic trypomastigotes in tsetse fly's midgut. Procyclic trypomastigotes multiply by binary fission.

⑦ Procyclic trypomastigotes leave the midgut and transform into epimastigotes.

⑧ Epimastigotes multiply in salivary gland. They transform into metacyclic trypomastigotes.

△ = Infective Stage
▲ = Diagnostic Stage

During a blood meal on the mammalian host, an infected tsetse fly (genus *Glossina*) injects metacyclic trypomastigotes into skin tissue. The parasites enter the lymphatic system and pass into the bloodstream in stege 1. Inside the host, they transform into bloodstream trypomastigotes in stge 2, are carried to other sites throughout the body, reach other blood fluids (*e.g.* lymph, spinal fluid) and continue the replication by binary fission in stage 3. The entire life cycle of African Trypanosomes is represented by extracellular stages.

The tsetse fly becomes infected with bloodstream trypomastigotes when taking a blood meal on an infected mammalian host in stage (4, 5). In the fly's midgut, the parasites transform into procyclic trypomastigotes, multiply by binary fission in stage 6, leave the midgutand transform into epimastigotes in stage 7. The epimastigotes reach the fly's salivary glands and continue multiplication by binary fission in stage 8. The cycle in the fly takes approximately 3 weeks. Humans are the main reservoir for *Trypanosoma brucei gambiense*, but this species can also be found in animals. Wild game animals are the main reservoir of *T. b. rhodesiense*.

1.5.1 Structure of *Trypanosoma*

The parasite has elongate, flat and fusiform body with an anterior flagellum, undulating membrane and a posterior basal granule. Undulating membrane helps in movement in viscous blood. The parasite lives in blood plasma of human beings, cause glandular swellings and fever. It later enters cerebro-spinal fluid and causes sleeping sickness. Reserve host is antelope. *Trypanosoma rhodeseinse* causes Rhodesian/East African meningo encephalitis or sleeping sickness. *Trypanosoma cruzi* produces Chaga's fever in children. Vector is blood sucking bug or tick like *Triatoma*. Parasite passes into liver, spleen, brain, spinal cord, heart and other muscles, blood, etc. It causes fever, swollen lymph glands, enlarged liver and spleen. The mitochondrial genome of the Trypanosoma as well as of other kinetoplastids known as kinetoplasts is made up of a highly complex series of catenated circles and minicircles and requires a cohort of protein for organization during cell division. *Trypanosoma* have parasitic absorptive nutrition.

1.5.2 Life cycle *Trypanosoma*

In the vertebrate hosts, most trypanosomes usually multiply by simple fission, although in some species, notably *Trypanosoma lewisi* of rats, division of the nuclei and kinetoplasts may outrun actual cell division early in an infection. The kinetoplast is the first structure to divide; next a new flagellum begins to grow out along the margin of the undulating membrane, then the nucleus divides and finally the body splits from the anterior end backwards.

Although usually regarded as blood parasites, most species are primarily parasites of the lymphatic system or of intercellular spaces or sometimes even of tissue cells, from which positions they secondarily invade the blood stream in large or small numbers. *T. cruzi* multiplies into swarms within tissue cells; the African polymorphic trypanosomes of man and animals are mainly parasites of the lymphatics and intercellular fluids; *T. equiperdum* thrives in edematous fluid of sex organs and skin; and some trypanosomes of birds apparently live mainly in the bone marrow. In many cases the favorite habitat is not known, only the blood forms having been recognized. In some species *e.g. T. lewisi* and the trypanosomes of sleeping sickness, numerous dividing parasites can be found in the blood during the height of an infection, whereas in others such dividing forms are rarely if ever found, presumably because division takes place elsewhere than in the blood stream. In some species at least *e.g. T. lewisi* of rats and *T. duttoni* of mice, an immune response which inhibits reproduction soon develops, in which case the coefficient of variation of the parasites quickly drops to a low level, but in some species dividing forms are found even late in the course of an infection. Trypanosomes are commonly spoken of as polymorphic or monomorphic, but these terms refer only to adult, non-dividing forms such as are found in a long established infection; polymorphic forms are those in which some individuals have a free flagellum and others do not *e.g. T. gambiense, T. brucei* and *T. rhodesiense*, while monomorphic forms may always have a free flagellum *e.g. T. lewisi, T. cruzi, T. vivax, T. evansi, T. equinum* and *T. equiperdumor* may always lack one *e.g. T. congolense, T. suis.*

lthough at least one trypanosome, *T. equiperdum,* has become completely independent of its ancestral invertebrate hosts and is transmitted directly from horse to horse during copulation and although other trypanosomes can live and multiply indefinitely in vertebrate hosts if artificially injected by the soiled proboscis of biting flies, the majority of them, when they reach a suitable invertebrate host, hark back to the traditions of their remote forebears and go through a cycle of development more or less like that of typical crithidias. Some, such as *T. cruzi* and *T. lewisi,* finding them in the ancestral home, revert almost completely. After being sucked into the stomach of an insect they assume the crithidial form, attach themselves to the epithelial cells' or enter them and multiply. Gradually they move backwards towards the rectum and the infective forms are voided with the feces. Infection occurs either by contamination of the bite with the feces, which probably the usual way in *T. cruzi;* by ingestion of the feces of the insect when licking the bites, as in the case of *T. lewisi;* or by ingestion of the whole insect. The reversion of *T. cruzi* to the crithidial condition is still more complete in that the infection commonly passes from insect to insect. Those trypanosomes which develop thus in the hindgut of invertebrates are said to develop in the posterior station. They are the conservatives. The trypanosomes of this group use a variety of invertebrates as intermediate hosts *e.g. T. lewisi* of rats develops in fleas, *T. melophagium* of sheep in sheep ticks, *T. theileri* of cattle, *T. cruzi* of man and other animals in triatomid bugs and African reptilian trypanosomes in tsetse flies. There are other trypanosomes, radicals, which after ingestion by their insect vectors develop in the anterior part of the alimentary canal and infect by way of the proboscis. So far as known at present this specialized procedure occurs only in Tse-Tse flies, which serve as transmitters of African mammalian trypanosomes and in leeches, which transmit the trypanosomes of aquatic animals. These trypanosomes are said to develop in the anterior station.

1.5.3 Pathogenicity of *Trypanosoma*

Trypanosoma brucei and its related subspecies are parasitic hemoflagellate protists that are implicated in a severe meningoencephalitic disease, African trypanosomiasis, more commonly known as sleeping sickness. Sleeping sickness itself is identified as a neurological disorder proceeded by an acute lymphatic infection. The disease garners its name from the effect it has of creating severe fatigue in a patient followed by bouts of mania and eventually causing coma and death. It is known to have affected up to 36 sub-Saharan countries with an estimated 300,000 new infections each year. A more complete understanding of the life cycle of this particularly fatal disease has been incited by organizations such as WHO in order to create novel treatments for the disease before it develops into a much more deadly issue. Trypanosomes in general exist in a very exposed and vulnerable ecological niche within their human hosts: the bloodstream. In this environment most pathogens would be susceptible to not only the damaging effects of the innate immune response such as inflammation, leukocytes, etc. but also the adaptive immune response such as antibodies, killer T cells, etc. Some hemolytic bacteria and protists have developed methods to avoid the innate immune response through the expression of a lipo-polysaccharide coat (gram negative bacteria only) or even thick cellular walls, but it is difficult for either of these methods to avoid the specific targeting mechanisms of the adaptive immune system. Trypanosomes have evolved to spoil the adaptive immune response of the host by maintaining a variant surface glycoprotein (VSG) coat which expresses one of 1500 surface glycoprotein genes. A new set of surface glycoprotein are expressed in *T. brucei* outer membranes in approximately 1 out of every 100 cell divisions. This ensures that once the host mounts an effective complementary immune response to the predominantly expressed VSG variant, the infection will persist into the next generation until the host mounts another complementary response. This variable expressive pattern is the main reason patients with chronic trypanosomiasis show cyclical bouts of infection followed by a period of relative latency. By the time the host's immune system identifies and synthesizes antibodies to combat certain trypanosomes, a percentage of the total trypanosome population has evaded detection and continued the infection.

Once a metacyclic *Trypanosoma brucei* enters the mammalian bloodstream, a regulated cascade of biochemical signals transforms the metacyclic trypanosome into the typical slender form of a trypanosome. This form flagellar, bloodborne pathogen alone causes the devastating effects of African trypanosomiasis and because of this; an incredible amount of research has developed to fully understand not only the disease itself but how the trypanosome itself traverses the various and complex labyrinth of the human body. There must be a distinction in the type of African trypanosomiasis as the *T. rhodosiense* subspecies and *T. gambiense* subspecies cause different symptoms altogether. Recall that *rhodosiense* infection is far more acute and severe and can quickly lead to death while *T. gambiense* is a more chronic and more actively employing the use of antigenic variation. Upon the site of metacyclic trypanosome injection, one of the first sign of trypanosome infection that occurs in the *T. rhodosiense* subspecies is the presence of deep lesions as the trypanosome tears its way through the capillary beds of the human skin and proceeds to infect larger and more favorable blood vessels. *Gambiense* infections do not cause the lesions of the rapidly spreading *T. rhodosiense*, but it indeed spreads throughout the capillary bed in a similar fashion and leads to the same large vasculature. These symptoms will persist for a few days and then, while the lymph node is draining from the infection, the trypanosome will pass through into the lymph node and begin infection of the lymphatic system. This infection causes severe bouts of headaches, fever and an increased level of fatigue in the patients. The trypanosome itself is digesting the cells of the lymphatic system systematically and causing the body to respond harshly. In the case of *T. rhodosiensis*, the effects of such an acute attack could cause the body to over respond in its attempts to rescue the body and possibly lead to edema, pancarditis and congestive heart failure. Fortunately, this form of trypanosomiasis is easily identified and diagnosable. If the disease is caught early within the hemolymphatic stage of the infection the risk involved with treatment is dramatically lowered. However, *T. gambiensis* does not show these severe symptoms of its brasher cousin, but it is far more insidious. It leads to a series of general immune responses and then, causes a swelling of the lymph nodes, which are both easily mistaken for other diseases. One unique symptom of *T. gambiense* infection is the presence of a swollen section of the lymph nodes of the trapezius region of the upper back that is known as winter bottom's sign.

The most deadly and serious symptoms of trypanosomiasis comes from when the trypanosomes invade the organ systems themselves. After a few weeks with rhodensiensis and after as much as a couple of years with gambiensis, evidence of increased immune response in tissues other than the blood begins to appear, signaling their infection. Trypanosomes have perhaps the most devastating effect on the human host by even attacking the central nervous system (CNS). Recent studies have shown that trypanosomes invade the central nervous system directly through the blood brain barrier (BBB) as well as through portions of the circum ventricular organs. Apparently, the trypanosomes somehow render themselves permissible through the BBB by expressing a parasite version of cysteine protease which increases the number of changes in the oscillatory patter of Calcium ions in the cell. As the meningo-encephalitic stage of the disease progresses, the patient will show a drastic change in their sleeping habits, where they sleep all day during the day and have intermittent periods of insomnia at night. Eventually in the most devastating periods of the disease, personality changes in the form of anger and depression can onset followed soon after by incapacitation of basic reasoning or mental processing. Severe ataxic dyskinesia eventually sets in and the patient can lose the ability to coordinate their actions at all. Beyond their pathogenic life cycles, the development of the stumpy trypanosomes is a potentially crucial part of the infective pathway of *T. brucei*. The stumpy trypanosomes develop from a quorum sensing apparatus that promotes several organelle rearrangements as well as an arrest of several mitotic gateways. The particular protein involved in the quorum sensing is an unknown theoretical molecule simply referred to as stumpy inducing factor. As the stumpy forms develop, they lose the ability to reproduce entirely and instead lie near the surface capillary beds to infect the blood meal of a potential insect vector. For a large period of time, it was assumed that differentiation of the slender form to the stumpy form was essential to the life cycle of *T. brucei*. However, recently a study has shown that both slender and stumpy forms of the trypanosome have the capacity to complete an entire life cycle throughout an insect vector, back into a mammalian host.

1.5.4 Diseases of *Trypanosoma*

Trypanosoma brucei causes African trypanosomiasis, commonly known as Sleeping Sickness in humans and Nagana (meaning loss of spirit' in the Zulu language) in cattle. *Trypanosoma cruzi* causes Chagas' Disease, a chronic human infection. There are two subspecies of the parasite *Trypanosoma brucei* that cause disease in humans. *T. b. rhodesiense* (East African sleeping sickness) is found in focal areas of eastern and southeastern Africa. *T. b. gambiense* (West African sleeping sickness) is found predominantly in central Africa and in limited areas of West Africa. Both forms of sleeping sickness are transmitted by the bite of the Tse-Tse fly (*Glossina* species). Tse-Tse flies inhabit rural areas, living in the woodlands and thickets that dot the East African savannah. The clinical features of the infection depend on the subspecies involved. The two subspecies are found in different regions of Africa. The clinical course of human African trypanosomiasis has two stages. In the first stage, the parasite is found in the peripheral circulation, but it has not yet invaded the central nervous system. Once the parasite crosses the blood-brain barrier and infects the central nervous system, the disease enters the second stage. The subspecies that cause African trypanosomiasis has different rates of disease progression and the clinical features depend on which form of the parasite (*T. b. rhodesiense* or *T. b. gambiense*) is causing the infection. However, infection with either form will eventually lead to coma and death if not treated. *T. b. rhodesiense* infection (East African sleeping sickness) progresses rapidly. In some patients, a large sore (chancre) will develop at the site of the tsetse bite. Most patients develop fever, headache, muscle and joint aches and enlarged lymph nodes within 1-2 weeks of the infective bite. Some people develop a rash. After a few weeks of infection, the parasite invades the central nervous system and eventually causes mental deterioration and other neurologic problems. Death ensues usually within months. *T. b. gambiense* infection (West African sleeping sickness) progresses more slowly. At first, there may be only mild symptoms. Infected persons may have intermittent fevers, headaches, muscle and joint aches and malaise. Itching of the skin, swollen lymph nodes and weight loss can occur. Usually, after 1-2 years, there is evidence of central nervous system involvement, with personality changes, daytime sleepiness with night-time sleep disturbance and progressive confusion. Other neurologic signs, such as partial paralysis or problems with balance or walking may occur, as well as hormonal imbalances. The course of untreated infection rarely lasts longer than 6-7 years and more often kills in about 3 years.

1.5.5 Causes, Symptoms and Control of *Trypanosoma*

The diagnosis of African Trypanosomiasis is made through laboratory methods, because the clinical features of infection are not sufficiently specific. The diagnosis rests on finding the parasite in body fluid or tissue by microscopy. The parasite load in *T. b. rhodesiense* infection is substantially higher than the level in *T. b. gambiense* infection. *T. b. rhodesiense* parasites can easily be found in blood. They can also be found in lymph node fluid or in fluid or biopsy of a chancre. Serologic testing is not widely available and is not used in the diagnosis, since microscopic detection of the parasite is straightforward. The classic method for diagnosing *T. b. gambiense* infection is by microscopic examination of lymph node aspirate, usually from a posterior cervical node. It is often difficult to detect *T. b. gambiense* in blood. Concentration techniques and serial examinations are frequently needed. All patients diagnosed with African trypanosomiasis must have their cerebrospinal fluid examined to determine whether there is involvement of the central nervous system, since the choice of treatment drug(s) will depend on the disease stage. The World Health Organization (WHO) criteria for central nervous system involvement include increased protein in cerebrospinal fluid and a white cell count of more than 5. Trypanosomes can often be observed in cerebrospinal fluid in persons with second stage infection. All persons diagnosed with African Trypanosomiasis should receive treatment. The specific drug and treatment course will depend on the type of infection (*T. b. gambiense* or *T. b. rhodesiense*) and the disease stage *i.e.* whether the central nervous system has been invaded by the parasite. Pentamidine, which is the recommended drug for first stage, the other drugs (suramin, melarsoprol, eflornithine and nifurtimox) used to treat African trypanosomiasis. After treatment patients need to have serial examinations of their cerebrospinal fluid for 2 years, so that relapse can be detected if it occurs.

There is no vaccine or drug for prophylaxis against African trypanosomiasis. Preventive measures are aimed at minimizing contact with tsetse flies. Local residents are usually aware of the areas that are heavily infested and they can provide advice about places to avoid. Other helpful measures include:

- *Clothing:* Wear long sleeved shirts and pants of medium weight material in neutral colors that blend with the background environment. Tse-tse flies are attracted to bright or dark colors and they can bite through lightweight clothing.

- *Inspect vehicles before entering*: The flies are attracted to the motion and dust from moving vehicles.

- *Avoid bushes:* The tsetse fly is less active during the hottest part of the day but will bite if disturbed.

- *Use insect repellent:* Permethrin-impregnated clothing and insect repellent have not been proved to be particularly effective against tsetse flies, but they will prevent other insect bites that can cause illness.

Control of African trypanosomiasis rests on two strategies: reducing the disease reservoir and controlling the tse tse fly vector. Because humans are the significant disease reservoir for *T. b. gambiense*, the main control strategy for this subspecies is active case finding through population screening, followed by treatment of the infected persons that are identified. Tse tse fly traps are sometimes used as an adjunct. Reducing the reservoir of infection is more difficult for *T. b. rhodesiense*, since there are a variety of animal hosts. Vector control is the primary strategy in use. This is usually done with traps or screens, in combination with insecticides and odors that attract the flies.

BOX 1.2

TRYPANOSOMIASIS (HUMAN AFRICAN SLEEPING SICKNESS)

Sleeping sickness occurs only in 36 sub-Saharan Africa countries where there are tsetse flies that transmit the disease. The people most exposed to the tsetse fly and therefore the disease live in rural areas and depend on agriculture, fishing, animal husbandry or hunting. *Trypanosoma brucei gambiense* accounts for more than 98% of reported cases of sleeping sickness. Diagnosis and treatment of the disease is complex and requires specifically skilled staff. Human African trypanosomiasis, also known as sleeping sickness, is a vector borne parasitic disease. It is caused by infection with protozoan parasites belonging to the genus *Trypanosoma*. They are transmitted to humans by tsetse fly (*Glossina* genus) bites which have acquired their infection from human beings or from animals harbouring the human pathogenic parasites. Tse-Tse flies are found just in sub-Saharan Africa though only certain species transmit the disease. For reasons that are so far unexplained, there are many regions where tsetse flies are found, but sleeping sickness is not. Rural populations living in regions where transmission occurs and which depend on agriculture, fishing, animal husbandry or hunting are the most exposed to the tsetse fly and therefore to the disease. The disease develops in areas ranging from a single village to an entire region. Within an infected area, the intensity of the disease can vary from one village to the next.

Forms of human African Trypanosomiasis

Human African trypanosomiasis takes two forms, depending on the parasite involved:·

Trypanosoma brucei gambiense is found in 24 countries in west and central Africa. This form currently accounts for over 98% of reported cases of sleeping sickness and causes a chronic infection. A person can be infected for months or even years without major signs or symptoms of the disease. When more evident symptoms emerge, the patient is often already in an advanced disease stage where the central nervous system is affected.·

Trypanosoma brucei rhodesiense is found in 13 countries eastern and southern Africa. Now-a-days, this form represents under 2% of reported cases and causes an acute infection. First signs and symptoms are observed a few months or weeks after infection. The disease develops rapidly and invades the central nervous system. Only Uganda presents both forms of the disease.Another form of trypanosomiasis occurs mainly in Latin America. It is known as American trypanosomiasis or Chagas disease. The causal organism is a different subgenus from those causing the African form of the disease.

Animal Trypanosomiasis

Other parasite species and sub-species of *Trypanosoma* genus are pathogenic to animals and cause animal trypanosomiasis in wild and domestic animals. In cattle the disease is called *Nagana*. Animals can host the human pathogen parasites, especially *T.b. rhodesiense*; thus domestic and wild animals are an important parasite reservoir. Animals can also be infected with *T.b. gambiense* and act as a reservoir. However the precise epidemiological role of the animal reservoir in the gambiense form of the disease is not yet well known. The disease in domestic animals, particularly cattle, is a major obstacle to the economic development of affected rural areas.

Distribution of Disease: Sleeping sickness threatens millions of people in 36 countries in sub-Saharan Africa. Many of the affected populations live in remote areas with limited access to adequate health services, which complicates the surveillance and therefore the diagnosis and treatment of cases. In addition, displacement of populations, war and poverty are important factors that facilitate transmission.

1. In 1998, almost 40 000 cases were reported, but estimates were that 300 000 cases were undiagnosed and therefore untreated.

2. During epidemic periods prevalence reached 50% in several villages in the Angola, Democratic Republic of Congoand South Sudan. Sleeping sickness was the first or second greatest cause of mortality in those communities, ahead of even HIV / AIDS.

3. In 2009, after continued control efforts, the number of cases reported dropped below 10 000 (9878) for first time in 50 years. This decline in number of cases has continued with 7216 new cases reported in 2012. However, the estimated number of actual cases is 20 000 and the estimated population at risk is 70 million people.

In 2000 and 2001, WHO established public-private partnerships with Aventis Pharma (Sanofi) and Bayer HealthCare which enabled the creation of a WHO led control and surveillance programme, providing support to endemic countries in their control activities and the supply of medicines free of charge. The partnership was renewed in 2006 and in 2011. The success in curbing the number of sleeping sickness cases has encouraged other private partners to sustain the WHO's initial effort towards eliminating the disease as a public health problem. In 2013, WHO and the Bill and Melinda Gates Foundation signed an agreement to support and implement innovative strategies for case finding and surveillance to reach the sustainable elimination of the gambiense form of the disease.**Current situation in Endemic Countries:** The prevalence of the disease differs from one country to another as well as in different parts of a single country.·

- In the last 10 years, over 70% of reported cases occurred in the Democratic Republic of Congo (DRC).·

- The DRC is the only country that has reported more than 1000 new cases annually and accounts for 83% of the cases reported in 2012.·

- Central African Republic, Chad and South Sudan declared between 100 and 500 new cases in 2012.
- Countries such as, Angola, Cameroon, Congo, Cote d'Ivoire, Equatorial Guinea, Gabon, Ghana, Guinea, Kenya, Malawi, Nigeria, Uganda, United Republic of Tanzania, Zambia and Zimbabwe are reporting fewer than 100 new cases per year.
- Countries like Benin, Botswana, Burkina Faso, Burundi, Ethiopia, Gambia, Guinea Bissau, Liberia, Mali, Mozambique, Namibia, Niger, Rwanda, Senegal, Sierra Leone, Swaziland and Togo have not reported any new cases for over a decade. Transmission of the disease seems to have stopped but there are still some areas where it is difficult to assess the exact situation because the unstable social circumstances and/or remote accessibility hinders surveillance and diagnostic activities.

Infection and Symptoms

The disease is mostly transmitted through the bite of an infected tsetse fly but there are other ways in which people are infected with sleeping sickness.

- *Mother to child infection:* The trypanosome can cross the placenta and infect the fetus.·
- *Mechanical Transmission:* Mechanical transmission through other blood sucking insects is possible. However, it is difficult to assess the epidemiological impact of transmission.·
- *Accidental infections:* Accidental infections have occurred in laboratories due to pricks from contaminated needles.

In the first stage, the trypanosomes multiply in subcutaneous tissues, blood and lymph. This is known as a first stage or haemolymphatic phase, which entails bouts of fever, headaches, joint pains and itching. In the second stage the parasites cross the blood-brain barrier to infect the central nervous system. This is known as the neurological or meningoencephalic phase. In general this is when more obvious signs and symptoms of the disease appear: changes of behaviour, confusion, sensory disturbances and poor coordination. Disturbance of the sleep cycle, which gives the disease its name, is an important feature of the second stage of the disease. Without treatment, sleeping sickness is considered fatal although cases of healthy carriers have been reported.

Disease management: Diagnosis

Disease management is made in three steps.

(a) Screening for potential infection. This involves using serological tests (only available for *T.b. gambiense*) and checking for clinical signs; generally swollen cervical glands.

(b) Diagnosing whether the parasite is present.

(c) Staging to determine the state of disease progression. This entails examining cerebrospinal fluid obtained by lumbar puncture and is also used to determine the outcome of treatment.

Diagnosis must be made as early as possible to avoid progressing to the neurological stage in order to elude complicated, difficult and risky treatment procedures. The long, relatively asymptomatic first stage of *T. b. gambiense* sleeping sickness is one of the reasons why an exhaustive, active screening of the population at risk is recommended, in order to identify patients at an early stage and reduce transmission. Exhaustive screenings require a major investment in human and material resources. In Africa such resources are often scarce, particularly in remote areas where the disease is mostly found. As a result, some infected individuals may die before they can ever be diagnosed and treated.

Treatment: The type of treatment depends on the stage of the disease. The drugs used in the first stage of the disease are of lower toxicity and easier to administer. The earlier the disease is identified, the better the prospect of a cure. Treatment success in the second stage depends on a drug that can cross the blood-brain barrier to reach the parasite. Such drugs are toxic and complicated to administer. Four drugs are registered for the treatment of sleeping sickness. These drugs are donated to WHO by manufacturers and distributed free of charge to countries endemic for the disease.

First stage treatment

- **Pentamidine:** Discovered in 1941, used for the treatment of the first stage of *T.b. gambiense* sleeping sickness. Despite non-negligible undesirable effects, it is in general well tolerated by patients.·

- **Suramin:** Discovered in 1921, used for the treatment of the first stage of *T.b. rhodesiense*. It provokes certain undesirable effects, in the urinary tract and allergic reactions.

Second stage treatment

- **Melarsoprol:** Discovered in 1949, it is used in both forms of infection. It is derived from arsenic and has many undesirable side effects. The most dramatic is reactive encephalopathy (encephalopathic syndrome) which can be fatal (3% to 10%). An increase in resistance to the drug has been observed in several foci particularly in central Africa.·

- **Eflornithine:** This molecule, less toxic than melarsoprol, was registered in 1990. It is only effective against *T.b. gambiense*. The regimen is strict and difficult to apply.·

- A combination treatment of nifurtimox and eflornithine was introduced in 2009. It simplifies the use of eflornithine in monotherapy, but unfortunately it is not effective for *T.b. rhodesiense*. Nifurtimox is registered for the treatment of American trypanosomiasis but not for human African trypanosomiasis. Nevertheless, after safety and efficacy data provided by clinical trials, its use in combination with eflornithine has been accepted and included in the WHO List of Essential Medicine and it is provided free of charge for this purpose by WHO to endemic countries.

1.6 Giardia

Giardia (Grand Old Man of Intestine) is a genus of anaerobic flagellated protozoan parasite that colonizes and reproduces in the small intestines of several vertebrates causing giardiasis. There life cycle consists of an actively swimming trophozoite and an infective, resistant cyst. *Giardia* was first described by the Dutch microscopist Antonie Van Leeuwenhoek in 1681.The genus is named after the French zoologist Alfred Mathiere Giard. *Giardia* is a microscopic parasite that causes the diarrheal illness known as giardiasis. *Giardia* (also known as *Giardia intestinalis, Giardia lamblia*or *Giardia duodenalis*) is found on surfaces or in soil, food or water that has been contaminated with feces (poop) from infected humans or animals. *Giardia* is protected by an outer shell that allows it to survive outside the body for long periods of time and makes it tolerant to chlorine disinfection. While the parasite can be spread in different ways, water (drinking water and recreational water) is the most common method of transmission.

1.6.1 Structure of *Giardia*

It is appear shaped flagellate (10-18 m) with an anterioventral attaching disc, two nuclei and four pairs of flagella (one anterior, one lateral, one ventral and one caudal). It is the first human protozoan parasite to be discovered. Giardia resides in the upper part of intestine. It is monogenetic parasite which spreads through contaminated water and food, occasionally from one person to another. Several animals also carry the parasite and contaminate streams, lakes and ponds *e.g.* cattle, Deer, Bear, Beaver, Dog. *Giardia lamblia/Giardia intestinalis* attaches to a cell of mucous membrane of intestinal wall with the help of its attaching disc which impairs fat absorption. These are saprozoic and absorb food materials present in the intestine through general surface. The parasite multiplies by binary fission and cysts. Cysts escape along with human faeces and are the source of fresh infection. Giardias like the other diplomonads have two nuclei, each with four associated flagella and lack mitochondria and golgiapparatus. However they possess a complex endomembrane system as well as mitochondrial relics, called mitosomes.

1.6.2 Life cycle of *Giardia*

Giardia intestinalis is a protozoan flagellate (Diplomonadida). This protozoan was initially namedCercomonas intestinalis by Lambl in 1859. It was renamed *Giardia lamblia* by Stiles in 1915 in honor of Professor A. Giard of Paris and Dr. F. Lambl of Prague.

Cysts are resistant forms and are responsible for transmission of giardiasis. Both cysts and trophozoites can be found in the feces (diagnostic stages) in stage 1. The cysts are hardy and can survive several months in cold water. Infection occurs by the ingestion of cysts in contaminated water, foodor by the fecal-oral route (hands or fomites) in stage 2.

In the small intestine, excystation releases trophozoites (each cyst produces two trophozoites) in stage 3. Trophozoites multiply by longitudinal binary fission, remaining in the lumen of the proximal small bowel where they can be free or attached to the mucosa by a ventral sucking disk in stage 4. Encystation occurs as the parasites transit toward the colon. The cyst is the stage found most commonly in nondiarrheal feces in stage 5. Because the cysts are infectious when passed in the stool or shortly afterward, person-to-person transmission is possible. While animals are infected with *Giardia*, their importance as a reservoir is unclear.

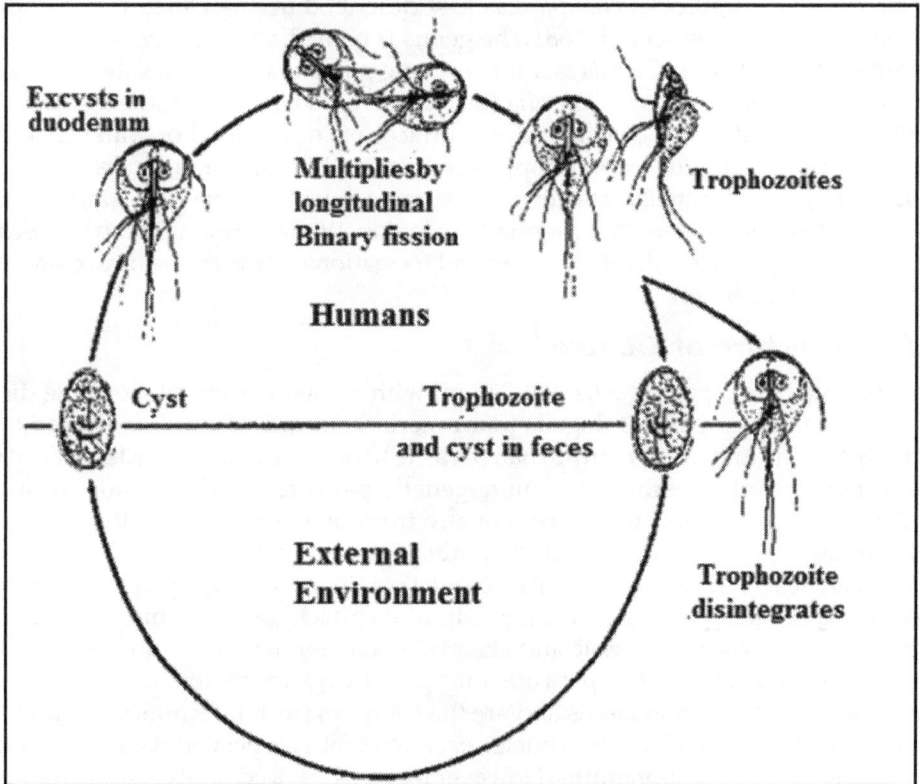

Figure 1.13: Life cycle of Giardia

1.6.3 Pathogenicity of *Giardia*

The majority of infections are asymptomatic. In symptomatic individuals, patients may experience nausea, chills, low grade fever, epigastric pain and sudden onset of watery diarrhea. Diarrhea is often explosive and presents a foul smell without the presence of blood, gas, bloating, mucusor cellular exudate. Most infections resolve spontaneously within six weeks. Chronic infections can occur and diarrhea leads to dehydration, mal-absorption, weight lost and impaired pancreatic function. Chronic infections can last from months to years. *G. lamblia* are usually found in the upper small intestine, but can be found in the gall bladder and in biliary drainage. Many infections are associated with mild to moderate mucosal damage which, in animal models of infection, has functional correlates. Possible mechanisms include direct physical injury, release of parasite products such as proteinases or lectin and mucosal inflammation associated with T cell activation and cytokine release. Other possible mechanisms of malabsorption include associated bacterial overgrowth and bile salt deconjugation, bile salt uptake by the parasite with depletion of intraluminal bile salts and inhibition of pancreatic hydrolytic enzymes. Thus, there is no single mechanism to explain the diarrhoea and mal-absorption caused by *Giardia*, which currently should be regarded as a multifactorial process. Giardiasis is a diarrheal disease caused by the microscopic parasite *Giardia*. A parasite is an organism that feeds off of another to survive. Once a person or animal (cats, dogs, cattle, deer and beavers) has been infected with *Giardia*, the parasite lives in the intestines and is passed in feces (poop). Giardiasis is a global disease. It infects nearly 2% of adults and 6% to 8% of children in developed countries worldwide. Nearly 33% of people in developing countries have had giardiasis. In the United States, Giardia infection is the most common intestinal parasitic disease affecting humans. People become infected with Giardia by swallowing Giardiacysts (hard shells containing Giardia) found in contaminated food or water. Cysts are instantly infectious once they leave the host through feces (poop). An infected person might shed 1-10 billion cysts daily in their feces (poop) and this might last for several months. However, swallowing as few as 10 cysts might cause someone to become ill. Giardia may be passed person-to-person or even animal-to-person. Alsooral-anal contact during sex has been known to cause infection. Symptoms of giardiasis normally begin 1 to 3 weeks after a person has been infected. Giardia infection rates have been known to go up in late summer.

Anyone may become infected with Giardia. However, those at greatest risk are:

- Travelers to countries where giardiasis is common,
- People in child care settings,
- Those who are in close contact with someone who has the disease,
- People who swallow contaminated drinking water,
- Backpackers or campers who drink untreated water from lakes or rivers,
- People who have contact with animals who have the disease,
- Men who have sex with men.

The risk of humans acquiring Giardia infection from dogs or cats is small. The exact type of Giardia that infects humans is usually not the same type that infects dogs and cats.

1.6.4 Diseases of *Giardia*

Signs and symptoms may vary and can last for 1 to 2 weeks or longer. In some cases, people infected with Giardia have no symptoms. Acute symptoms include:

- Diarrhea,
- Gas,
- Greasy stools that tend to float,
- Stomach or abdominal cramps,
- Upset stomach or nausea/vomiting,
- Dehydration (loss of fluids).

Other, less common symptoms include itchy skin, hives and swelling of the eye and joints. Sometimes, the symptoms of giardiasis might seem to resolve, only to come back again after several days or weeks. Giardiasis can cause weight loss and failure to absorb fat, lactose, vitamin A and vitamin B_{12}. In children, severe giardiasis might delay physical and mental growth, slow development and cause malnutrition.

1.6.5 Causes, Symptoms and Control of *Giardia*

The parasite that causes giardiasis lives in the intestines of infected humans and animals. It enters the soil, water, foodor other surfaces after bowel movements. The most frequent method of infection is by drinking contaminated water. However, people may also become infected through hand-to-mouth transmission. This involves eating contaminated food or touching contaminated surfaces and unknowingly swallowing the parasite. The parasites produce cysts (resistant forms of the parasite), which are swallowed. The cysts then reproduce in the intestines causing the signs and symptoms of giardiasis. The parasites then form new cysts that are passed in the stool, continuing the life cycle of the parasite. Ingestion of as little as 10 cysts is enough to cause illness. Giardia infection can cause a variety of intestinal symptoms, which include:

- Diarrhea,
- Gas or flatulence,
- Greasy stool that can float,
- Stomach or abdominal cramps,
- Upset stomach or nausea,
- Dehydration.

These symptoms may also lead to weight loss. Some people with Giardia infection have no symptoms at all. Giardiasis can be spread by:

- Swallowing Giardia picked up from surfaces such as bathroom handles, changing tables, diaper pails or toys that contain stool from an infected person or animal.
- Drinking water or using ice made from water sources where Giardia may live *e.g.* untreated or improperly treated water from lakes, streams or wells.
- Swallowing water while swimming or playing in water where Giardia may live, especially in lakes, rivers, springs, ponds and streams.
- Children in child care settings, especially diaper-aged children
- Eating uncooked food that contains Giardia organisms.
- Having contact with someone who is ill with giardiasis.
- Traveling to countries where giardiasis is common.
- People exposed to human feces (poop) through sexual contact.

Anything that comes into contact with feces (poop) from infected humans or animals can become contaminated with the Giardia parasite. People become infected when they swallow the parasite. It is not possible to become infected through contact with blood. Symptoms of giardiasis normally begin 1 to 3 weeks after becoming infected. In otherwise healthy people, symptoms of giardiasis may last 2 to 6 weeks. Occasionally, symptoms last longer. Medications can help decrease the amount of time symptoms last. Though giardiasis is commonly thought of as a camping or backpacking-related disease and is sometimes called Beaver Fever, anyone can get giardiasis.

Many prescription drugs are available to treat giardiasis. Although the *Giardia* parasite can infect all people, infants and pregnant women may be more likely to experience dehydration from the diarrhea caused by giardiasis. To prevent dehydration, infants and pregnant women should drink a lot of fluids while ill. Dehydration can be life threatening for infants, so it is especially important that parents talk to their health care providers about treatment options for their infants.

To prevent and control infection with the Giardia parasite, it is important to:

- Practice good hygiene.
- Avoid water (drinking or recreational) that may be contaminated.
- Avoid eating food that may be contaminated.
- Prevent contact and contamination with feces (poop) during sex.

Several drugs can be used to treat *Giardia* infection. Effective treatments include metronidazole, tinidazoleand nitazoxanide. Alternatives to these medications include paromomycin, quinacrineand furazolidone. Different factors may shape how effective a drug regimen will be, including medical history, nutritional status and condition of the immune system. Therefore, it is important to discuss treatment options with a health care provider.

1.7 Wuchereria

Wuchereria bancrofti is a filarial nematode that, as an adult, is a thread-like worm. The female nematodes are 10 cm long and 0.2 mm wide, while the males are only about 4 cm long. The adults reside and mate in the lymphatic system where they can produce up to 50 000 microfilaria per day. The microfilaria is 250-300 μm long, 8 μm wide and circulates in the peripheral blood. They can live in the host as microfilaria for up to 12 months. Adult worms take 6 to 12 months to develop from the larval stage and can live between 4 and 6 years. Wucheria (Filarial Worm) causes filariasis or elephantiasis in human beings. Another related genus *Brugia malayi* causes filariasis in Malayan Region and *Brugia timori*, human filarial parasitic nematode (roundworm) which causes the disease Timor filariasis. The parasite is digenetic, where primary host is human where it resides in lymph vessels and lymph nodes.The life cycle of this worm involves a secondary host, which is female of species mosquito of genus Culex, Aedes or Anopheles depending on the region it is found. The adult parasite is found in lymph vessels and lymph nodes while the larvae called microfilariae, occurs in blood and develop in mosquito females. The generic name of this worm is named after Wucherer who first reported it in 1866. The species *Wucheria bancrofti* is named after Bancroft who discovered the adult females in human lymph in 1876. Male worm is smaller (about 4 cm long) and female is larger (8 cm long) and ovoviviparous. Life span is of 4-5 years.

1.7.1 Structure of *Wuchereria*

An **Adult** female *Wuchereria bancrofti* is about 80–100 mm long and 0.24–0.30 mm in diameter, whereas a male is about 40 mm long and 0.1 mm in diameter. A microfilaria is about 240–300 µm (micrometers) long and 7.5–10 µm thick. It is sheathed and has nocturnal periodicity, except the South Pacific microfilaria which does not have marked periodicity. It has a gently curved body and a tail that is tapered to a point. The nuclear column (cells that constitute its body) is loosely packed. The cells can be seen individually under a microscope and do not extend to the tip of the tail.

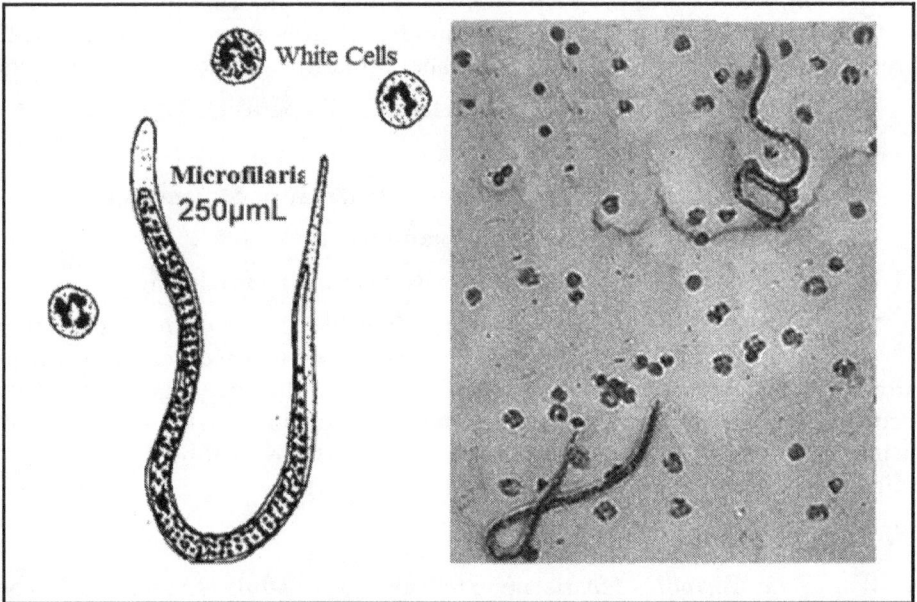

Figure 1.14: Structure of *Wuchereria*

A mosquito is the intermediate host and carrier. The most common vectors/carriers are:

- *Anopheles* species in Africa.
- *Culex quinquefasciatus* in the America.
- *Mansonia* and *Aedes* species in the Pacific and in Asia.

1.7.2 Life cycle of *Wuchereria*

The **life cycle** of *Wuchereria bancrofti* starts, when a male and a female mate inside lymphatic vessels of an infected human. The female releases thousands of microfilariae (prelarval eggs) into the bloodstream. When the host is awake, the microfilariae tend to stay in deep blood vessels. During the sleep they travel near the surface in peripheral blood vessels. This behaviour enables them to get ingested by the night biting mosquito. When ingested by the mosquito, the microfilariae migrate through the wall of the proventriculus and cardiac portion of the midgut eventually reaching the thoracic muscles. Within 1–2 weeks they mature into first-stage larvae and eventually into infective third-stage larvae which migrate through the hemocoel to the mosquito's prosbocis. When the mosquito bites another person, the larvae are injected into the human skin. They migrate to the lymph vessels and mature into adults within six months. Adult females can live up to seven years.

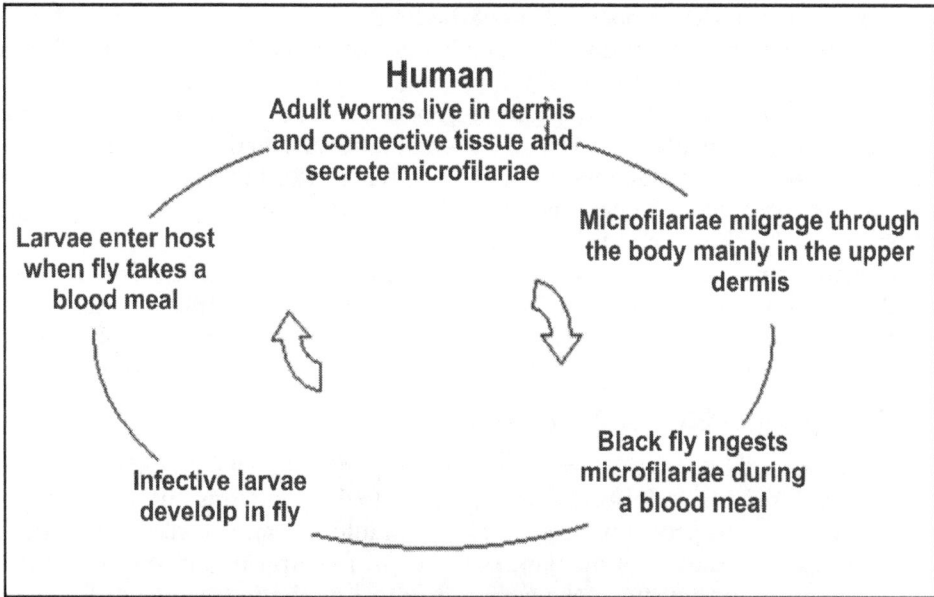

Figure 1.15: Life cycle of *Wuchereria*

Different species of the following genera of mosquitoes are vectors of *W. bancrofti* filariasis depending on geographical distribution. Among them are *Culex* (*C. annulirostris, C. bitaeniorhynchus, C. quinquefasciatus* and *C. pipiens*), *Anopheles* (*A. arabinensis, A. bancroftii, A. farauti, A. funestus, A. gambiae, A. koliensis, A. melas, A. merus, A. punctulatus* and *A. wellcomei*), *Aedes* (*A. aegypti, A. aquasalis, A. bellator, A. cooki, A. darlingi, A. kochi, A. polynesiensis, A. pseudoscutellaris, A. rotumae, A. scapularis* and *A. vigilax*), *Mansonia* (*M. pseudotitillans, M. uniformis*), *Coquillettidia* (*C. juxtamansonia*). During a blood meal, an infected mosquito introduces third-stage filarial larvae onto the skin of the human host, where they penetrate into the bite wound.

They develop in adults that commonly reside in the lymphatics. The female worms measure 80 to 100 mm in length and 0.24 to 0.30 mm in diameter, while the males measure about 40 mm by 1 mm. Adults produce microfilariae measuring 244 to 296 im by 7.5 to 10 im, which are sheathed and have nocturnal periodicity, except the South Pacific microfilariae which have the absence of marked periodicity. The microfilariae migrate into lymph and blood channels moving actively through lymph and blood. A mosquito ingests the microfilariae during a blood meal. After ingestion, the microfilariae lose their sheaths and some of them work their way through the wall of the proventriculus and cardiac portion of the mosquito's midgut and reach the thoracic muscles. There the microfilariae develop into first stage larvae and subsequently into third-stage infective larvae. The third-stage infective larvae migrate through the hemocoel to the mosquito's prosbocis and can infect another human when the mosquito takes a blood meal. Repeated mosquito bites during several months are usually needed to develop lymphatic filariasis. In some cases lymphedema (swollen tissue caused by obstruction of the lymph fluid) may develop within six months and elephantiasis within a year. Citizens of tropical and subtropical areas have the biggest risk whereas tourists have a very low risk. *Wuchereria bancrofti* infection is usually asymptomatic. Some people can develop lymphedema, swelling, which is prevalent in the legs, but sometimes also in the arms, genitalia and breasts. The swelling and decreased flow of the lymph fluid will expose the body to skin and lymph system infections. Over time the disease causes thickening and hardening of the skin, a condition called elephantiasis which can be fatal. Filarial infection might also cause pulmonary tropical eosinophilia syndrome, which is mostly found in patients living in Asia. Pulmonary tropical eosinophilia syndrome can cause: cough, shortness of breathand wheezing. In addition to eosinophilia there might be high levels of IgE (Immunoglobulin E) and antifilarial antibodies.

1.7.3 Pathogenicity of *Wuchereria*

In filarial endemic areas, there are three groups of patients recognized. The first group, considered endemic normals, are exposed to the nematode but have not been infected. The second group have been exposed, infected and have microfilaria in their peripheral circulatory system, but remain asymptomatic. Asymptomatic infections can go undetected for years and with lymphatic filariasis (LF) it may eventually result in internal damage which is not easily diagnosed. The third group is those who are chronically infected and present with lymphoedema (which affects 16 million people), hydrocoele and elephantiasis. Acute (bacterial) dermato-lymphangio-adenitis (ADLA), another condition that can result from infection, presents with fever, chills, swelling and lymphoedema. ADLA usually occurs when an adult worm dies and the lymph vessels surrounding it are inflamed due to the host's immunological response. ADLA normally occurs in older children and youth and remains with the infected individual throughout life. Chronic ADLA attacks can cause renal disease, haematuria, proteinuria, chyluria, nephritic syndrome and glomerulanephritis. Patients with LF can also have rheumatic problems, cystitis with urethral obstruction, fibrosing mediastinitis, tropical vaginal hydroceles and bladder pseudo-tumors.

Another indication of LF is pulmonary eosinophila which is characterized by paroxysmal cough and wheezing and, even though the patient harbours adult worms, there are no microfilarias in the blood. The most disabling of health problems caused by LF is elephantiasis, a permanent swelling of limb usually lower limbs although it can effect arms, breasts and genitalia. *Streptococci* bacteria can infect the affected limb, worsening the condition. Certain markers predispose patients to chronic filarial disease, including a high dose of the infectious agent, a pre-existing bacterial infection or a specific host response. Infection with *W. bancrofti* occurs in tropical and subtropical areas and is endemic in central Africa, along the Mediterranean coast and in many parts of Asia, including China, Korea, Japan and the Philippines. It is also present in Haiti, Trinidad, Surinam, Panama, Costa Rica and Brazil. No animal reservoir has been identified. *B. malayi* is found primarily in Malaysia, India, Thailand, Vietnamand parts of China, Korea, Japanand many Pacific islands. Animal reservoirs, such as cats and monkeys, are recognized.

1.7.4 Diseases of *Wuchereria*

Humans are the only known host for Wuchereria. Infection usually involves numerous exposures to this organism. It is not uncommon that an individual receive 2700 to 1,000,000 bites from infected mosquitoes (approximately equivalent to 10 to 20 years of exposure) before becoming infected. The disease is usually transmitted through the bite of an infectious mosquito. Overall there are 6 genera and 70 species of mosquitoes responsible for the spread of *Wuchereria bancrofti*. The incubation period is variable and often difficult to determine. Both microfilaria and adult worms have been observed in patients as early as 6 months and as late as 12 months after infection. This disease is not transmitted from person-to-person. Mosquitoes can be infected by humans if they ingest microfilaria during a blood meal of an infected individual. The mosquito remains infectious for only 10-14 days after consuming an infected blood meal. Mosquitoes are the vector for this nematode and certain genera and species appear to transmit the infectious agent in particular geographical locations. Although the parasite damages the lymph system, most infected people have no symptoms and will never develop clinical symptoms.

These people do not know they have lymphatic filariasis unless tested. A small percentage of persons will develop lymphedema. This is caused by fluid collection because of improper functioning of the lymph system resulting in swelling. This mostly affects the legs, but can also occur in the arms, breastsand genitalia. Most people develop these symptoms years after being infected. The swelling and the decreased function of the lymph system make it difficult for the body to fight germs and infections. These people will have more bacterial infections in the skin and lymph system. This causes hardening and thickening of the skin, which is called elephantiasis. Many of these bacterial infections can be prevented with appropriate skin hygiene and exercise. Men can develop hydrocele or swelling of the scrotum due to infection with one of the parasites that causes LF specifically *W. bancrofti*. Filarial infection can also cause tropical pulmonary eosinophilia syndrome, although this syndrome is typically found in persons living with the disease in Asia. Symptoms of tropical pulmonary eosinophilia syndrome include cough, shortness of breathand wheezing. The eosinophilia is often accompanied by high levels of IgE (Immunoglobulin E) and antifilarial antibodies.

1.7.5 Causes, Symptoms and Control of *Wuchereria*

Diagnosis for lymphatic filariasis is traditionally done from a blood sample by microscopic examination. The sample has to be taken during the night to ensure the microfilariae are present in the bloodstream. The blood can also be check for the presence of antibodies (antifilarial IgG) that the human body develops to fight against antigens excreted by adult female *Wuchereria bancrofti* worms. A new method of a highly sensitive card test has been developed to detect antigens without laboratory equipment using finger-prick blood droplets taken anytime of the day. Molecular diagnosis by polymerase chain reaction (PCR) is possible, too. Treatment for infected patients is usually done using a drug called diethylcarbamazine (DEC). The medicine kills the microfilariae in the bloodstream and sometimes adult worms in the lymph vessels. It has some side effects which include: dizziness, fever, headache, nausea and muscle and joint pain. DEC should only be used, if *Wuchereria bancrofti* has been identified. This is because most people with lymphedema are not infected with parasites. DEC can worsen Onchocerciasis (an eye disease caused by *Onchocerca volvulus*) and can cause encephalopathy (brain disease) and death in people who are infected with *Loa loa*. Another drug, Ivermectin, can also be used, although it only kills microfilariae. In some cases lymphedema can be prevented from getting worse by exercising the swollen leg or arm to improve the lymph flow. The swollen skin is vulnerable to bacterial infections because immune defenses cannot work properly due to the impaired flow of fluids. That is why the skin must be kept clean. According to recent studies *Wolbachia* bacteria are in symbiosis with *Wuchereria bancrofti*. The bacteria live inside the worm. If the bacteria are killed with antibiotics, *Wuchereria bancrofti* dies, too. DEC is effective against adults and microfilariae; however, destruction of the parasites may induce severe allergic reactions that require treatment with corticosteroids. Albendazole or ivermectin has been shown to be effective in reducing microfilarial loads. Surgical removal of worms migrating across the eye or bridge of the nose can be accomplished by immobilizing the worm with instillation of a few drops of 10% cocaine. Education regarding the infection and its vector, especially for people entering the known endemic areas, is essential. Protection from fly bites by using screening, appropriate clothing and insect repellents, along with treatment of cases, is also critical in reducing the incidence of infection. However, the presence of disease in animal reservoirs *e.g.* monkeys limits the feasibility of controlling this disease. To prevent new infections, avoid infective mosquitoes between dusk and dawn, the time when they mostly feed. A mosquito net can be applied all around your bed. Mosquito repellent applied on your skin or the use of long trousers and sleeves might keep the mosquitoes away. Mass treatments are given to whole communities in some endemic countries. Programmes to eliminate lymphatic filariasis in more than forty countries are decreasing the risk of infection.

The best way to prevent lymphatic filariasis is to avoid mosquito bites. The mosquitoes that carry the microscopic worms usually bite between the hours of dusk and dawn.

At night

- Sleep in an air-conditioned room,
- Sleep under a mosquito net.

Between dusk and dawn

- Wear long sleeves and trousers,
- Use mosquito repellent on exposed skin.

Another approach to prevention includes giving entire communities medicine that kills the microscopic worms and controlling mosquitoes. Annual mass treatment reduces the level of microfilariae in the blood and thus, diminishes transmission of infection. This is the basis of the global campaign to eliminate lymphatic filariasis. Experts consider that lymphatic filariasis, a neglected tropical disease (NTD), can be eradicated and a global campaign to eliminate lymphatic filariasis as a public health problem is under way. The elimination strategy is based on annual treatment of whole communities with combinations of drugs that kill the microfilariae. As a result of the generous contributions of these drugs by the companies that make them, tens of millions of people are being treated each year. Since these drugs also reduce levels of infection with intestinal worms, benefits of treatment extend beyond lymphatic filariasis.

Summary

1. Parasitology is the study of parasites and their relationships to their hosts.

2. Parasitology is an applied field of biology dedicated to the study of the biology, ecology and relationships which parasites are involved in with other organisms known as the host.

3   Parasites are an extremely varied group. They range from flies, such as the blood sucking mosquitoes, nematodes such as the heartworm of dogs, liver flukes of cattle and sheep, fleas commonly found on dogs and cats, lice and ticks found on almost all domestic animals and protozoa such as Giardia which are found in most domestic animals but are of particular significance in cattle and dogs.

4. A definitive host is the host in which the parasite becomes sexually mature. An intermediate host is a temporary environment for the parasite, but is nonetheless necessary for the parasite to complete its life cycle.

5. A carrier is an animal or man which has a light infection with a parasite but is not harmed by it, usually due to immunity resulting from previous infection, but which serves as a source of infection for susceptible animals or men.

6. The study of parasites that cause economic losses in agriculture or aquaculture operations or which infect companion animals. This is becoming particularly important as emerging diseases threatens global food security.

7. Parasites are dynamic in their distribution; some are endemic while many are ubiquitous. The environment plays a key role in their survival and transmission.

8. Nematode parasites of domestic vertebrate animals are managed by strategies that include control of secondary hosts or vectors and the use of chemical anthelminthics.

9. Helminth infections of wild animals are not managed, except by attrition of infected individuals.

10. The word helminth is a general term meaning worm, but there are many different types of worms.

11. Nematodes (roundworms) have long thin un-segmented tube like bodies with anterior mouths and longitudinal digestive tracts.

12. Two classes of nematodes are recognized on the basis of the presence or absence of special chemoreceptors known as phasmids; Secernentea (Phasmidea) and Adenophorea (Aphasmidea).

13. Two subclasses of cestodes are differentiated on the basis of the numbers of larval hooks, the Cestodaria being decacanth (10 hooks) and Eucestoda being hexacanth (6 hooks).

14. Trypanosoma is a group of unicellular parasitic flagellate heteroxenous protozoan, requiring more than one obligate host to complete life cycle and are transmitted via vector.

15. In 1902, Forde and Dutton discovered the presence of trypanosomes in human blood in a case of Gambia fever, the preliminary stage of sleeping sickness.

16. In the vertebrate hosts, most trypanosomes usually multiply by simple fission, although in some species, notably *Trypanosoma lewisi* of rats, division of the nuclei and kinetoplasts may outrun actual cell division early in an infection.

17. *Trypanosoma brucei* and its related subspecies are parasitic hemoflagellate protists that are implicated in a severe meningoencephalitic disease, African trypanosomiasis, more commonly known as sleeping sickness.

18. *Trypanosoma brucei* causes African trypanosomiasis, commonly known as Sleeping Sickness in humans and Nagana (meaning loss of spirit' in the Zulu language) in cattle. *Trypanosoma cruzi* causes Chagas' Disease, a chronic human infection.

19. The diagnosis of African Trypanosomiasis is made through laboratory methods, because the clinical features of infection are not sufficiently specific.

20. There is no vaccine or drug for prophylaxis against African trypanosomiasis. Preventive measures are aimed at minimizing contact with tsetse flies. Local residents are usually aware of the areas that are heavily infested and they can provide advice about places to avoid.

21. *Giardia* (Grand Old Man of Intestine) is a genus of anaerobic flagellated protozoan parasite that colonizes and reproduces in the small intestines of several vertebrates causing giardiasis.

22. *Giardia intestinalis* is a protozoan flagellate (Diplomonadida). This protozoan was initially named *Cercomonas intestinalis* by Lambl in 1859.

23. The risk of humans acquiring Giardia infection from dogs or cats is small. The exact type of Giardia that infects humans is usually not the same type that infects dogs and cats.

24. The parasite that causes giardiasis lives in the intestines of infected humans and animals. It enters the soil, water, food or other surfaces after bowel movements.

25. Many prescription drugs are available to treat giardiasis. Although the *Giardia* parasite can infect all people, infants and pregnant women may be more likely to experience dehydration from the diarrhea caused by giardiasis.

26. *Wuchereria bancrofti* is a filarial nematode that, as an adult, is a thread-like worm. The female nematodes are 10 cm long and 0.2 mm wide, while the males are only about 4 cm long.

27. An Adult female *Wuchereria bancrofti* is about 80–100 mm long and 0.24–0.30 mm in diameter, whereas a male is about 40 mm long and 0.1 mm in diameter.

28. The life cycle of *Wuchereria bancrofti* starts, when a male and a female mate inside lymphatic vessels of an infected human. The female releases thousands of microfilariae (prelarval eggs) into the bloodstream.

29. In filarial endemic areas, there are three groups of patients recognized. The first group, considered endemic normals, are exposed to the nematode but have not been infected. The second group have been exposed, infected and have microfilaria in their peripheral circulatory system, but remain asymptomatic.

30. Humans are the only known host for Wuchereria. Infection usually involves numerous exposures to this organism. It is not uncommon that an individual receive 2700 to 1,000,000 bites from infected mosquitoes (approximately equivalent to 10 to 20 years of exposure) before becoming infected.

31. Diagnosis for lymphatic filariasis is traditionally done from a blood sample by microscopic examination. The sample has to be taken during the night to ensure the microfilariae are present in the bloodstream.

32. The best way to prevent lymphatic filariasis is to avoid mosquito bites.

Chapter 2
Vectors and Pests

2.1 Introduction

A pest is an organism with characteristics that people see as damaging or unwanted, as it harms agriculture through feeding on crops or parasitizing livestock. An animal can also be a pest when it causes damage to a wild ecosystem or carries germs. A pest is a plant or animal detrimental to humans or human concerns. When pests such as insects attack us by biting or stinging, disease symptoms may result. Some animal species harbor pathogenic microbial organisms such as bacteria or viruses. If an animal transmits such an organism to a person and the person becomes ill, then the animal has served as a disease vector. Some organisms are included as public health pests not because they directly attack or annoy us, but because they help produce situations favoring the growth of pests or vectors. Of all the insect species now living on earth, at least half of them (4,00,000 -5,00,000) feed directly on the tissues of living plants or animal. It is probably no exaggeration to claim that every plant species on earth serves as food for at least one species of insect. No parts of a plant are immune from attack; insect herbivores chew the leaves, suck the sap, mine the cambium, gather the pollen, invade the buds, destroy the flowers and devour the fruit. Even plants that manufacture potent insecticides such as the nicotine in tobacco, pyrethrum in chrysanthemums or rotenone in tropical legumes have insect pests that are especially adapted to feed on their tissues and detoxify their chemical defenses. Herbivores with chewing mouthparts consume a plant directly. They use mandibles to masticate (knead), triturate (grind) or abrade (scrape) plant tissue into manageable bites. Most species consume entire roots, stems, leaves, buds, flowers, fruit and/or seeds. All members of the orders Orthoptera and Phasmida feed in this manner, as do nearly all larvae of Lepidoptera. Chewing herbivores are also found in the order Diptera *e.g.* larvae of Tephritid fruit flies, in the Coleoptera *e.g.* larvae and adults of weevils, scarab beetles, leaf beetles and many others and in the Hymenoptera (ants, some bees and the larvae of all sawflies). Immatures of aquatic orders, such as Trichoptera, Plecoptera and Ephemeroptera, also feed by chewing plant tissues but they are seldom regarded as major pests. Not all chewing herbivores consume entire portions of their host plant. Leaf miners represented by several families in the Diptera and Lepidoptera are specialized herbivores that excavate galleries in mesophyll, the inner layer of cells between a leaf's upper and lower epidermis. Other species concentrate on epidermal cells. The pear slug (immature sawfly) skeletonizes the leaves of its host plant by abrading only cells from the lower epidermal surface. Many bark beetles feed only in cambium, the layer of cells just beneath the bark of a tree or shrub.

Plant tissue is also damaged by herbivores with piercing-sucking mouthparts. Some species *e.g.* stink bugs stab their feeding stylets into individual plant cells, inject digestive enzymes to liquify the substrate and then suck out the partially digested food. Other species *e.g.* aphids thread their stylets delicately through intercellular spaces, tap into the plant's vascular system and feed by withdrawing sap from the phloem. Most pest species with piercing-sucking mouthparts belong to the orders Hemiptera (Heteroptera and Homoptera) and Thysanoptera. Damage from these insects is often less visible than that of chewing insects, but it may still result in severe injury to the plant. Gall making insects are herbivores that live within the tissues of a plant. They secrete a hormone like substance that stimulates growth in surrounding plant tissue and induces the host plant to produce a specialized shelter (gall) that nourishes and protects the herbivore inside. Gall making insects sometimes called Cecidozoa include species in the orders Hemiptera, Hymenoptera, Lepidoptera and Diptera. Gall formation is also induced by certain species of mites, fungi and bacteria. Gall makers are highly specialized herbivores; each species is narrowly adapted to its host plant and produces a distinctively shaped gall. Herbivores may also injure their host plants during oviposition; females often cut holes or slits in plant tissues as they deposit their eggs. Oviposition scars from cicadas, crickets and katydids may be severe enough to kill twigs or stems. This problem is most troublesome in nurseries and greenhouses where ornamental plants with obvious injury are less marketable. Many insects that feed on plants also serve as vectors of plant diseases. All major taxa of plant pathogens are spread by insects, including viruses, mycoplasma, bacteria, protozoa, fungi and nematodes. Plant pathogens may be carried externally on a vector's feet, mouthparts or ovipositors. This mechanical transmission has been well-documented in vectors representing at least eight arthropod orders such as Hemiptera (both suborders), Thysanoptera orthoptera, Diptera, Coleoptera, Hymenoptera, Lepidoptera, plus Acarina (mites).

Some pathogens even provide symbiotic advantages for their insect vectors. Bark beetles infect trees with a pathogenic fungus whenever they establish new colonies. As the fungus becomes established in each new tree, it changes the micro-environment of the wood and improves reproductive success for the bark beetles. A blue-stain fungus carried by *Ips sp.* bark beetles and Dutch elm disease spread by *Scolytus* sp. bark beetles are examples of this type of symbiotic relationship between pathogen and vector. Plant pathogens may also be carried internally in the salivary glands, digestive tract or reproductive system of insect vectors (biological transmission). These pathogens are usually inoculated into new hosts during feeding or ovi-position, but they may also be spread through the insect's feces. Several families of vectors show strong affinity for biological transmission of pathogens in specific taxonomic groups. Thrips, aphids and whiteflies, tend to be vectors of virus pathogens, whereas leafhoppers are more likely to transmit mycoplasma like organisms (MLOs). Invertebrate animals include millions of animals that are not pests, such as sponges, starfish, earthworms and squid. Nearly all the public health invertebrate pests are in the Phylum Arthropoda and are called arthropods. The arthropods of public health importance are primarily the insects and their close arachnid relatives' ticks, mites and spiders. There are well over one million species of insects, which means that there are more kinds of insects than any other kind of organism. Insects may cause diseases or annoyance to people in many ways, including:

- Causing allergic reactions,
- Causing fright and annoyance,
- Crawling, scraping, biting, bloodsucking and other ways of attacking people,
- Invading body tissues or organs of people,
- Stinging people,
- Transmitting disease organisms,
- Serving as hosts to disease organisms.

2.2 Vectors

A vector is an organism that carries a pathogen with it. An example would be malaria-carrying mosquito. Pests are in themselves the problem and usually refer to insects or animals that destroy crops. Integrated pest management (IPM) techniques are necessary to reduce the number of pests that threaten human health and property. The term vector refers to any arthropod that transmits a disease through feeding activity. Vectors typically become infected by a disease agent while feeding on infected vertebrates *e.g.* birds, rodents, other larger animals or humans and then pass on the microbe to a susceptible person or other animal. In almost all cases, an infectious microbe must infect and multiply inside the arthropod before the arthropod is able to transmit the disease through its salivary glands. A vector is any arthropod, insect, rodent or other animal of public health significance capable of harboring or transmitting the causative agents of human disease *e.g.* malaria, plague to humans. Under certain circumstances, insects or other arthropods that cause human discomfort or injury, but not disease, are sometimes referred to as vectors. Vector-borne disease is the term commonly used to describe an illness caused by an infectious microbe that is transmitted to people by blood sucking arthropods. The arthropods (insects or arachnids) that most commonly serve as vectors include blood sucking insects such as mosquitoes, fleas, lice, biting flies and bugs and blood sucking arachnids such as mites and ticks.

In ancient times, insects were very important in the transmission of communicable diseases. The definition of vector was related mostly to insects. Later on the term vector has been used more widely to include other non-human animals including snails, dogs and rats. Alternative definitions are found. For example, vectors can be defined as arthropods and other invertebrates which transmit infection by inoculation into or through the skin or mucous membrane by biting or by deposit of infective materials on the skin or on food or other objects.

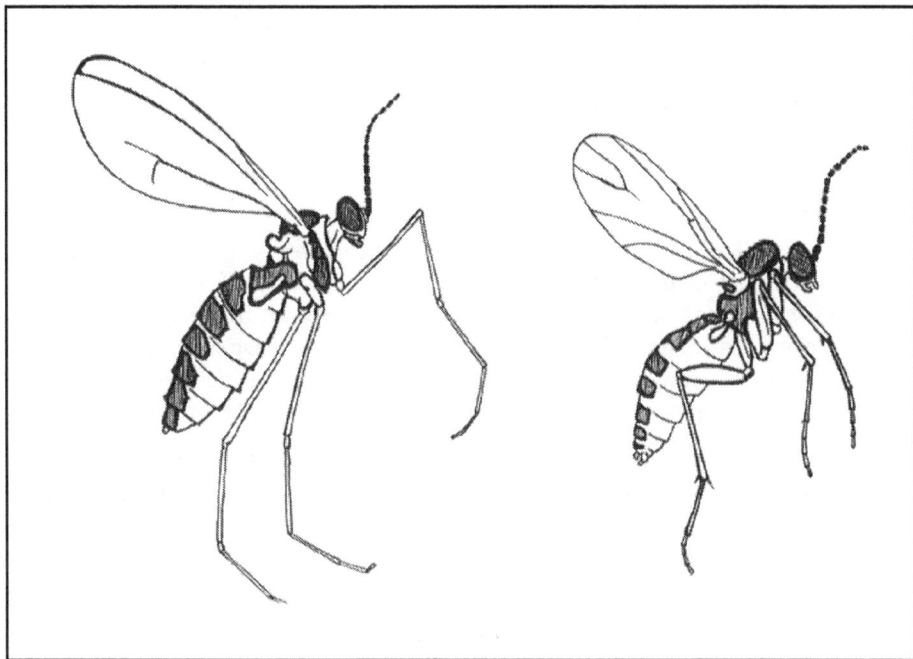

Figure 2.1: Vector

This classical definition considers mainly the arthropods which include insects and other organisms such as mites. It shows the mechanisms of transmission as inoculation (biting) and depositing infective materials (pathogenic organisms such as bacteria) on skin and food. Vectors can also be defined as any non-human carriers of pathogenic organisms that can transmit these organisms directly to humans. Vertebrates, such as dogs and rodents and invertebrates, such as insects, can all be vectors of disease. This second definition focuses on the range of living things involved. Knowing this definition is helpful in the design of preventive measures for controlling living organisms such as insects and rats which carry the disease agent (bacteria, virus) from an infected person to a healthy person. Malaria, yellow fever, typhus fever, epidemic typhus, malaria, onchocerciasis, leishmaniasis, rabies and schistosomiasis are all communicable diseases that are prevalent. All of these are transmitted by vectors. A number of diarrhoeal diseases (acute watery diarrhoea, dysentery, typhoid fever) can also be transmitted by vectors and are commonly observed among children in areas where sanitation is very poor. Diarrhoea alone kills many children before they get to their fifth year. Vector borne diseases not only cause illness, they also act as a barrier to development. Irrigation and dam workers will not be productive if they get malaria or schistosomiasis (bilharzia or snail fever). A person with malaria will need healthcare and will lose productive days at work. Some diseases like onchocerciasis (river blindness) have a devastating health impact. If onchocerciasis is left untreated the person could go blind. Additionally, vectors like rats destroy food and household materials and weevils damage cereals.

The public health importance of vectors can be summarized as follows:

- They cause illness that could be fatal or restrict working capacity.
- They damage food and household goods.
- They are a barrier to development.

2.3 Pests

Human civilization has been competing with insects, rodents, diseases and weeds for survival throughout its history. Historical records of plagues, famine and pestilence fill volumes of texts. Modern man has, through his technology, created tools to combat these pests. The use of a tool, such as a pesticide, depends on the applicators ability to know when they are needed. Proper identification of the problem is the first step to proper application. A pest is considered to be anything that:

- Injures humans, animals, crops, structures or possessions.
- Competes with humans, domestic animals or crops for food, feed or water.
- Spreads disease to humans, domestic animals or crops.

Pests can be placed into four main categories:

- Insects and closely related animals,
- Plant diseases,
- Weeds,
- Vertebrates.

2.3.1 Insects

Insects, as a class of animals, outnumber all other living animals on earth. There are three times as many insects as there are animals in the rest of the animal kingdom. Insects are found everywhere; in snow, water, air, soil, hot springs and in or on plants and animals. They compete with man and animals for food and are also considered food for a significant number of other animals. Some insects survive solely by feeding on man, for example human lice and cannot survive for long if removed from the human body. Insects are an extremely important part of the earth's ecosystem and despite our dread of insects we could not survive without them. Insects can be divided into three groups by their importance:

- **Species not considered pests:** About 99% of all insect species are in this group. They are food for other animals (birds, fish, mammals, reptiles and other insects). Some insects like butterflies are considered pleasant to look at.
- **Beneficial insects:** This important group includes predators and parasites that feed on pest insects, mites and weeds. Good examples are ladybird beetles (lady bugs) and praying mantids. Pollinating insects are also very important, such as honey bees, bumble bees, moths, butterflies and beetles. Honey bees make food for humans and animals. Some other benefits derived from insects are silk from the cocoons of silkworms or dyes for paints made from insect secretions.

- **Pest insects.** This group includes the smallest number of species. These insects feed on, cause injury to or transmit disease to humans, animals, plants, food, fiber and structures. Some examples of pest insects are mosquitoes, fleas, termites, aphids and beetles.

Insect Body Characteristics

All adult insects have two characteristics in common; they have three pairs of jointed legs and they have three body regions; head, thorax and abdomen.

Head: Attached to the insect head are the antennae, eyes and mouthparts. All of these parts vary in size and shape and can be helpful in identifying some pest insects.

Antennae: Antennae are paired appendages usually located between or below the eyes. Antennae vary greatly in size and form and are used in classifying and identifying insects. Some of the common antennae types are:

- **Filiform:** Threadlike; the segments are nearly uniform in size and shaped like a cylinder (ground beetle, cockroach).

- **Moniliform:** Look like a string of beads; the segments are similar in size and round in shape (termites).

- **Serrate:** Sawlike; the segments are more or less triangular (Click beetle).

- **Clubbed:** Segments increase in diameter away from the head (Japanese beetle).

- **Plumose:** Feathery; most segments with whorls of long hair (Male mosquito).

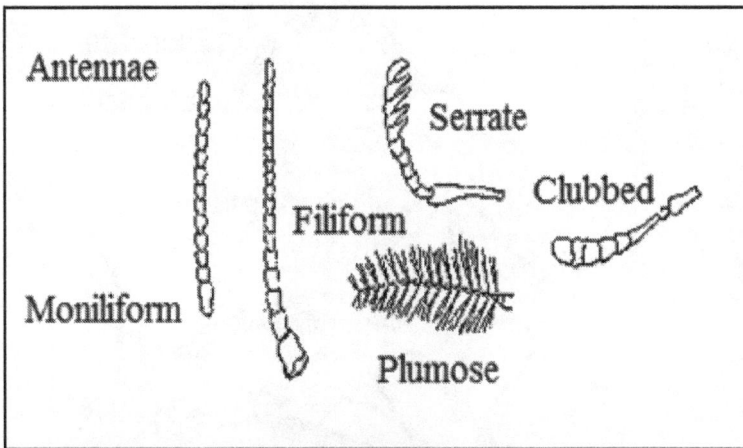

Figure 2.2: Insect Body Parts

Mouthparts: Mouthparts are different in various insect groups and are often used in classification and identification. The type of mouthpart determines how the insect feeds and what sort of damage it does. There are mainly four types of mouthparts categorized:

i.   Chewing mouthparts have toothed jaws that bite and tear the food. Example includes beetles, cockroaches, ants, caterpillars and grasshoppers.

ii.   Piercing-sucking mouthparts are usually long slender tubes that are forced into plant or animal tissue to suck out fluids or blood. Example includes mosquitoes, aphids.

iii. Sponging mouthparts are tongue like structures that have spongy tips to suck up liquids or food that can be made liquid by the insect's vomit. Example includes house flies, blow flies.

iv.   Siphoning mouthparts are long tubes used for sucking nectar such as butterflies, moths.

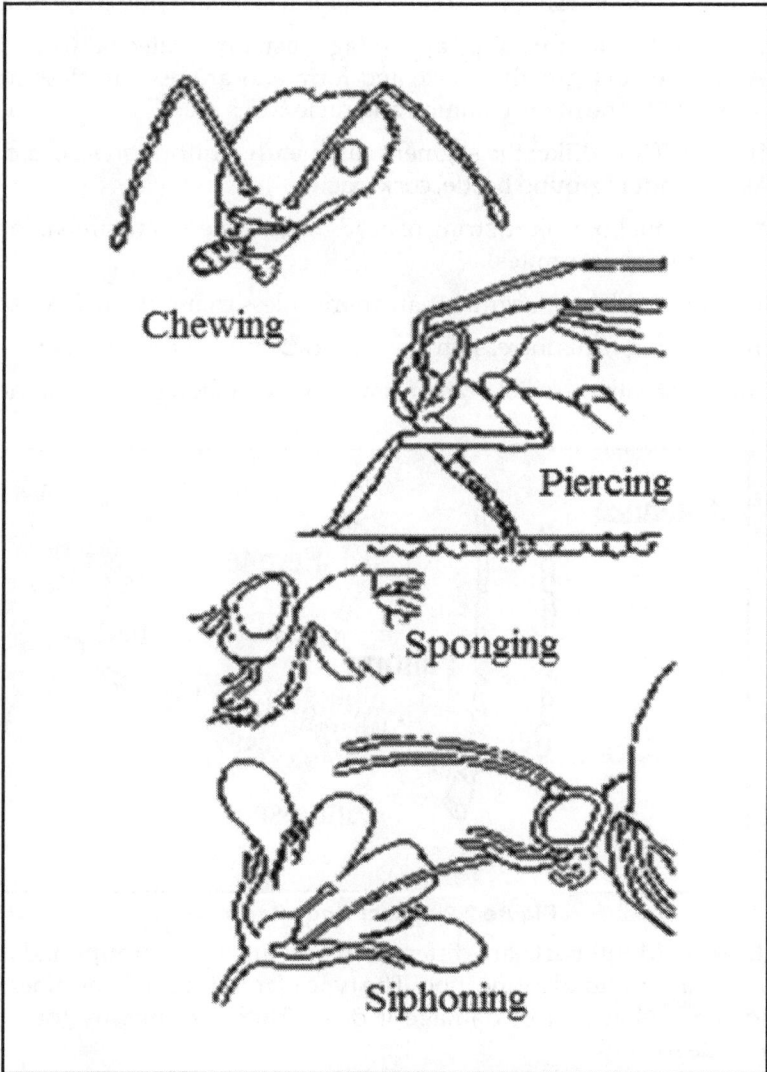

Figure 2.3: Activity of Mouth Part of Insects

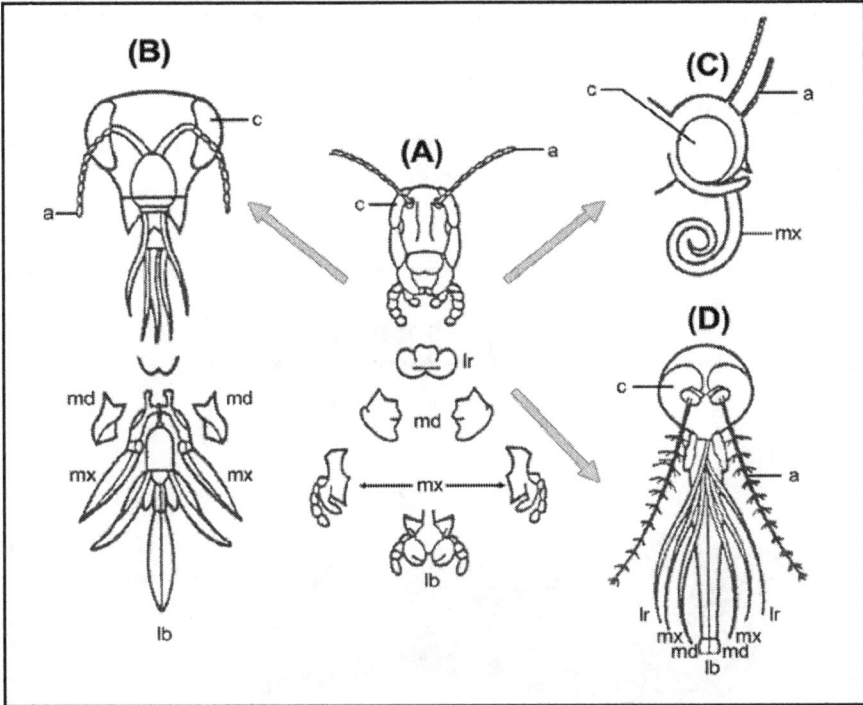

Figure 2.4: Mouthparts of Insects

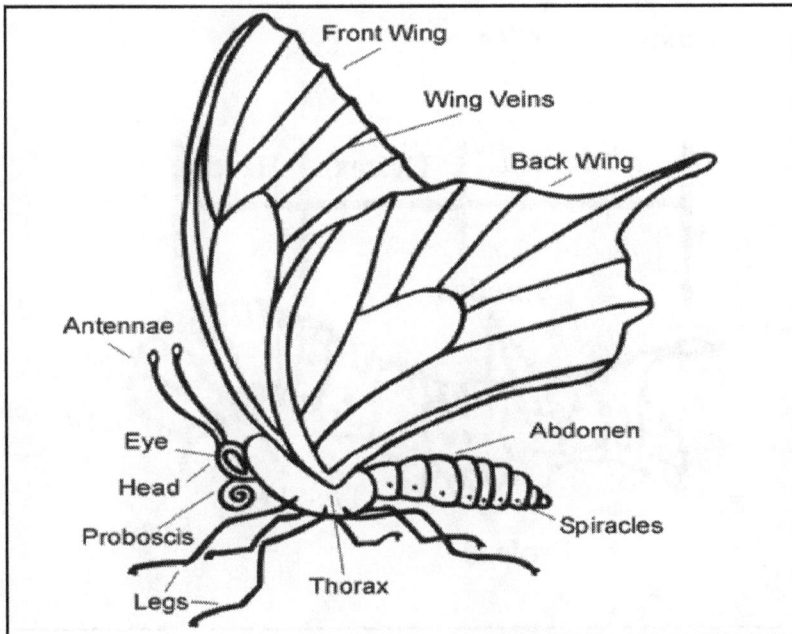

Figure 2.5: Parts of Butterfly

Thorax: The thorax or middle body segment has three pair of legs and sometimes one or two pair of wings (forewings, hind wings). Legs come in many sizes, shapes and functions and are helpful in identifying insects. Used for walking, running, jumping and climbing, legs have become very specialized in some insects like the large jumping leg in the grasshopper. Crickets and long horned grasshoppers have an eardrum at the base of one of their leg segments.

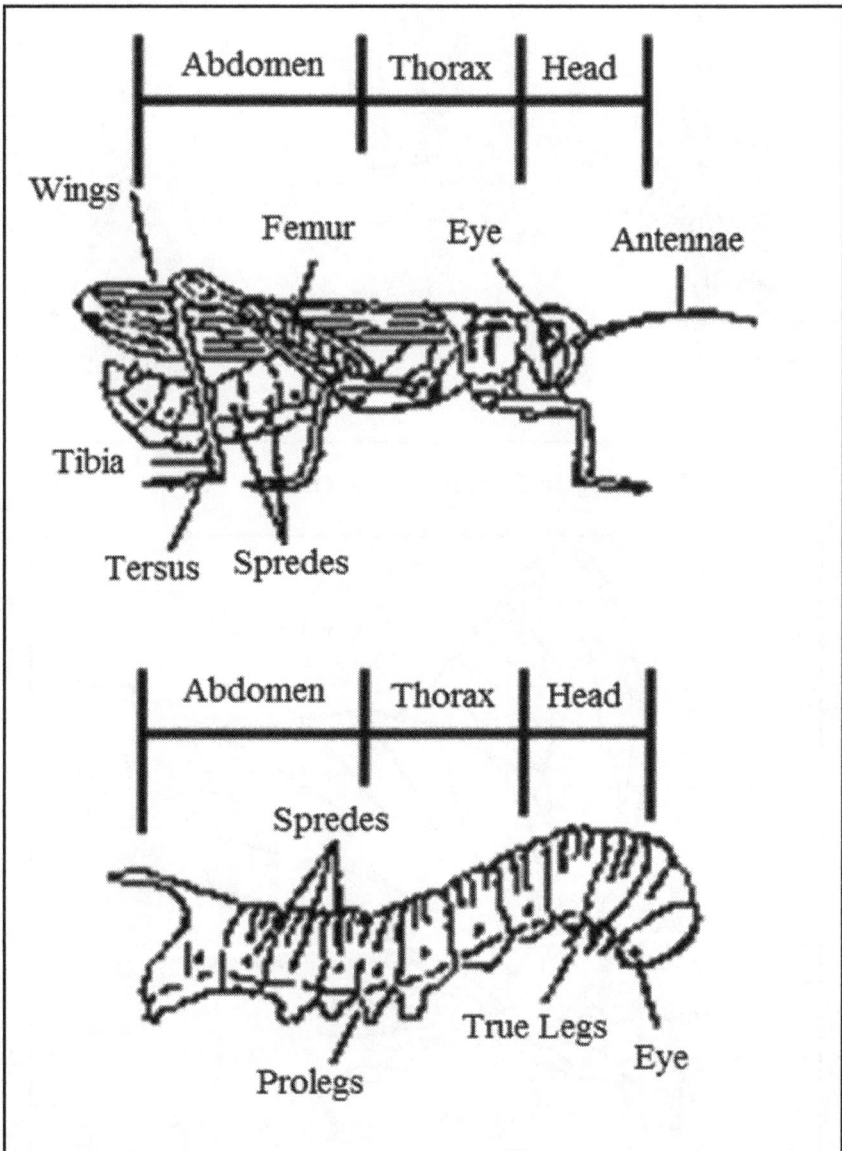

Figure 2.6: Structure of Insect

Wings also vary in size, shape and texture. The pattern of veins on the wings of an insect are often used to identify insect species. Forewings in some insects are hard and shell like, as in beetles. The grasshoppers have forewings that are leathery. The forewings of flies are thin, clear and like membranes. The wings of moths, butterflies and mosquitoes are membranous and are also covered with scales.

Wings also vary in size, shape and texture. The pattern of veins on the wings of an insect are often used to identify insect species. Forewings in some insects are hard and shell like, as in beetles. The grasshoppers have forewings that are leathery. The forewings of flies are thin, clear and like membranes. The wings of moths, butterflies and mosquitoes are membranous and are also covered with scales.

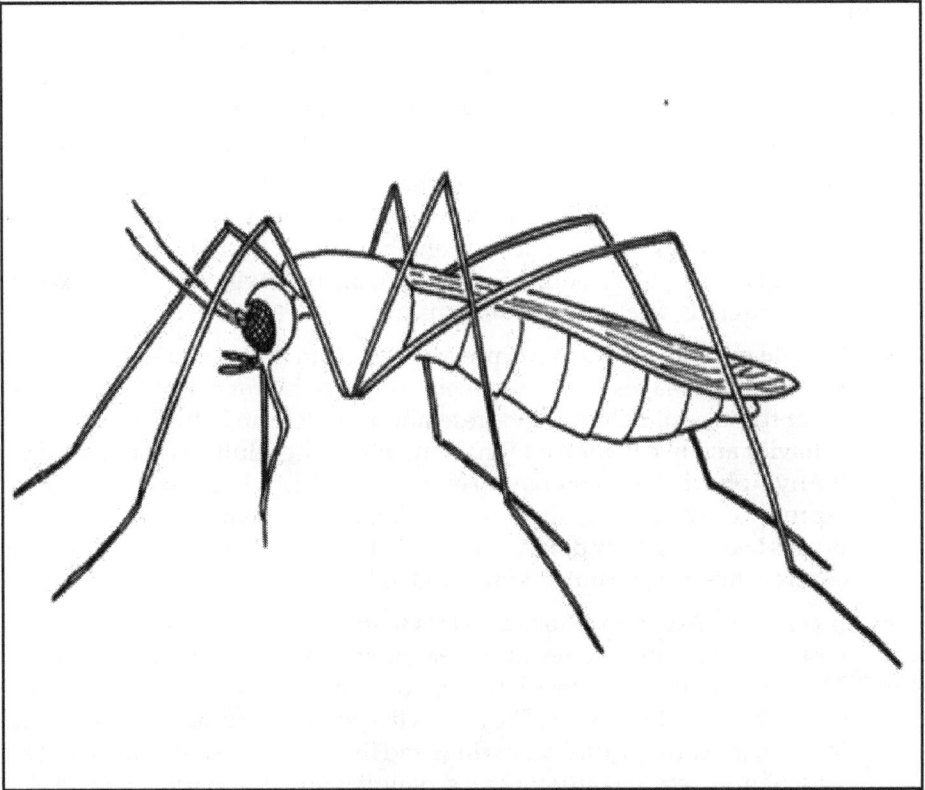

Figure 2.7: Mosquito

Insect Reproduction and Development

Insect Reproduction: In most insects, reproduction results from the males fertilizing females. The females then lay the eggs. This is the pattern of life for most insects, but there are a few interesting variations. For example, some parasitic wasps produce eggs without ever mating. In some of these species, males are unknown.

There are a few insects that give birth to live young, without the egg stage. Egg hatching is affected by temperature, humidity and light. Eggs come in several shapes (round, oval, flat and elongate) and sizes. They are laid one at a time, in groups and in floating rafts. Some insects lay eggs in capsules containing several eggs, then carry them until hatching to be sure of the survival of their young (German cockroach). Sometimes eggs are placed inside the bodies of animals, trees and green plants. In some species, the eggs are used to identify the adult. For example, the egg capsules of cockroaches can be used to identify an infesting species of cockroach.

Insect Metamorphosis (Development): Insects go through a series of changes as they develop from the egg to adulthood. This process of growth is called metamorphosis. After hatching from an egg, the young insect is called a larva, nymph or naiad. The young feed for a while and grow. When they grow to a point where the skin cannot stretch further, the young insect molts and a new skin is formed. These stages of growth and skin shedding called instars differ from insect to insect and sometimes may vary with the temperature, humidity and food supply. Generally, the heaviest feeding occurs in the last two instars. There are four types of metamorphosis:

- **No Metamorphosis:** A few insects change very little except in size between hatching and reaching adulthood. The insect grows larger with each instar until it reaches maturity. The food and habitats of the nymphs are similar to those of the adult. The adults and nymphs are both wingless. Some examples are springtails, firebrats and silverfish.

- **Simple or Gradual Metamorphosis:** Insects in this group mature through three distinct stages of development before reaching maturity such as egg, nymph and adult. The nymphs resemble the adults in both form and feeding behavior and live in the same environment. If the adult has compound eyes, the nymph will have compound eyes. However, nymphs will not be able to reproduce. The body matures gradually, with the wings and reproductive organs becoming fully developed only in the adult stage. Some examples are: cockroaches, lice, termites, scales and aphids.

- **Incomplete Metamorphosis:** Insects with incomplete metamorphosis also pass through three stages of development such as egg, naiad and adult. There are some similarities between the adult and naiad, but there are also some dramatic differences. The naiads live in the water (aquatic) and breathe through gills. The adults have wings and live near the water, but do not have gills. Some examples are stoneflies, mayflies and dragonflies.

- **Complete Metamorphosis:** This is a four stage development process, consisting of stages called egg, larva, pupa and adult. The young are called larvae and are familiar to everyone as caterpillars, maggots or grubs and are entirely different from the adults. The larvae and the adults usually live in different habitats and eat different food. For example, caterpillars may live on a plant and eat leaves, while the adult butterfly flies freely, sipping nectar for food.

The larvae hatch from an egg. As they grow larger they molt and pass through one to several instars.

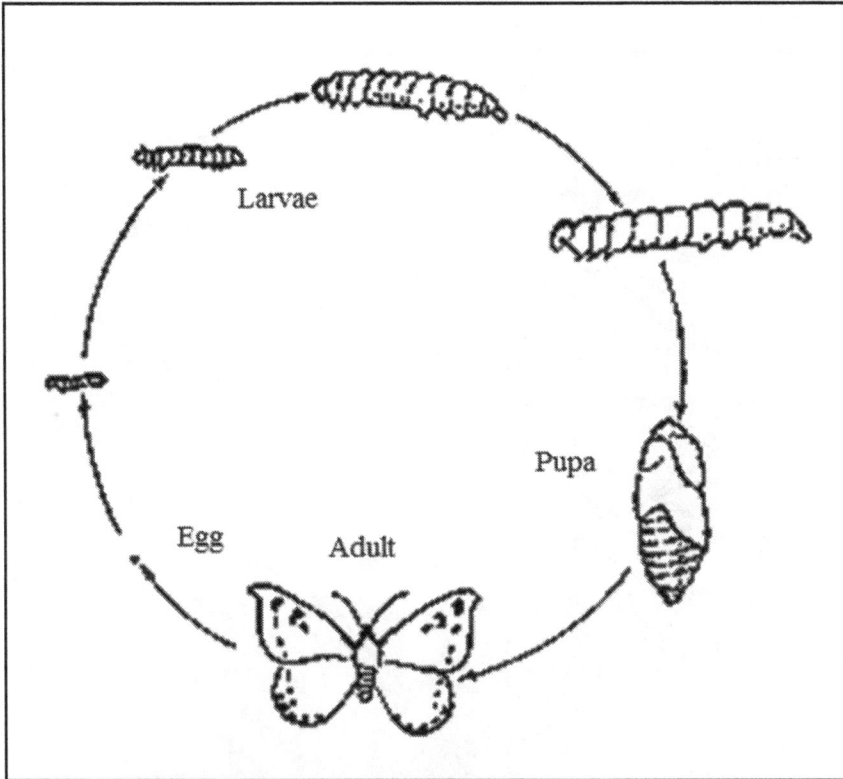

Figure 2.8: Complete Metamorphosis

Larvae come in several forms, shapes and sizes such as caterpillars with many legs to maggots which are legless. The pupa is often called the resting stage, but the insect is doing anything but resting. While in this stage, the larvae changes into an adult with legs, wings, antennae and a fully functional reproductive system.

2.3.2 Insect like Pests

Spiders, ticks, mites, sowbugs, pillbugs, millipedes and centipedes resemble insects in habit, appearance, life cycle and size. Although they are not insects, they are often mistaken for them.

Centipedes and Millipedes

Centipedes are flat, long, worm like animals, with each body segment having one pair of legs. They have chewing mouthparts. Some can give painful bites to humans. Centipedes are found in protected places under tree bark or in rotting logs. They are very fast and predaceous, capturing and feeding on insects, spiders and other small animals. All centipedes have poisonous jaws. Millipedes have a cylindrical shape, like an earthworm and have many legs, two pair on each body segment. The mouth parts are adapted to feeding on decaying organic material.

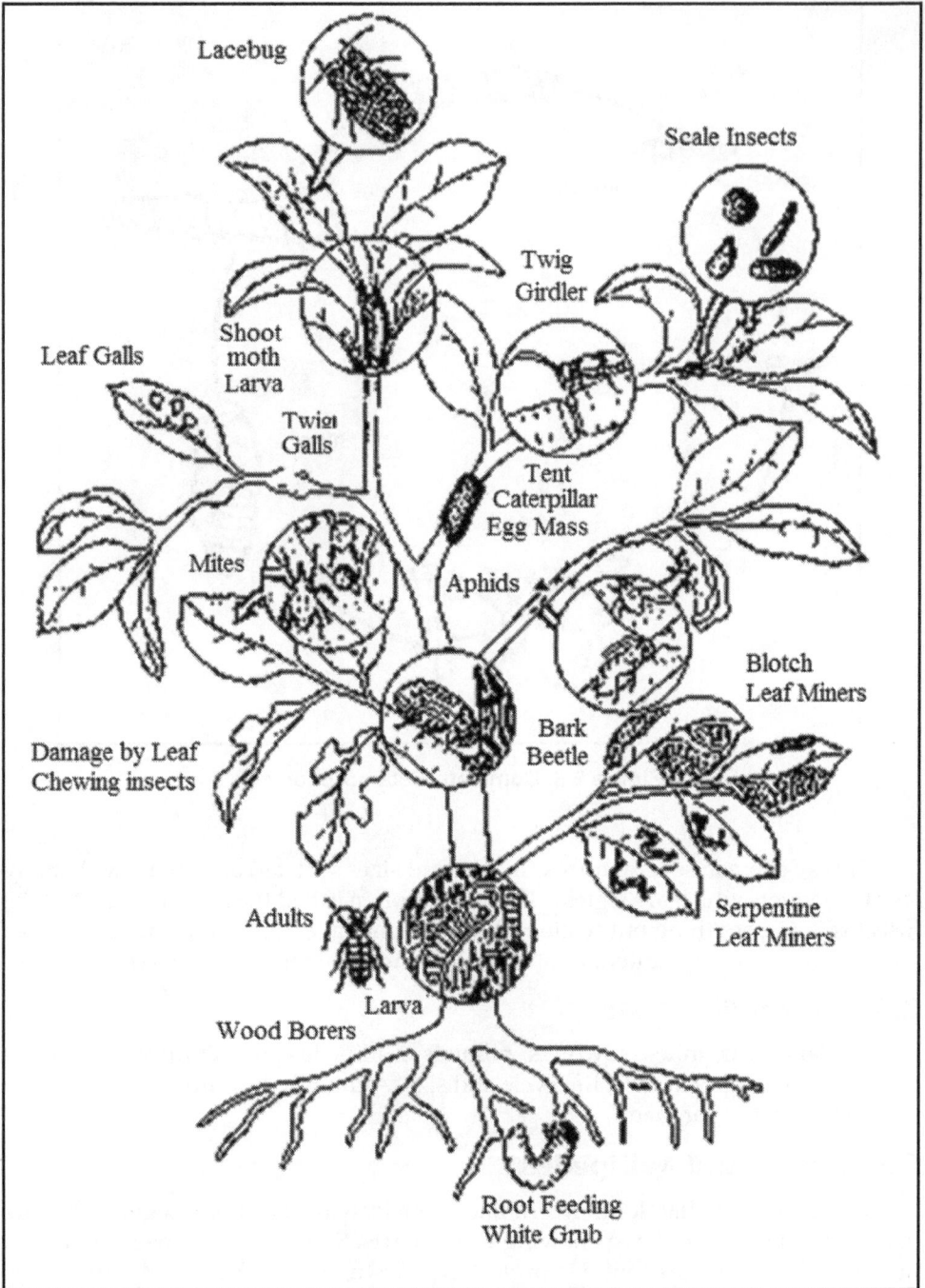

Figure 2.9: Insects and Injury

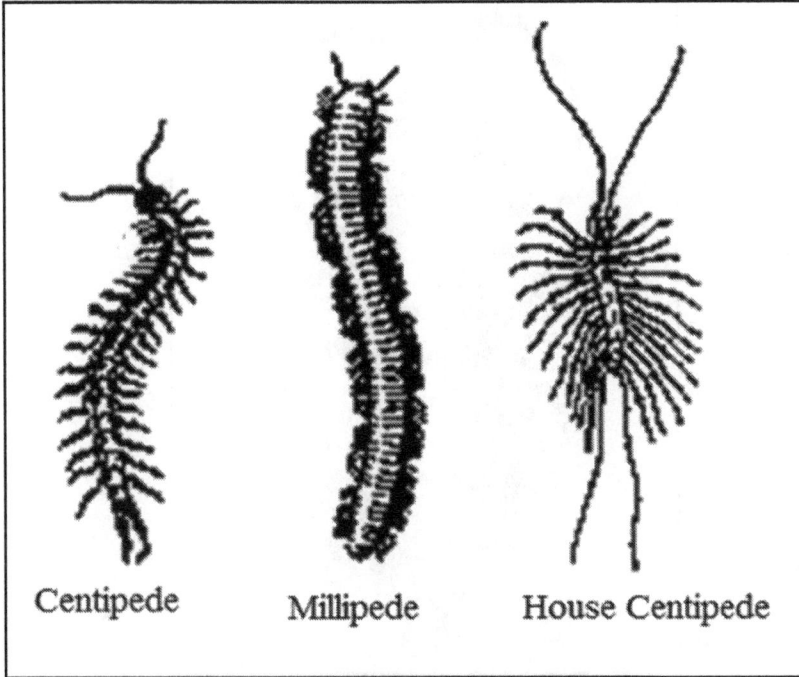

Figure 2.10: Centipede and Millipede

Thus, they are found in decaying leaf litter, rotting logs and near damp debris near foundations. Millipedes and centipedes have no metamorphosis. They only change in size between hatching from the egg and reaching the adult stage.

2.3.3 Insects and Injury

- **Crustaceans:** This class of animals (lobsters, shrimp) is nearly all aquatic (living in water) but there are members living on land that may become pests and are often thought to be insects. Sowbugs (called pillbugs) are black, gray or brown and are capable of rolling up into a ball. Sowbugs are found in damp decaying wood or under objects such as stones, boards or blocks. There have been cases when crustaceans have been considered pests of cultivated plants in some areas, but usually are found living in damp basements or garages where people do not want them.

- **Arachnids:** This group, which consists of spiders, mites, ticks and scorpions all, has eight legs and only two body regions. Arachnids are wingless and lack antennae. They mature through gradual metamorphosis that includes both larval and nymphal stages. Eggs hatch into larvae (six legs) which molt into nymphs (eight legs) and then adults. Spiders and scorpions have chewing mouthparts. Ticks and mites have a modified version of piercing-sucking mouthparts. Ticks are of particular interest because they sometimes transmit diseases such as Lyme disease and Rocky Mountain spotted fever to man during feeding.

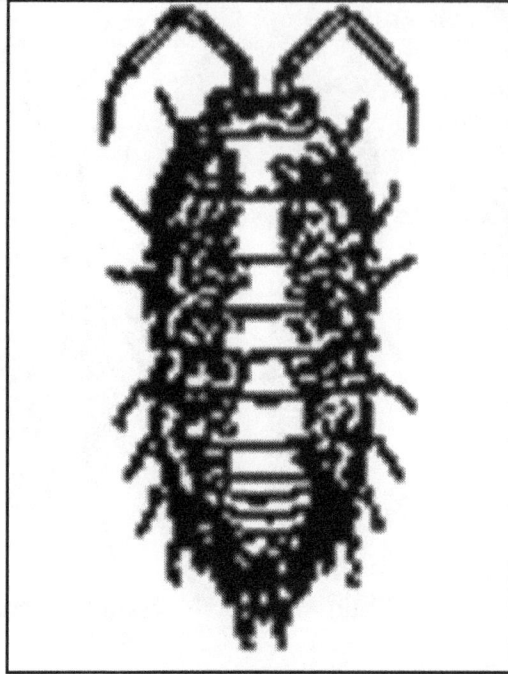

Figure 2.11: Sowbug

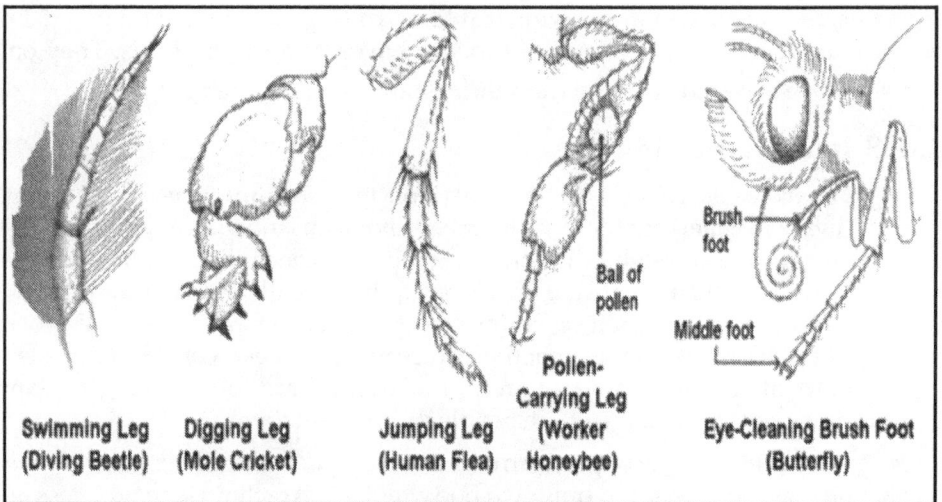

Swimming Leg (Diving Beetle)   Digging Leg (Mole Cricket)   Jumping Leg (Human Flea)   Pollen-Carrying Leg (Worker Honeybee)   Eye-Cleaning Brush Foot (Butterfly)

Figure 2.12: Different types of Legs of Insects

2.3.4 Plant Diseases

A plant disease is any harmful condition that alters a plants growth, appearance or function. Diseases are caused by biological agents called pathogens. They are of interest to pesticide applicators because some diseases can be cured with pesticides, while other pesticides can prevent the pathogen from infecting the host plant. Pathogens include bacteria, fungi, viruses and nematodes. They are spread by wind, rain, insects, birds, snails, slugs and earthworms. In addition, pathogens can be carried by transplanted soil, nursery grafts, vegetative propagation, contaminated equipment and tools, infected seed, pollen, dust storms, irrigation water and people. Plant pathogens are parasites which live and feed on the host plant. In order for a disease to develop, a pathogen must be present, the host plant must be susceptible and the environment must be favorable for development of the pathogen. Temperature and moisture are especially important to the success of the pathogen. The disease starts with the arrival of the pathogen on the plant. If the parasite can get into the plant, the infection starts. Three main ways a plant responds to a disease are:

- Overdevelopment of tissue, galls, swellings and leaf curls.

- Underdevelopment of tissue, stunting, lack of chlorophyll and incomplete development of organs.

- Death of tissue, blights, leaf spots, wilting and cankers.

Bacteria: Bacteria are microscopic can only be seen with a microscope, one-celled organisms that reproduce by single cell division. Bacteria numbers multiply quickly under warm, humid weather conditions. Bacteria may attack any part of a plant, either above or below the soil surface. Several of the leaf spot and rot diseases are caused by bacteria.

Fungi: Fungi are plants that lack chlorophyll and cannot make their own food. Fungi are the most frequent pathogens on plants. They feed off other living organisms or live on dead or decaying organic matter. Most of the time fungi are beneficial because they help release nutrients from dead plants and animals, adding to the fertility of the soil. Fungi reproduce with spores, which function about the same way seeds do. Fungus spores are usually microscopic and are produced in high numbers. Most spores die because they do not find a host to feed on, though some can survive for months without a host. High humidity (above 90%) is essential for spore germination and active growth. Mildew and smut are good examples of fungal diseases.

Viruses: Viruses are tiny organisms smaller than bacteria and cannot be seen with an ordinary microscope. Viruses are usually recognized from the symptoms they induce on the infected plant. They depend on other living organisms for food and cannot live long on their own. Viruses invade healthy plants through wounds or during pollination. Insects that feed with piercing-sucking mouthparts (aphids, whiteflies, leafhoppers), as well as chewing insects (beetles) can transmit viruses while feeding. Viruses can also be spread by nematodes. Practically all plants can be infected by viruses. Mycoplasma are the smallest known independently living organisms. Unlike viruses, they can exist apart from the host organism. Mycoplasma obtain their food from plants. Yellows disease and some stunts are caused by mycoplasmas.

Nematodes: Nematodes are tiny (microscopic) eel or worm like organisms. Nematodes destroy root systems while feeding, which causes a loss in the uptake of water and minerals by the plant, thus weakening the plant. Common symptoms are wilting, stunting and lack of vigorous growth under good growing conditions. Nematodes may also spread plant diseases while feeding. Nematodes feed by sucking the contents of a cell through a hypodermic like mouth inserted into a cell. Not all nematodes feed on roots. Some foliar feeding nematodes attack chrysanthemums and leave triangles of brown, dried tissue that develop on the leaves late in the season. Some nematodes are parasitic to insects.

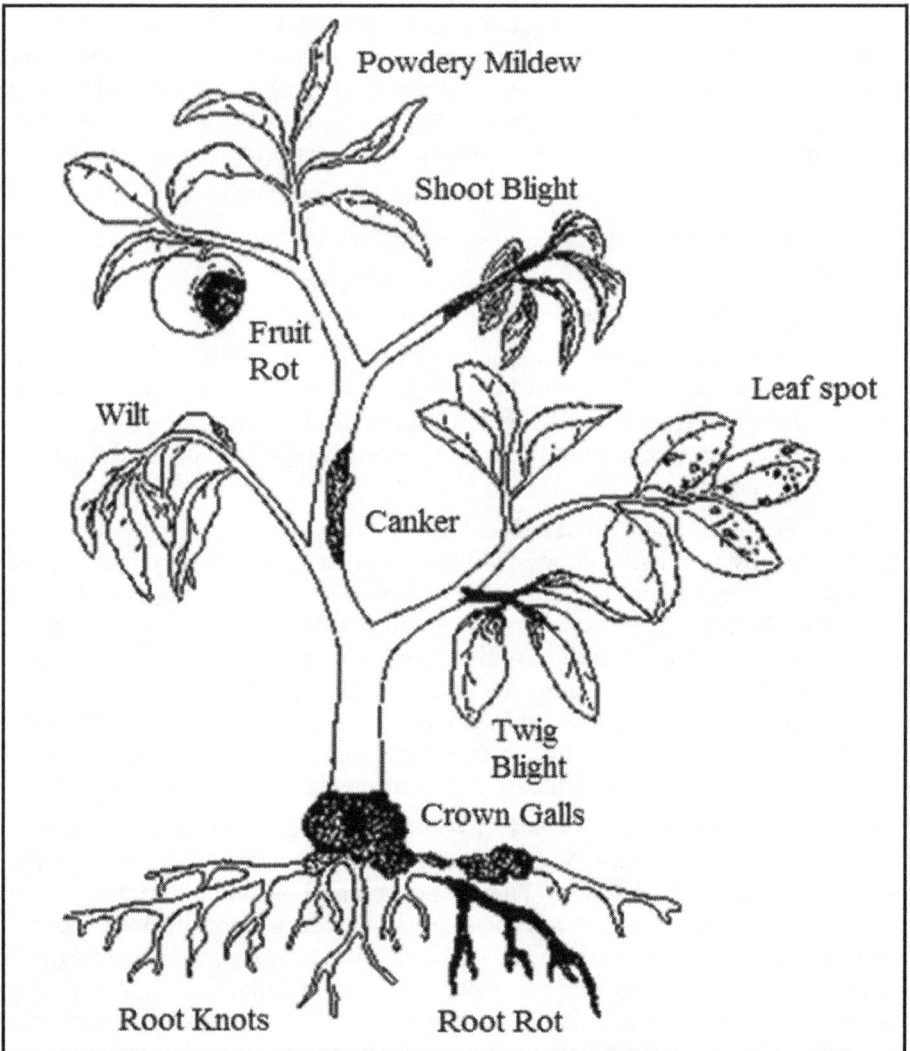

Figure 2.13: Disease Symptoms

2.3.5 Weeds

Any plant can be considered a weed when it is growing where it is not wanted. This is a very broad definition, but considers the following problems caused by weeds.

Weeds can harm man by:

- Causing skin irritation (poison ivy).
- Causing hay fever (ragweed).
- Harboring pests such as rodents, ticks or insects.

Weeds can harm desirable plants by releasing toxins in the soil which inhibit the growth of desirable plants.

- Contaminating the product at harvest.
- Competing for water, nutrients, light and space.
- Harboring pest insects, mites, vertebrates or plant disease agents.

Weeds can harm grazing animals by:

- Poisoning.
- Causing an off-flavor in milk and meat.

Weeds may become pests in water by:

- Hindering fish growth and reproduction.
- Increasing mosquito reproduction.
- Hindering boating, fishing and swimming.
- Clogging irrigation ditches, drainage ditches and channels.

Weeds are dangerous and undesirable on rights of way because they:

- Block vision, road signs and crossroads.
- Increase road maintenance costs.

Plant Development Stages: After a plant seed has germinated, development can be separated into four stages:

- **Seedling:** Very small, very vulnerable plantlets.
- **Vegetative:** Rapid growth, root stems and foliage produced. Nutrients and water move rapidly throughout the plant.
- **Seed production:** Becomes the priority for energy use. Water and nutrient uptake are slow and directed to flower, fruit and seed production.
- **Maturity:** Movement of water and nutrients slow down, energy production is low.

Duration of Weed

i. Annuals: Plants that grow from seed mature and produce seed for the next generation in one year or less are called annuals. This group has many grass-like weeds (crabgrass) and broadleaved (pigweed) members. There are two basic types of annual weeds:

- **Summer annuals** grow from seeds that sprout in the spring. These weeds grow, mature, produce seed and die before winter. Some examples are foxtail, pigweed, lambs quarters and crabgrass.

- **Winter annuals** grow from seeds which sprout in the fall. These weeds mature, produce seed and die before the next summer. Some examples are henbit, common chickweed and annual bluegrass.

ii. Biennials: These plants have a two-year life cycle. During the first year, they grow from seed and develop a heavy root and compact cluster of leaves called a rosette. During the second year, they mature, produce seed and die. Some examples are bull thistle and burdock.

iii. Perennials: When plants live more than two years they are called perennials. Perennials may mature and reproduce in the first year, but they will repeat the cycle for several years or maybe indefinitely. Some perennial plants die back each winter. Others, such as trees, may lose their leaves but do not die back. Most perennials grow from seed and many produce tubers, bulbs, rhizomes (below ground root like stems) or stolons (above-ground stems that produce roots).

- **Simple perennials** usually reproduce with the use of seeds. They also may reproduce when root pieces are cut by cultivation. The pieces then grow into new plants. Examples include trees, shrubs, plantain and dandelions.

- **Bulbous perennials** may reproduce by seed bulblets or bulbs. Wild garlic produces seed and bulblets above ground and bulbs below ground.

- **Creeping perennials** produce seed, rhizomes (below ground stems) or stolons (above ground stems that can produce roots). Examples include Johnson grass, field bindweed and Bermuda grass.

Weed Identification

(a) Arrangement of Leaves

- **Alternate:** One leaf found at each level on the stem.
- **Opposite:** Two leaves opposite each other or paired.
- **Whorled:** Three or more leaves at each level on the stem.

(b) Leaf Structure

- **Simple:** The leaf blade is a single piece and not divided into separate leaflets.
- **Compound:** The leaf blade is divided into several leaf-like parts called leaflets.

(c) Leaf Shape

- **Ovate:** Egg-shaped, elliptical, broadest at the base.
- **Lanceolate:** Lance-shape, are longer than ovate and usually pointed at the tip.
- **Linear:** Long and narrow with parallel sides (grasses).

(d) Arrangement of the Flowers

- **Inflorescence:** In a definite cluster, usually at the top of the plant.
- **Auxiliary:** Along the stem of the plant in the angles (leaf axils) between the foliage, leaves and the stem.

(e) Flower Parts

- **Petals:** The expanded and usually colorful parts of the flower.
- **Sepals:** The greenish hull surrounding the flower when it is budding.

Major Classes of Weeds

  i. Grasses: Leaves of grasses are narrow, stand upright and have parallel veins. When the seedlings sprout, they have only one leaf. Grasses grow from a point (growing point) located below the soil surface, thus the growing point is sheltered. This is why grass can be mowed without killing the plant. Most grasses have fibrous root systems. Grasses have both annual and perennial species.

  ii. Sedges: These are similar to grasses, but they have triangular stems and three rows of leaves. They are sometimes listed under grasses on the pesticide label. These plants often are found in wet places, but are principal pests in fertile, well drained soils. Yellow and purple nuts edge is perennial weed species and produce rhizomes and tubers.

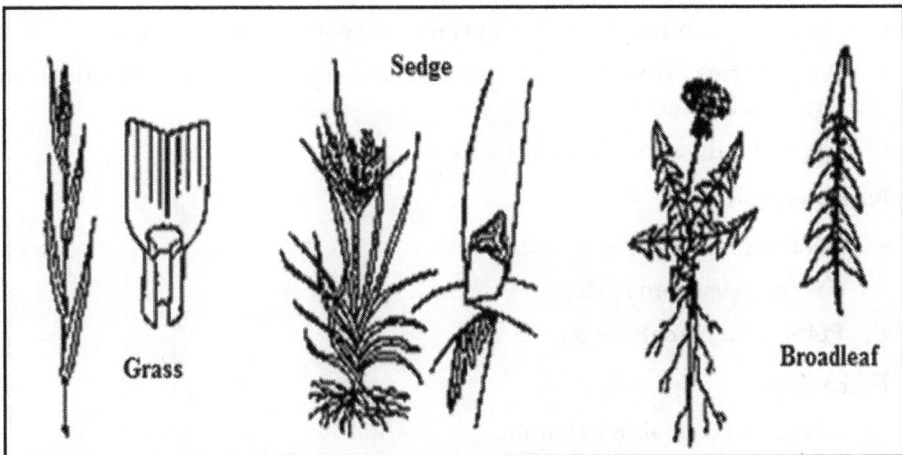

Figure 2.14: Types of Leaf of Weeds

iii. Broadleaves: Seedlings of broadleaves have two leaves that emerge from the seed. The veins of their leaves are netlike. Broadleaves usually have a taproot and their root system is relatively coarse. All broadleaf plants have exposed growing points that are at the end of each stem and in each leaf axial. The perennial broadleaf plants may also have growing points on roots and stems above and below the surface of the soil. The broadleaves have species with annual, biennial and perennial life cycles.

2.3.6 Vertebrate Pests

Vertebrate animals all have a jointed backbone. Humans are vertebrates, as are mammals, birds, reptiles, amphibians and fish. Like insects, most vertebrate animals are not pests and can be an enjoyable part of our environment. There are situations when vertebrates can be pests. Sometimes birds, rodents, raccoons or deer may damage crops or ornamentals. Birds and rodents eat the same food as humans and often ruin more food than they eat. Mammal and bird predators of livestock and poultry cause financial losses to farmers and ranchers each year. Great flocks of roosting birds can soil buildings. There are also those in the vertebrate group particularly rodents that are a hazard to public health when they are in homes, restaurants, offices or warehouses. Rodents, other mammals and some birds are potential reservoirs of serious diseases of humans and domestic animals. Some examples are: rabies, plague and tularemia.

(a) Insects

- Ants, cockroaches, flies and wasps are household pests, as they typically consume human food,
- Aphids, larvae, grasshoppers and crickets cause damage to crop plants,
- Lice, fleas and bed bugs can all cause skin irritation,
- Mosquitoes, tsetse flies and kissing bugs cause irritation and carry disease,
- Termites, woodworm and wood ants cause structural damage,
- Bookworms, silverfish, carpet beetles and clothes moths cause non-structural damage,
- Gypsy moths attack hardwood trees.

(b) Nematodes

- Root-knot nematode,
- Soybean cyst nematode,
- Potato cyst nematode.

(c) Parasites

- Chiggers cause skin irritation,
- *Sarcoptes scabiei* causes scabies,
- Ticks and mites cause irritation and can spread disease.

(d) Gastropods

Some slugs are pests in both agriculture and gardens. Their significance is increasing drastically. *Deroceras reticulatum* is a worldwide distributed slug pest. Local importance slug pests include: *Deroceras* sp., *Milax* sp. *Tandonia* sp., *Limax* sp. *Arion* sp. and some species of Veronicellidae *Veronicella sloanei*. Land snail pests include:

- *Helix aspersa* damages citrus fruits,

- *Cernuella virgata*, *Theba pisana* and *Cochlicella* sp. decrease quality of grains when harvested with the product.

- *Achatina fulica* damages vegetables and ornamental plants.

- *Succinea costaricana* damages ornamental plants.

- *Ovachlamys fulgens* damages ornamental plants and orchids.

- Other species considered to be pests include *Amphibulima patula dominicensis*, *Zachrysia provisoria* and *Bradybaena similaris*.

Freshwater snail pests include:

- *Pomacea canaliculata* damages rice.

- *Bulinus* sp., *Biomphalaria* sp. and *Oncomelania* sp. are intermediate hosts of schistosomes causing schistosomiasis.

- Various species in Lymnaeidae are intermediate hosts of fasciolosis.

2.4 Life cycle and Control of Pests

Structural pest control is the control of household pests (including but not limited to rodents, vermin and insects) and wood-destroying pests and organisms or such other pests which may invade households or structures, including railroad cars, ships, docks, trucks, airplanes or the contents thereof. The practice of structural pest control includes the engaging in, offering to engage in soliciting or the performance of identification of infestations or infections; the making of an inspection for the purpose of identifying or attempting to identify infestations or infections of household or other structures by such pests or organisms; the making of inspection reports; recommendations, estimates and bids, whether oral or written, with respect to such infestation or infections and the making of contracts or the submitting of bids for or the performance of any work including the making of structural repairs or replacements or the use of pesticides, insecticides, rodenticides, fumigants or allied chemicals or substances or mechanical devices for the purpose of eliminating, exterminating, controlling or preventing infestations or infections of such pests or organisms.

2.5 Gundhi bug

2.5.1 Systematic Position

Phylum- Arthropoda

Class - Insecta

Order - Hemiptera

Genus - *Leptocorisa*

Species - *varicornis*

Gundhi Bug (*Leptocorisa varicornis*) is a serious pest of paddy which sucks the juice of developing (milk grain stage) grains and reduces the yield and hence called Paddy Bug. The insect emits an unpleasant smell from abdominal scent glands. The insect is a pest of paddy and hibernates during cold months and feeds on other plants like grasses, sugarcane, maize, millets, sorghum, etc. during non-paddy season. It is green to light brown in colour, 1.5-2.0 cm in length which is active during morning and evening. Legs are long and antennae are 4-jointed. Tarsi are 3-joined. Mouthparts are sucking types. The body is slender and anterior wings are thick and tough while posterior one is membranous. The adults and nymphs suck the juice from the developing grains in the early stage of grain formation. Young succulent leaves and shoots are also attacked before the grain formation stage. Infestation is characterized by the presence of some empty or ill-formed grains in the panicles. Many grasses and even dicotyledonous plants have been listed as hosts. Of the different grasses, *Echinochloa colona* has been found to be a potential host for successful survival and multiplication.

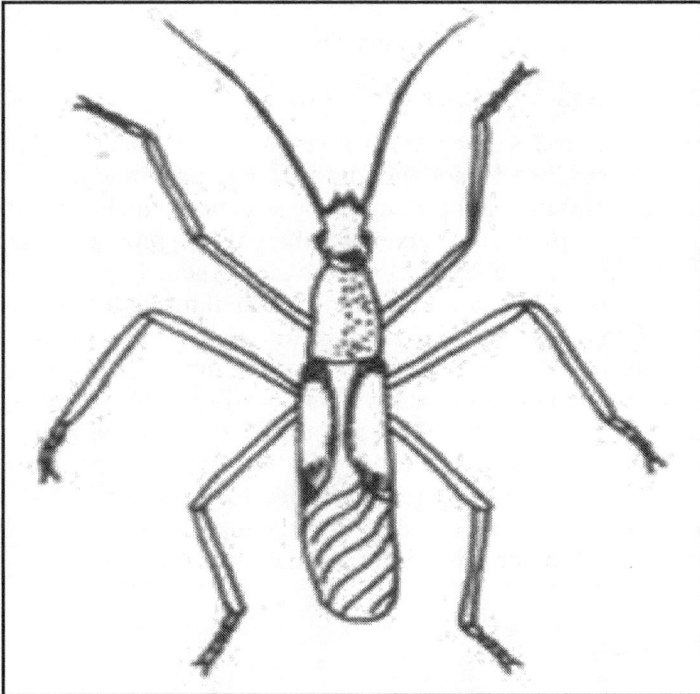

Figure 2.15: *Leptocorisa varicornis* (adult)

2.5.2 Life cycle of Gundhi bug

After copulation female lay eggs symmetrically, into two or three rows. Eggs are dark coloured, oval in outline and flattened at the top. Eggs hatch in about a week. The young nymphs have slender green body and longer legs. These nymphs generally take about twenty days to attain full maturity. All stages of developing bug clusters round the riping ears and suck out the juice. This pest is more common during July to November. During winter their breeding rate is lowered much and the adults manage to tide over the cold on several species of grasses. On paddy it has five broods during the season.

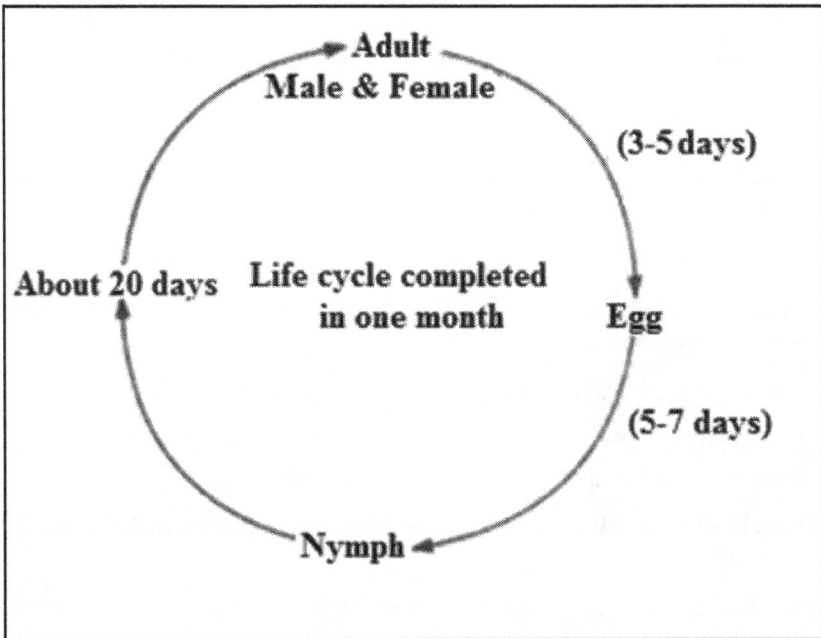

Figure 2.16: Life cycle of Gundhi bug

- The female moth is bigger than the male and its forewings are bright yellowish brown with a distinct black spot in the center.

- The abdomen is wide, the tip being covered with tufts of yellowish hairs.

- The male moth is pale yellow; the abdomen is slender and the anal end has a thin hairy covering dorsally.

- Spots on the forewings are not conspicuous.

- The female moth laid eggs near the top of the leaf blade early at night in small masses covered with hairs and scales derived from the anal tuff.

- The ovi-position occurs upto 5 nights from emergence. The moths are short-lived and die 2 to 3 days after ovi-position.

- The fecundity of the moth varies from 100 to 150 eggs. The eggs are creamy white, flattened, oval and scale like. Egg period is 5 to 8 days.

- The first instar larvae are about 1.5 mm long and 0.5 mm wide. Pale yellow in colour with dark brown prothoraxic shield and orange head.

- Larvae crawl upward towards the tip of the plant during roaming period many larvae die.

- Remaining larvae descend towards the base of the plant and crawl between leaf sheath and stem.

- They enter into leaf sheath and feed on tissue for about a week and bore into stem through nodal region.

- In mature rice plants the caterpillars bore into the stalk region just below the ear head.

- Larval period lasts for 30 days.

- Pupation takes place inside the stem mostly in the lowest node of the plant and just above water level

- In seedling stage, pupation takes place in the root region.

- In single cropped areas mature larvae diapauses in rice stubbles after harvest in December.

- Larvae pupate and emerge as moths after the monsoon rains.

- Egg development takes place at about 16°C with an optimum temperature of 24 to 29°C and relative humidity of 90 to 100%.

- Hatching is drastically reduced at low temperatures of 13°C and relative humidity of 70%.

- The rate of larval development is positively correlated to temperature range from 17 to 35°C.

- The threshold for pupal development is 15 to 16°C.

2.5.3 Control of Gundhi bug

Biological Control

- A number of natural enemies including parasites and predators are known to attack the rice bug at various stages.

- Small scelionid wasps *Gryon nixoni* (Masner) parasitize the eggs of *Leptocorisa* spp.

- Several species of parasitic wasps attack stink bugs.

- The meadow grasshopper *Conocephalus longipennis* (Haan) preys on rice bug eggs; several species of spiders *e.g.* Neo.

Chemical Control

- Dust Malathion or Carbaryl at rate of 30 kg of the formulation/ha

- Spray monocrotophos 36 WSC at rate of 1500 ml ha^{-1} or endosulfan 35 EC at rate of 1500 ml ha-1 or carbaryl 50 WP at rate of 1500 g ha^{-1} or dust malathion or carbaryl at rate of 30 kg of the formulation per hectare.

- Insecticide application should be done if the population reaches ETL of 1 nymph or adult/ hill.

Cultural Control

- Delayed, but synchronous, planting of early-maturing varieties is suggested so that all crops ripen at the same time.

- Weed sanitation and eradication of alternate hosts from rice fields and surrounding areas can help prevent the multiplication of the bug

- Mechanical control measures such as smoking the field, hand-picking of bug, etc.

2.6 Sugarcane Leafhopper

Sugarcane leafhopper (*Pyrillaper pusilla*) is a serious pest of sugar cane in northern India where it also feeds on maize, millets, rice, barley, oats, sorghum, bajra and wild grasses. The pest is found throughout the Indian subcontinent from Afghanistan to Burma and Thailand. Sugarcane leafhopper is piercing and sucking insects. Adults are long, slender, hair like and whitish cream in colour. The male measures 2.5-4 cm in length and females are of 8-10 cm. Posterior end of male has a curved tail contains rows of genital papillae, caudalalae on the lateral side and two unequal copulatory spicules projecting from cloaca, whereas females have a narrow and abruptly pointed tail and an anus before the tip of the tail. The female genital pore or vulva is located ventrally on the anterior two third of the body. Adult hoppers are straw coloured to brownish, 7-8 mm long, with a pointed snout bearing piercing and sucking mouth parts. They are found gregariously and jump of readily when being disturbed. Adult insects are active fliers, migrating from one crop to another and breed throughout the year. Eggs are light yellowish in colour, oval, one mm long and laid on the lower surface of the leaf, near the midrib in groups of about 20 eggs. Eggs hatch of approximately in 6-15 days depending upon the temperature. Hoppers are found in a very large number on the under surface of the leaves where they suck up plant sap that causes yellowing and eventually drying of leaves. Photosynthesis is reduced resulting in the reduction of sucrose content of the juice by up to 30%. The pests secrete a sweet substance called honey dew that costs the leaves and attracts a blackish fungus, which reduces photosynthesis which results in the yield loss.

2.6.1 Life cycle of Sugarcane Leafhopper

Adult hoppers are straw coloured to brownish, 7-8 mm long, with a pointed snout bearing piercing and sucking mouthparts. They are found gregariously and jump off readily when disturbed. Adults are active fliers, migrating from one crop to another and breed throughout the year. Eggs are light yellowish in colour, oval, one mm long and laid on the lower surface of the leaf, near the midrib in groups of about 20 eggs, which hatch in 6-15 days depending on temperature. Nymphs are initially greenish, later turn pale brownish, wingless and with a pair of anal filaments covered with whitish fluffy waxy material. There are 5 nymphal instars which take 40-60 days to complete development. Multiplication of the pest is favoured by high humidity and luxuriant plant growth as in heavily manured and irrigated field or in rainy season.

2.6.2 Control of Sugarcane Leafhopper

The parasite can be controlled by spraying 0.05% of parathion, malathion, thiodon, fenithrothion or rogor. Dusting plants with 10% aldrin or dieldrin also helps. Conservation of the following natural enemies helps in controlling the pests.

2.7 Rodents and their Control

Rodents destroy property, spread disease, compete for human food sources and are aesthetically displeasing. Rodent-associated diseases affecting humans include plague, murine typhus, leptospirosis, rickettsial pox and rat-bite fever. The three primary rodents of concern to the homeowner are the roof rat (*Rattus rattus*), Norway rat (*Rattus norvegicus*) and the house mouse (*Mus musculus*). The term commensal is applied to these rodents, meaning they live at people's expense. The roof rat is a slender, graceful and very agile climber. The roof rat prefers to live aboveground: indoors in attics, between floors, in walls or in enclosed spaces; and outdoors in trees and dense vine growth. Contrasted with the roof rat, the Norway rat is at home below the ground, living in a burrow. The house mouse commonly is found living in human quarters, as suggested by its name. Signs indicative of the presence of rodents, aside from seeing live or dead rats and hearing rats are rodent droppings, runways and tracks. Other signs include nests, gnawings, food scraps, rat hair, urine spots and rat body odors. The waste droppings from rodents are often confused with cockroach egg packets, which are smooth, segmented and considerably smaller than a mouse dropping. The first of four basic strategies for controlling rodents is to eliminate food sources. To accomplish this, it is imperative for the occupants or occupant to do a good job of solid waste management. This requires proper storing, collecting and disposing of refuse. The second strategy is to eliminate breeding and nesting places. This is accomplished by removing rubbish from near the home, including excess lumber, firewood and similar materials.

These items should be stored above ground with 18 inches of clearance below them. This height does not provide a habitat for rats, which have a propensity for dark, moist places in which to burrow. Wood should not be stored directly on the ground and trash and similar rubbish should be eliminated. The third strategy is to construct buildings and other structures using rat-proofing methods. Tactics for rodent exclusion include building or covering doors and windows with metal. Rats can gnaw through wooden doors and windows in a very short time to gain entrance. All holes in a building's exterior should be sealed. Rats are capable of enlarging openings in masonry, especially if the mortar or brick is of poor quality. All openings more than ¾-inch wide should be closed, especially around pipes and conduits.

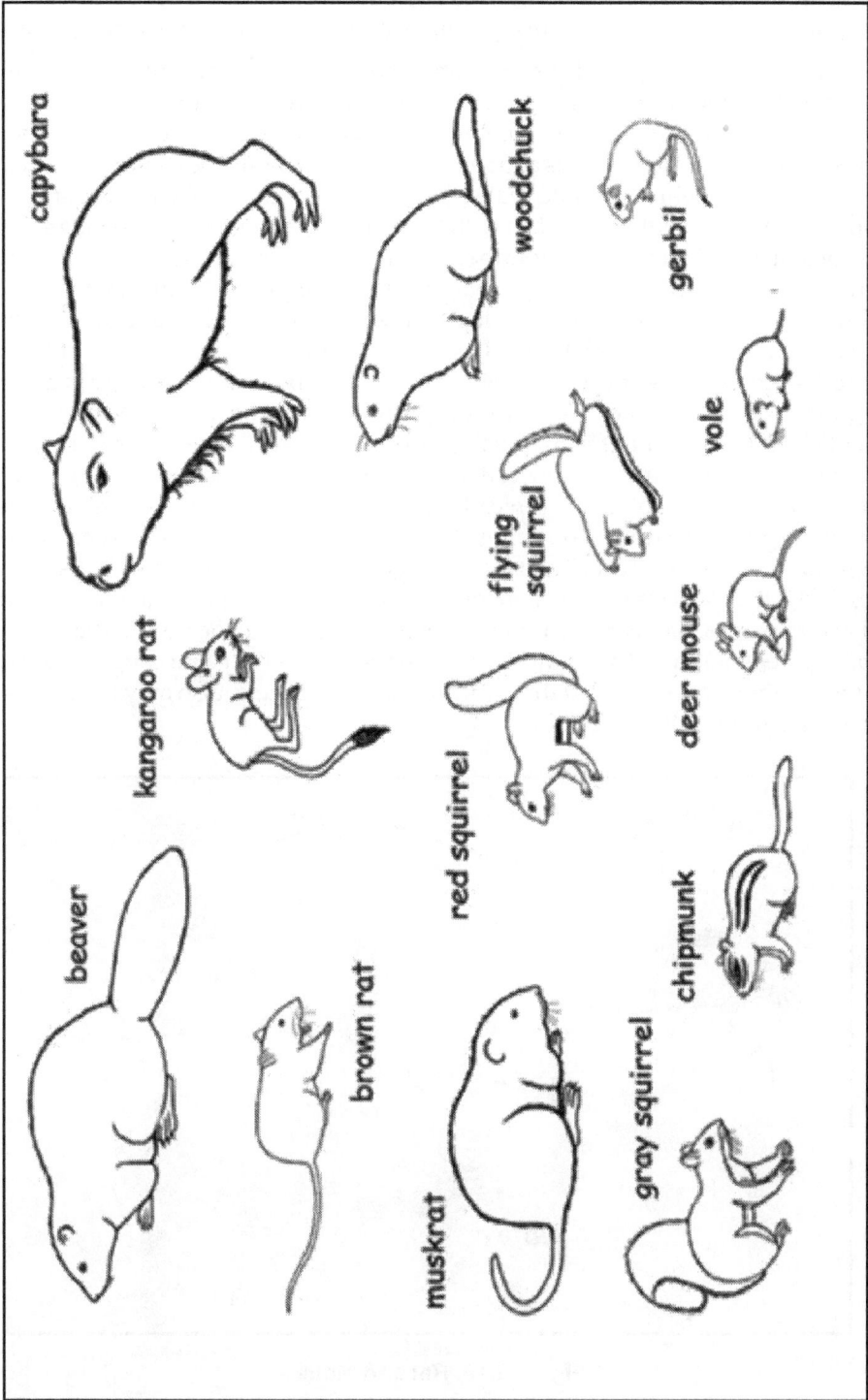

Figure 2.17: Rodents

Cracks around doors, gratings, windows and other such openings should be covered if they are less than 4 feet above the ground or accessible from ledges, pipes or wires.

Additional tactics include using proper materials for rat proofing. For example, sheet metal of at least 26-gauge, ¼ inch or ½ inch hardware cloth and cement are all suitable rat-resistant materials. However, ½ inch hardware cloth has little value against house mice. Tight fittings and self-closing doors should be constructed. Rodent runways can be behind double walls; therefore, spaces between walls and floor supporting beams should be blocked with fire stops. A proper rodent-proofing strategy must bear in mind that rats can routinely jump 2 feet vertically, dig 4 feet or more to get under a foundation, climb rough walls or smooth pipes up to 3 inches in diameter and routinely travel on electric or telephone wires. The first three strategies, good sanitation techniques, habitat denial and rat proofing, should be used initially in any rodent management program. Should they fail, the fourth strategy is a killing program, which can vary from a family cat to the professional application of rodenticides. Cats can be effective against mice, but typically are not useful against a rat infestation. Over the counter rodenticides can be purchased and used by the homeowner or occupant. These typically are in the red squill or wayfaring groups. A more effective alternative is trapping. There is a variety of devices to choose from when trapping rats or mice. The two main groups of rat and mouse traps are live traps and kill traps. Traps usually are placed along walls, near runways and burrows and in other areas. Bait is often used to attract the rodents to the trap. To be effective, traps must be monitored and emptied or removed quickly. If a rat caught in a trap is left there, other rats may avoid the traps. A trapping strategy also may include using live traps to remove these vermin.

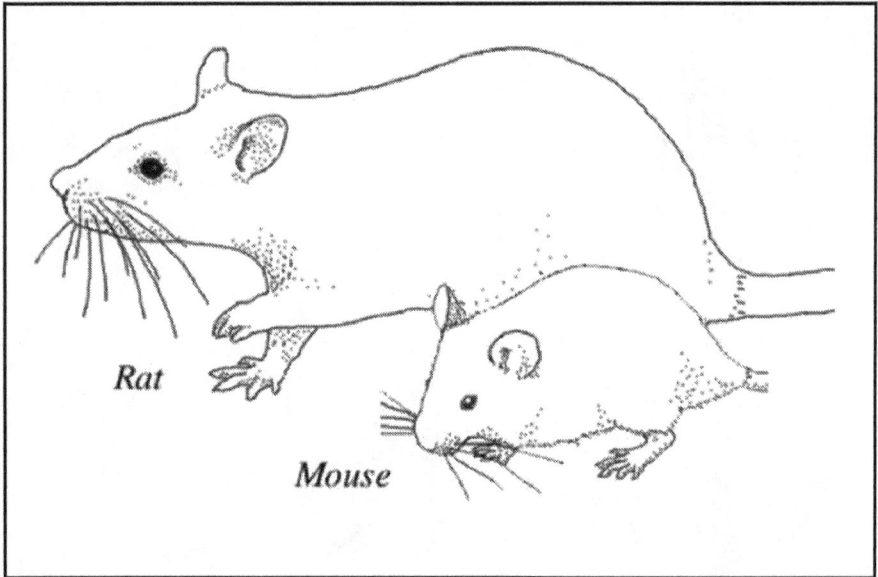

Figure 2.18: Rat and Mouse

2.8 Termites and their Control

Termites (*Microtermes obesi*) constitute a large group of social insects with some 2000 species. They live in tunnels dug in logs, furniture, trees or specially built nest called termitarium. A termitarium can be under ground or above ground earthen mound having chambers for different castes and storage. A termite colony may have from a few hundred to several thousand members' divisible in castes such as the king, the queen, supplementary kings, supplementary queens, workers and soldiers. Soldiers constitute about 2-3% of population. Kings and queens are initially winged with yellow-brown or black colour. They are produced in large number during rainy season. They come out towards evening, swarm, shed their wings, seek safer places, copulate and produce a new colony. With time, the queen becomes very large and continues to lay eggs and produce off springs. Workers are sterile, wingless and blind and perform all the duties of searching and collecting food feeding young ones, building nests, attending to queen etc. Cellulose is the common food of termites. The digested food is brought in the nest and shared. Soldiers are larger than workers and defend the colony against intruders. Some soldiers have long conical snout and are known as nasutes. Nasutes often produces an offensive sticky substance capable of dissolving hard substances. Termites eat away any wood articles, paper, plants and animal products. They destroy doors, windows, cupboards, almirahs etc.

Termites consume wood and other cellulose products, such as paper, cardboard and fiberboard. They will also destroy structural timbers, pallets, crates, furniture and other wood products. In addition, they will damage many materials they do not normally eat as they search for food. The tunneling efforts of subterranean termites can penetrate lead and plastic covered electric cable and cause electrical system failure. In nature, termites may live for years in tree stumps or lumber beneath concrete buildings before they penetrate hairline cracks in floors and walls, as well as expansion joints, to search for food in areas such as interior door frames and immobile furniture. Termite management costs to homeowners are exceeded only by cockroach control costs. Typical signs of termite infestations occur in March through June and in September and October. Swarming is an event where a group of adult males and female reproductive leave the nest to establish a new colony. If the emergence happens inside a building, flying termites may constitute a considerable nuisance. These pests can be collected with a vacuum cleaner or otherwise disposed of without using pesticides. Each homeowner should be aware of the following signs of termite infestation:

- Pencil-thin mud tubes extending over the inside and outside surfaces of foundation walls, piers, sills, joists and similar areas.

- Presence of winged termites or their shed wings on windowsills and along the edges of floors.

- Damaged wood hollowed out along the grain and lined with bits of mud or soil.

Differentiating the ant from the dark brown or black termite reproductive can be accomplished by noting the respective wings and body shape. The primary reproductive (alates) vary in color from pale yellow-brown to coal black, are ½-inch to

\!-inch in length, are flattened dorsa-ventrally and have pale or smoke-gray to brown wings. The secondary reproductive have short wing buds and are white to cream colored. The workers are the same size as the primary reproductive and are white to grayish-white, with a yellow-brown head and are wingless. In addition, the soldiers resemble workers, in that they are wingless, but soldiers have large, rectangular, yellowish and brown heads with large jaws.

There are five families of termites found in the world. The families are *Hodotermitidae* (rotten-wood termites), *Kalotermitidae* (dry-wood termites), *Rhinotermitidae* (subterranean termites) and *Termitidae* (desert termites) are common. Subterranean termites typically work in wood aboveground, but must have direct contact with the ground to obtain moisture. Nonsubterranean termites colonize above the ground and feed on cellulose; however, their life cycles and methods of attack and consequently methods of control, are quite different. Nonsubterranean termites commonly called dry wood termites. Dry-wood termites (*Cryptotermes spp.*) live entirely in moderately to extremely dry wood. They require contact with neither the soil nor any other moisture source and may invade isolated pieces of furniture, fence posts, utility poles, firewood and structures. Dry-wood termite colonies are not as large as other species, so they can occupy small wooden articles, which are one way these insects spread to different locations. Dry-wood termites are slightly larger than most other species, ranging from ½ inch to]! inch long and are generally lighter in color. Damp-wood termites do not need contact with damp ground like subterranean termites do, but they do require higher moisture content in wood. However, once established, these termites may extend into slightly drier wood. Termites of minor importance are the tree-nesting groups. The nests of these termites are found in trees, posts and, occasionally, buildings.

Occupants can reduce the risk for termite attack by adhering to the following suggestions:

- **Eliminate wood contact with ground:** Earth to wood contact provides termites with simultaneous access to food, moisture and shelter in conjunction with direct, hidden entry into the structure. In addition, the occupants or occupant should be aware that pressure-treated wood is not immune to termite attack because termites can enter through the cut ends and build tunnels over the surfaces.

- **Do not allow moisture to accumulate near home's foundation:** Proper drainage, repair of plumbing and proper grading will help to reduce the presence of moisture, which attracts termites.

- **Reduce humidity in crawl spaces:** Most building codes state that crawl space area should be vented at a rate of 1 square foot per 150 square feet of crawl space area. This rate can be reduced for crawl spaces equipped with a polyethylene or equivalent vapor barrier to 1 square foot per 300 to 500 square feet of crawl space area. Vent placement design includes positioning one vent within 3 feet of each building corner. Trimming and controlling shrubs so that they do not obstruct the vents is imperative. Installing 4 to 6 mil polyethylene sheeting over a minimum of 75% of the crawl space will reduce the crawl-space moisture. Covering the entire floor of the crawl space with such material can reduce two potential home problems at one time: excess moisture and radon. The barrier will reduce the absorption of moisture from the air and the release of moisture into the air in the crawl space from the underlying soil.

- **Never store firewood, lumber or other wood debris against the foundation or inside the crawl space:** Termites are both attracted to and fed by this type of storage. Wood stacked in contact with a dwelling and vines, trellises and dense plant material provide a pathway for termites to bypass soil barrier treatment.

- **Use decorative wood chips and mulch sparingly:** Cellulose containing products attract termites, especially materials that have moisture-holding properties, such as mulch. The occupants should never allow these products to contact wood components of the home. The use of crushed stone or pea gravel is recommended as being less attractive to termites and helpful in diminishing other pest problems.

- **Have the structure treated by a professional pest control treatment:** The final and most effective, strategy to prevent infestation is to treat the soil around and beneath the building with termiticide. The treated ground is then both a repellant and toxic to termites.

Aalternative Termite Control Measures

- **Nematodes:** Certain species of parasitic round worms (nematodes) will infest and kill termites and other soil insects. Varying success has been experienced with this method because it is dependent on several variables, such as soil moisture and soil type.

- **Sand as a physical barrier:** This would require preconstruction planning and would depend on termites being unable to manipulate the sand to create tunnels. Some research in California and Hawaii has indicated early success.

- **Chemical baits:** This method uses wood or laminated texture-flavored cellulose impregnated with a toxicant and/or insect growth regulator. The worker termite feeds on the substance and carries it back to the nest, reducing or eliminating the entire colony.

Generally, termites invade homes by way of the foundation, either by crawling up the exterior surface where their activity is usually obvious or by traveling inside hollow block masonry. One way to deter their activity is to block their access points on or through the foundation. Metal termite shields have been used for decades to deter termite movement along foundation walls and piers on up to the wooden structure. Metal termite shields should extend 2 inches from the foundation and 2 inches down. Improperly installed *i.e.* not soldered/sealed properly, damaged or deteriorated termite shields may allow termites to reach parts of the wooden floor system. Shields should be made of non-corroding metal and have no cracks or gaps along the seams.

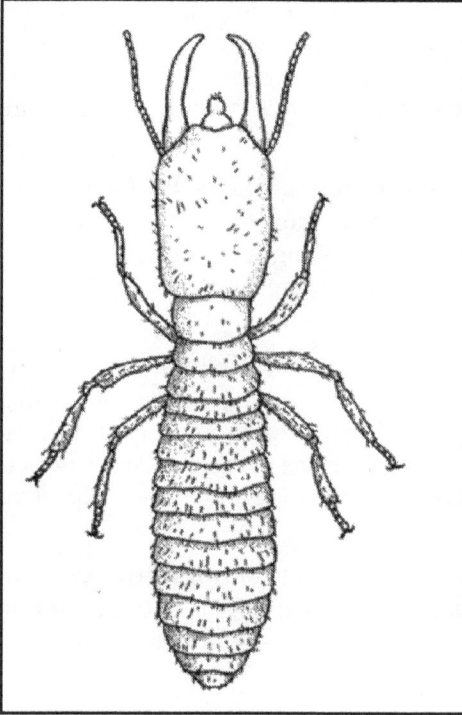

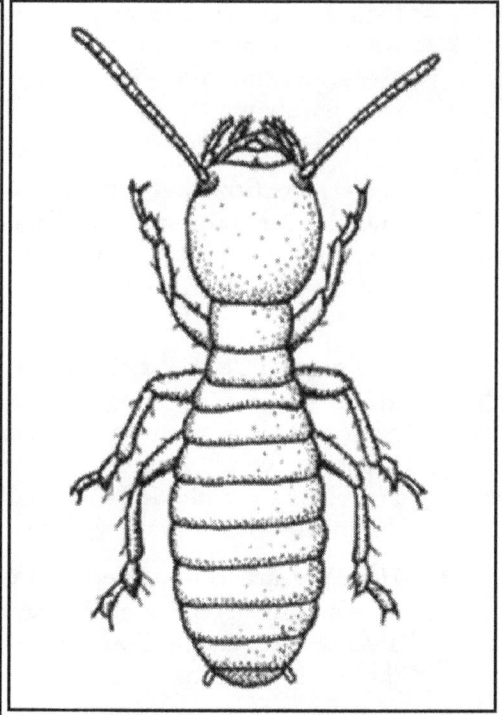

Figure 2.19a: Subterrain Termite   **Figure 2.19b: Worker Termite**

If a house is being built with metal termite shielding, the shielding should extend at least 2 inches out and 2 inches down at a 45° angle from the foundation wall. An alternative to using termite shields on a hollow block foundation is to fill the block with concrete or put in a few courses of solid or concrete filled brick which is often done anyway to level foundations. These are referred to as masonry caps. The same approach can be used with support piers in the crawl space. Solid caps *i.e.* a continuously poured concrete cap are best at stopping termites, but are not commonly used. Concrete-filled brick caps should deter termite movement or force them through small gaps, thus allowing them to be spotted during an inspection.

Control of Termites

Pressure impregnation of creosote, coal tar, zincchloride, mercuricchloride, sodiumfluosilicates, dieldrinetc helps to get rid of them. Wool can be immersed in the insecticide solution for 24 hours to make it termite resistant. Soil treatment with dieldrin or BHC before construction of house should be done to keep termites away from the buildings. Termite nest can be destroyed by pouring in them a mixture of dieldrin and kerosene.

2.9 Mosquitoes and their Control

Mosquito borne diseases, such as malaria, dengue and yellow fever, have plagued civilization for thousands of years. New threats include Lyme disease and West Nile Virus. The frequency and extent of these diseases depend on a complex series of factors. Mosquito control agencies and health departments cooperate in being aware of these factors and reducing the chance for disease. It is important to recognize that young adult female mosquitoes taking their first blood meal do not transmit diseases. It is instead the older females, who, if they have picked up a disease organism in their first blood meals, can then transmit the disease during the second blood meal. The proper method to manage the mosquito problem in a community is through an organized integrated pest management system that includes all approaches that safely manage the problem. The spraying of toxic agents is but one of many approaches. All mosquitoes have four stages of development, egg, larva, pupa and adult and spend their larval and pupal stages in water. The females of some mosquito species deposit eggs on moist surfaces, such as mud or fallen leaves that may be near water but dry. Later, rain or high tides reflood these surfaces and stimulate the eggs to hatch into larvae. The females of other species deposit their eggs directly on the surface of still water in such places as ditches, street catch basins, tire tracks, streams that are drying up and fields or excavations that hold water for some time. This water is often stagnant and close to the home in discarded tires ornamental pools, unused wading and swimming pools, tin cans, bird baths, plant saucers and even gutters and flat roofs. The eggs soon hatch into larvae. In the hot summer months, larvae grow rapidly, become pupae and emerge 1 week later as flying adult mosquitoes. A few important spring species have only one generation per year. However, most species have many generations per year and their rapid increase in numbers becomes a problem.

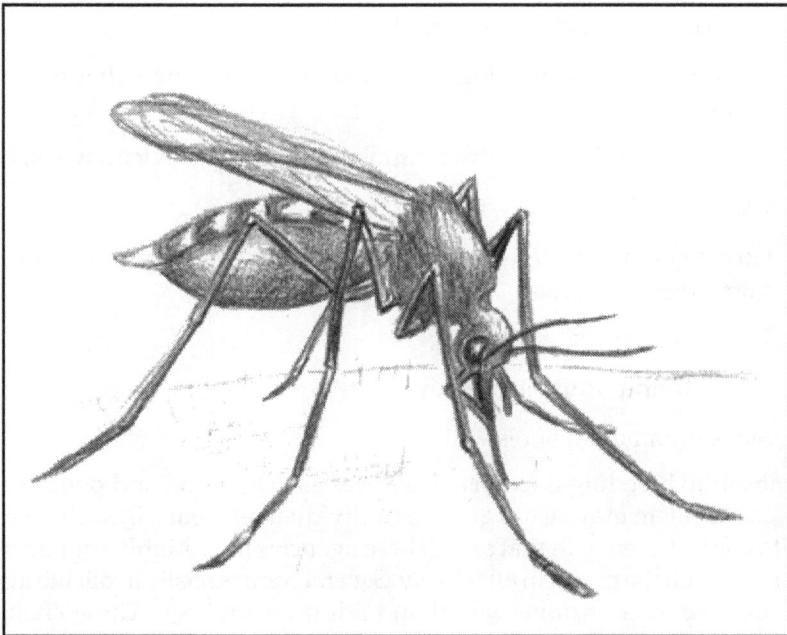

Figure 2.20: Mosquito- Sucking the blood

When adult mosquitoes emerge from the aquatic stages, they mate and the female seeks a blood meal to obtain the protein necessary for the development of her eggs. The females of a few species may produce a first batch of eggs without this first blood meal. After a blood meal is digested and the eggs are laid, the female mosquito again seeks a blood meal to produce a second batch of eggs. Depending on her stamina and the weather, she may repeat this process many times without mating again. The male mosquito does not take a blood meal, but may feed on plant nectar. They live for only a short time after mating. Most mosquito species survive the winter or overwinter, in the egg stage, awaiting the spring thaw, when waters warm and the eggs hatch. A few important species spend the winter as adult, mated females, resting in protected, cool locations, such as cellars, sewers, crawl spaces and well pits. With warm spring days, these females seek a blood meal and begin the cycle again. Only a few species can overwinter as larvae.

Reduction of Mosquito Population

The most efficient method of controlling mosquitoes is by reducing the availability of water suitable for larval and pupal growth. Large lakes, ponds and streams that have waves, contain mosquito-eating fish and lack aquatic vegetation around their edges do not contain mosquitoes; mosquitoes thrive in smaller bodies of water in protected places. Examine the home and neighborhood and take the following precautions:

- Dispose of unwanted tin cans and tires,
- Clean clogged roof gutters and drain flat roofs,
- Turn over unused wading pools and other containers that tend to collect rainwater,
- Change water in birdbaths, fountains and troughs twice a week,
- Clean and chlorinate swimming pools,
- Cover containers tightly with window screen or plastic when storing rainwater for garden,
- Use during drought periods,
- Flush sump-pump pits weekly,
- Stock ornamental pools with fish.

If mosquito breeding is extensive in areas such as woodland pools or roadside ditches, the problem may be too great for individual residents. In such cases, call the mosquito control agency in that area. These agencies have highly trained personnel who can deal with the problem effectively. Several commercially available insecticides can be effective in controlling larval and adult mosquitoes. These chemicals are considered sufficiently safe for use by the public. Select a product whose label states that the material is effective against mosquito larvae or adults. For safe and effective use, read the label and follow the instructions for applying the material. The label lists those insects that the EPA agrees are effectively controlled by the product. For use against adult mosquitoes, some liquid insecticides can be mixed according to direction and sprayed lightly on building foundations, hedges, low shrubbery, ground covers and grasses. Do not over apply liquid insecticides, excess spray dips from the sprayed surfaces to the ground, where it is ineffective. The purpose of such sprays is to leave a fine deposit of insecticide on surfaces where mosquitoes rest. Such sprays are not effective for more than 1 or 2 days. Some insecticides are available as premixed products or aerosol cans. These devices spray the insecticide as very small aerosol droplets that remain floating in the air and hit the flying mosquitoes. Apply the sprays upwind, so the droplets drift through the area where mosquito control is desired. Rather than applying too much of these aerosols initially, it is more practical to apply them briefly but periodically, thereby eliminating those mosquitoes that recently flew into the area.

Various commercially available repellents can be purchased as a cream or lotion or in pressurized cans, then applied to the skin and clothing. Some manufacturers also offer clothing impregnated with repellents; coarse, repellent bearing particles to be scattered on the ground and candles whose wicks can be lit to release a repellent chemical. The effectiveness of all repellents varies from location to location, from person to person and from mosquito to mosquito. Repellents can be especially effective in recreation areas, where mosquito control may not be conducted. All repellents should be used according to the manufacturers' instructions. Mosquitoes are attracted by perspiration, warmth, body odor, carbon dioxide and light. Mosquito control agencies use some of these attractants to help determine the relative number of adult mosquitoes in an area. Several devices are sold that are supposed to attract, trap and destroy mosquitoes and other flying insects. However, if these devices are attractive to mosquitoes, they probably attract more mosquitoes into the area and may, therefore, increase rather than decrease mosquito annoyance.

2.10 Cockroaches

Cockroaches have become well adapted to living with and near humans and their hardiness are legendary. In light of these facts, cockroach control may become a homeowner's most difficult task because of the time and special knowledge it often involves. The cockroach is considered an allergen source and an asthma trigger for residents. Although little evidence exists to link the cockroach to specific disease outbreaks, it has been demonstrated to carry *Salmonella typhimurium*, *Entamoeba histolytica* and the poliomyelitis virus. In addition, Kamble and Keith note that most cockroaches produce a repulsive odor that can be detected in infested areas. The sight of cockroaches can cause considerable psychologic or emotional distress in some individuals. They do not bite, but they do have heavy leg spines that may scratch. Cockroaches will eat a great variety of materials, including cheese and bakery products, but they are especially fond of starchy materials, sweet substances and meat products. Cockroaches are primarily nocturnal. Daytime sightings may indicate potentially heavy infestations. They tend to hide in cracks and crevices and can move freely from room to room or adjoining housing units via wall spaces, plumbing and other utility installations. Entry into homes is often accomplished through food and beverage boxes, grocery sacks, animal food and household goods carried into the home. The species of public health interest that commonly inhabit human dwellings include brown cockroach (*Periplaneta brunnea*), German cockroach (*Blattella germanica*), American cockroach (*Periplaneta americana*), Oriental cockroach (*Blatta orientalis*), brown banded cockroach (*Supella longipalpa*); Australian cockroach (*Periplaneta australasiae*) and smoky-brown cockroach (*Periplaneta fuliginosa*).

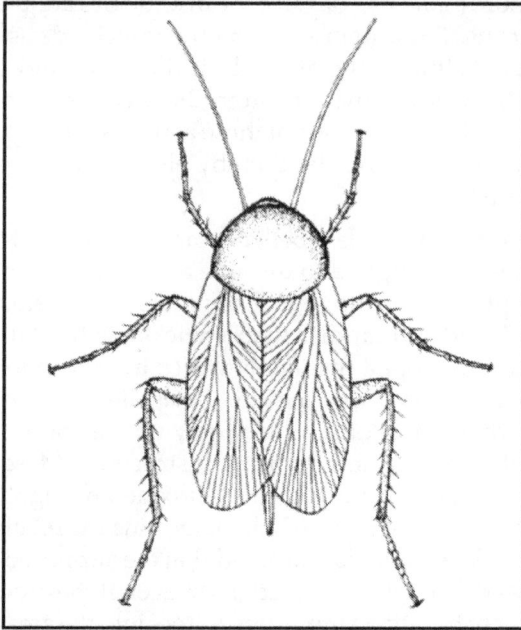

Figure 2.21: Outer Structure of Cockroach

Four management strategies exist for controlling cockroaches. The first is prevention. This strategy includes inspecting items being carried into the home and sealing cracks and crevices in kitchens, bathrooms, exterior doors and windows. Structural modifications would include weather stripping and pipe collars. The second strategy is sanitation. This denies cockroaches' food, water and shelter. These efforts include quickly cleaning food particles from shelving and floors; timely washing of dinnerware; and routine cleaning under refrigerators, stoves, furniture and similar areas. If pets are fed indoors, pet food should be stored in tight containers and not left in bowls overnight. Litter boxes should be cleaned routinely. Access should be denied to water sources by fixing leaking plumbing, drains, sink traps and aquaria. Elimination of shelter can be partially accomplished by purging clutter, such as papers and soiled clothing and rags. The third strategy is trapping. Commercially available cockroach traps can be used to capture roaches and serve as a monitoring device. The most effective trap placement is against vertical surfaces, primarily corners and under sinks, in cabinets, basements and floor drains. The fourth strategy is chemical control. The use of chemicals typically indicates that the other three strategies have been applied incorrectly. Numerous insecticides are available and appropriate information is obtainable from EPA.

2.11 Fleas and Flies

2.11.1 Fleas

The most important fleas as disease vectors are those that carry murine typhus and bubonic plague. In addition, fleas serve as intermediate hosts for some species of dog and rodent tapeworms that occasionally infest people. They also may act as intermediate hosts of filarial worms (heartworms) in dogs. The most important disease related to fleas is the bubonic plague. This is primarily a concern of residents in the southwestern and western parts of the country. Of approximately 2,000 species of flea, the most common flea infesting both dogs and cats is the cat flea *Ctenocephalides felis*. Although numerous animals, both wild and domestic, can have flea infestations, it is from the exposure of domestic dogs and cats that most homeowners inherit flea infestation problems. Fleas tend to be host-specific, thus feeding on only one type of host. However, they will infest other species in the absence of the favored host. They are found in relative abundance on animals that live in burrows and sheltered nests, while mammals and birds with no permanent nests or that are exposed to the elements tend to have light infestations. Flea eggs usually are laid singly or in small groups among the feathers or hairs of the host or in a nest. They are often laid in carpets of living quarters if the primary host is a household pet. Eggs are smooth, spherical to oval, light colored and large enough to be seen with the naked eye. An adult female flea can produce up to 2,000 eggs in a lifetime. Flea larvae are small (2 to 5 millimeters), white and wormlike with a darker head and a body that will appear brown if they have fed on flea feces. This stage is mobile and will move away from light, thus they typically will be found in shaded areas or under furniture. In 5 to 12 days, they complete the three larval stages; however, this may take several months depending on environmental conditions. The larvae, after completing development, spin a cocoon of silk encrusted with granules of sand or various types of debris to form the pupal stage. The pupal stage can be dormant for 140 to 170 days. The fleas can actually survive through the winter. The pupae, after development, are stimulated to emerge as adults by movement, pressure or heat. The pupal form of the flea is resistant to insecticides. An initial treatment, while killing egg, larvae and adult forms, will not kill the pupae. Therefore, a reapplication will be necessary. The adult forms are usually ready to feed about 24 hours after they emerge from the cocoon and will begin to feed within 10 seconds of landing on a host. Mating usually follows the initial blood meal and egg production is initiated 24 to 48 hours after consuming a blood meal. The adult flea lives approximately 100 days, depending on environmental conditions. Following are some guidelines for controlling fleas:

(a) The most important principle in a total flea control program is simultaneously treating all pets and their environments (indoor and outdoor).

(b) Before using insecticides, thoroughly clean the environment, removing as many fleas as possible, regardless of the form. This would include indoor vacuuming and carpet steam cleaning. Special attention should be paid to "source points" where pets spend most of their time.

(c) Outdoor cleanup should include mowing, yard raking and removing organic debris from flowerbeds and under bushes.

(d) Insecticide should be applied to the indoor and outdoor environments and to the pet.

(e) Reapplication to heavily infested source points in the home and the yard may be needed to eliminate pre-emerged adults.

2.11.2 Flies

The public health view is to classify flies as biting or nonbiting. Biting flies include sand flies, horseflies and deerflies. Non-biting flies include houseflies, bottle flies and screwworm flies. The latter group is referred to as synanthropic because of their close association with humans. In general, the presence of flies is a sign of poor sanitation. The primary concern of most homeowners is non-biting flies. The housefly (*Musca domestica*) is one of the most widely distributed insects and is usually the predominant fly species in homes and restaurants. *M. domestica* is also the most prominent human-associated (synanthropic) fly. Because of its close association with people, its abundance and its ability to transmit disease, it is considered a greater threat to human welfare than any other species of nonbiting fly. Each housefly can easily carry more than 1 million bacteria on its body. Some of the disease-causing agents transmitted by houseflies to humans are *Shigella* sp. (dysentery and diarrhea = shigellosis), *Salmonella* sp. (typhoid fever), *Escherichia coli*, (traveler's diarrhea) and *Vibrio cholera* (cholera). Sometimes these organisms are carried on the fly's tarsi or body hairs and frequently they are regurgitated onto food when the fly attempts to liquefy it for ingestion. Favorite breeding sites include garbage, animal manure, spilled animal feed and soil contaminated with organic matter. Favorable environmental conditions will result in the eggs hatching in 24 hours or less. Normally, a female fly will produce 500 to 600 eggs during her lifetime.

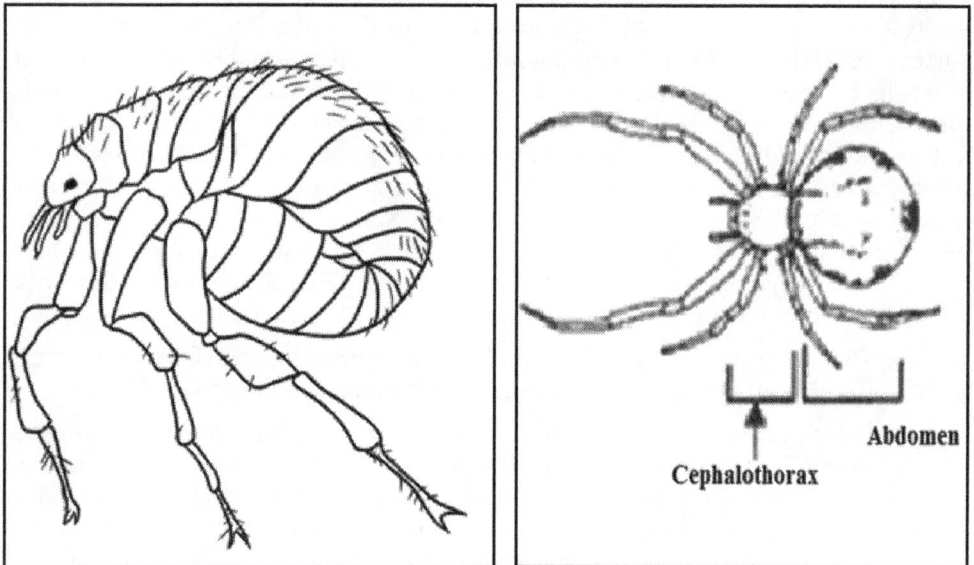

Figure 2.22a: Fleas and flies

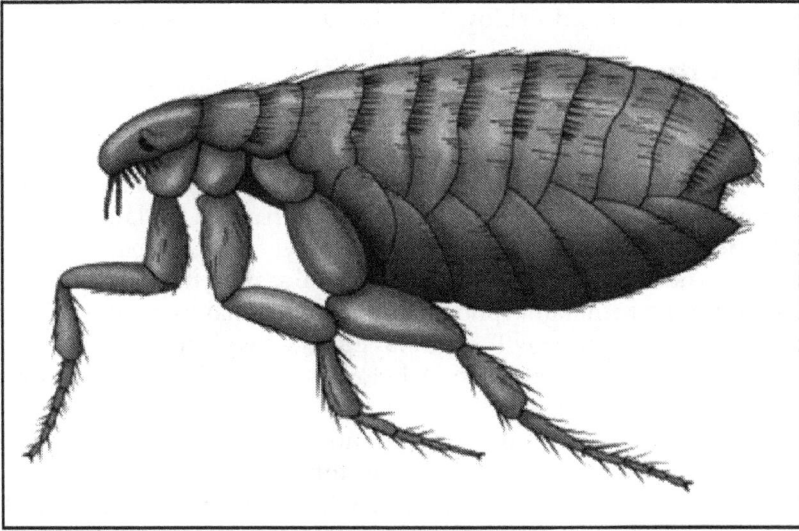

Figure 2.22b: Flea

The creamy, white larvae (maggots) are about ½ inch long when mature and move within the breeding material to maintain optimum temperature and moisture conditions. This stage lasts an average of 4 to 7 days in warm weather. The larvae move to dry parts of the breeding medium or move out of it onto the soil or sheltered places under debris to pupate, with this stage usually lasting 4 to 5 days. When the pupal stage is accomplished, the adult fly exits the puparium, dries, hardens and flies away to feed, with mating occurring soon after emergence. The control of the housefly is hinged on good sanitation (denying food sources and breeding sites to the fly). This includes the proper disposal of food wastes by placing garbage in cans with close-fitting lids. Cans need to be periodically washed and cleaned to remove food debris. The disposal of garbage in properly operated sanitary landfills is paramount to fly control. The presence of adult flies can be addressed in various ways. Outside methods include limited placement of common mercury vapor lamps that tend to attract flies. Less-attractive sodium vapor lamps should be used near the home. Self-closing doors in the home will deny entrance, as will the use of proper-fitting and well maintained screening on doors and windows. Larger flies use homes for shelter from the cold, but do not reproduce inside the home. Caulking entry points and using fly swatters is effective and much safer than the use of most pesticides. Insecticide bombs can be used in attics and other rooms that can be isolated from the rest of the house. However, these should be applied to areas away from food, where flies rest. The blowfly is a fairly large, metallic green, gray, blue, bronze or black fly. They may spend the winter in homes or other protected sites, but will not reproduce during this time. Blowflies breed most commonly on decayed carcasses *e.g.* dead squirrels, rodents, birds and in droppings of dogs or other pets during the summer; thus, removal of these sources is imperative. Small animals, on occasion, may die inside walls or under the crawl space of a house. A week or two later, blowflies or maggots may appear. The adult blowfly is also attracted to gas leaks.

2.12 Fire Ants

Ants are one of the most numerous species on earth. Ants are in the same order as wasps and bees and, because of their geographic distribution, they are universally recognized. The life cycle of the fire ant begins with the mating of the winged forms (alates) some 300 to 800 feet in the air, typically occurring in the late spring or early summer. The male dies after the mating; and the newly mated queen finds a suitable moist site, drops her wings and burrows in the soil, sealing the opening behind her. Ants undergo complete metamorphosis and, therefore, have egg, larval, pupal and adult stages. The new queen will begin laying eggs within 24 hours. Once fully developed, she will produce approximately 1,600 eggs per day over a maximum life span of 7 years. Soft, whitish, legless larvae are produced from the hatching. These larvae are fed by the worker ants. Pupae resemble adults in form, but are soft, non-pigmented and lack mobility. There are at least three distinct castes of ants; workers, queens and males. Typically, the males have wings, which they retain until death. Queens, the largest of the three castes, normally have wings, but lose them after mating. The worker, which is also a female, is never winged, except as a rare abnormality. Within this hierarchy, mature colonies contain males and females that are capable of flight and reproduction. These are known as reproductive and an average colony may produce approximately 4,500 of these per year. A healthy nest usually produces two nuptial flights of reproductive each year and a healthy, mature colony may contain more than 250,000 ants. Though uncommon among ants, multiple queen colonies (10 to 100) occur somewhat frequently in fire ants, resulting in more numerous mounds per acre.

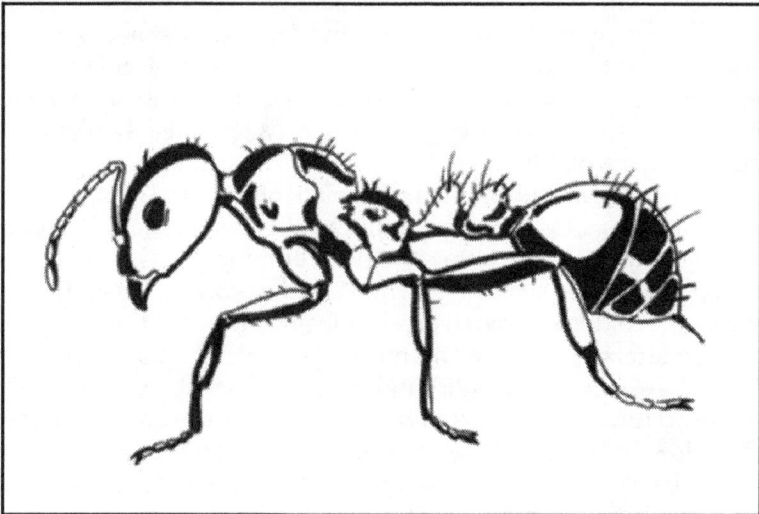

Figure 2.23: Red Imported Fire Aunt

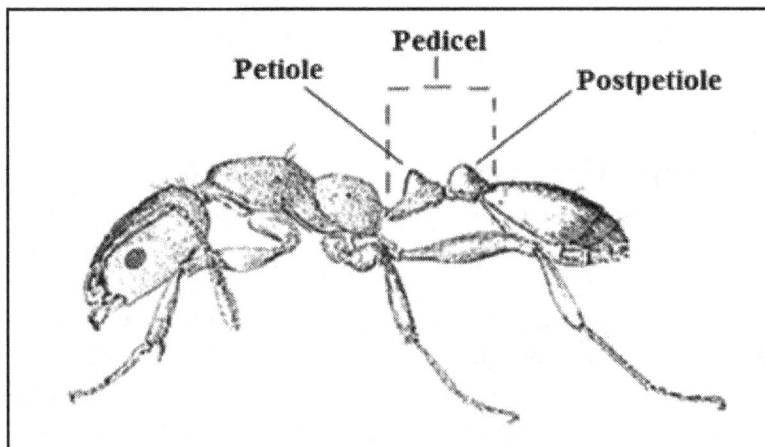

Figure 2.24: Fire Aunts

The most important are four species in the genus *Solenopsis*. Of these, the number one fire ant pest is the red imported fire ant (RIFA) *Solenopsis invicta*. The second most important species is the black imported fire ant, *S. richteri*. There are two native species of fire ants; the tropical fire ant *S. geminata* and the Southern fire ant *S. xyloni*. The most important extension of the RIFA range is thought to have occurred during the 1950s housing boom as a result of the transportation of sod and nursery plants. RIFAs prefer open and sun exposed areas. They are found in cultivated fields, cemeteries, parks and yards and even inside cars, trucks and recreational vehicles. RIFAs are attracted to electrical currents and are known to nest in and around heat pumps, junction boxes and similar areas. They are omnivorous; thus they will attack most things, living or dead. Their economic effects are felt by their destruction of the seeds, fruit, shoots and seedlings of numerous native plant species. Fire ants are known to tend pests, such as scale insects, mealy bugs and aphids, for feeding on their sweet waste excretion (honeydew). RIFAs transport these insects to new feeding sites and protect them from predators. The positive side of RIFA infestation is that the fire ant is a predator of ticks and controls the ground stage of horn flies. The urban dweller with a RIFA infestation may find significant damage to landscape plants, with reductions in the number of wild birds and mammals. RIFAs can discourage outdoor activities and be a threat to young animals or small confined pets. RIFA nests typically are not found indoors, but around homes, roadways and structures, as well as under sidewalks. Shifting of soil after RIFAs abandon sites has resulted in collapsing structures. The medical complications of fire ant stings have been noted in the literature since 1957. People with disabilities, reduced feeling in their feet and legs, young children and those with mobility issues are at risk for sustaining numerous stings before escaping or receiving assistance. Fatalities have resulted from attacks on the elderly and on infants. Control of the fire ant is primarily focused on the mound by using attractant bait consisting of soybean oil, corn grits or chemical agents. The bait is picked up by the worker ants and taken deep into the mound to the queen. These products typically require weeks to work. Individual mound treatment is usually most effective in the spring. The key is to locate and treat all mounds in the area to be protected. If young mounds are missed, the area can become reinfested in less than a year.

Summary

1. A pest is a plant or animal detrimental to humans or human concerns.

2. Some pathogens even provide symbiotic advantages for their insect vectors. Bark beetles infect trees with a pathogenic fungus whenever they establish new colonies.

3. A vector is an organism that carries a pathogen with it. An example would be malaria-carrying mosquito.

4. In ancient times, insects were very important in the transmission of communicable diseases. The definition of vector was related mostly to insects.

5. Human civilization has been competing with insects, rodents, diseases and weeds for survival throughout its history. Historical records of plagues, famine and pestilence fill volumes of texts.

6. All adult insects have two characteristics in common; they have three pairs of jointed legs and they have three body regions; head, thorax and abdomen.

7. Mouthparts are different in various insect groups and are often used in classification and identification.

8. The thorax or middle body segment has three pair of legs and sometimes one or two pair of wings (forewings, hind wings).

9. The abdomen of the insect is built of segments. Along the side of the segments are openings, called spiracles, which the insect uses to breathe.

10. In most insects, reproduction results from the males fertilizing females. The females then lay the eggs. This is the pattern of life for most insects, but there are a few interesting variations.

11. Insects go through a series of changes as they develop from the egg to adulthood. This process of growth is called metamorphosis.

12. Insects with incomplete metamorphosis also pass through three stages of development such as egg, naiad and adult.

13. Spiders, ticks, mites, sowbugs, pillbugs, millipedes and centipedes resemble insects in habit, appearance, life cycle and size.

14. Centipedes are flat, long, worm like animals, with each body segment having one pair of legs. They have chewing mouthparts. Some can give painful bites to humans.

15. A plant disease is any harmful condition that alters a plants growth, appearance or function. Diseases are caused by biological agents called pathogens.

16. Bacteria are microscopic can only be seen with a microscope, one-celled organisms that reproduce by single cell division. Bacteria numbers multiply quickly under warm, humid weather conditions. Bacteria may attack any part of a plant, either above or below the soil surface. Several of the leaf spot and rot diseases are caused by bacteria.

17. Fungi are plants that lack chlorophyll and cannot make their own food. Fungi are the most frequent pathogens on plants. They feed off other living organisms or live on dead or decaying organic matter.

18. Viruses are tiny organisms smaller than bacteria and cannot be seen with an ordinary microscope. Viruses are usually recognized from the symptoms they induce on the infected plant.

19. Nematodes are tiny (microscopic) eel or worm like organisms. Nematodes destroy root systems while feeding, which causes a loss in the uptake of water and minerals by the plant, thus weakening the plant.

20. Vertebrate animals all have a jointed backbone. Humans are vertebrates, as are mammals, birds, reptiles, amphibians and fish.

21. Structural pest control is the control of household pests (including but not limited to rodents, vermin and insects) and wood-destroying pests and organisms or such other pests which may invade households or structures, including railroad cars, ships, docks, trucks, airplanes or the contents thereof.

22. Gundhi Bug (*Leptocorisa varicornis*) is a serious pest of paddy which sucks the juice of developing (milk grain stage) grains and reduces the yield and hence called Paddy Bug.

23. After copulation female Gundi bug lay eggs symmetrically, into two or three rows. Eggs are dark coloured, oval in outline and flattened at the top. Eggs hatch in about a week. The young nymphs have slender green body and longer legs. These nymphs generally take about twenty days to attain full maturity.

24. During winter their breeding rate is lowered much and the adults manage to tide over the cold on several species of grasses. On paddy it has five broods during the season.

25. Sugarcane leafhopper (*Pyrillaper pusilla*) is a serious pest of sugar cane in northern India where it also feeds on maize, millets, rice, barley, oats, sorghum, bajra and wild grasses.

26. Adult hoppers are straw coloured to brownish, 7-8 mm long, with a pointed snout bearing piercing and sucking mouthparts.

27. The parasite Sugarcane leafhopper can be controlled by spraying 0.05% of parathion, malathion, thiodon, fenithrothion or rogor. Dusting plants with 10% aldrin or dieldrin also helps. Conservation of the following natural enemies helps in controlling the pests.

28. Rodents destroy property, spread disease, compete for human food sources and are aesthetically displeasing.

29. Termites (*Microtermes obesi*) constitute a large group of social insects with some 2000 species. They live in tunnels dug in logs, furniture, trees or specially built nest called termitarium.

30. Termites consume wood and other cellulose products, such as paper, cardboard and fiberboard. They will also destroy structural timbers, pallets, crates, furniture and other wood products.

31. Generally, termites invade homes by way of the foundation, either by crawling up the exterior surface where their activity is usually obvious or by traveling inside hollow block masonry.

32. Mosquito borne diseases, such as malaria, dengue and yellow fever, have plagued civilization for thousands of years.

33. A few important species of mosquito spend the winter as adult, mated females, resting in protected, cool locations, such as cellars, sewers, crawl spaces and well pits. With warm spring days, these females seek a blood meal and begin the cycle again. Only a few species can overwinter as larvae.

34. Cockroaches have become well adapted to living with and near humans and their hardiness are legendary.

35. The most important fleas as disease vectors are those that carry murine typhus and bubonic plague.

36. The flies as biting or nonbiting. Biting flies include sand flies, horseflies and deerflies. Non-biting flies include houseflies, bottle flies and screwworm flies. The latter group is referred to as synanthropic because of their close association with humans. The housefly (*Musca domestica*) is one of the most widely distributed insects and is usually the predominant fly species in homes and restaurants.

37. Ants are one of the most numerous species on earth. Ants are in the same order as wasps and bees and, because of their geographic distribution, they are universally recognized. The life cycle of the fire ant begins with the mating of the winged forms (alates) some 300 to 800 feet in the air, typically occurring in the late spring or early summer.

38. The most important are four species in the genus *Solenopsis*. Of these, the number one fire ant pest is the red imported fire ant (RIFA) *Solenopsis invicta*. The second most important species is the black imported fire ant, *S. richteri*.

Chapter 3
Animal Breeding and Culture

3.1 Introduction

From the very early days human beings depend on animals and animal products for food and other requirements. In dairy and poultry farms high yielding animals are nurtured. These high yielding animals are produced by hybridization experiments. Previously the animals were developed basing on unscientific methods. Before the discovery of principles of heredity human beings have selected the animals with required characters and learned to develop the plants having the selected characters. This phenomenon is called artificial selection. However, an increased knowledge of biology, especially genetics, has helped in improving the quality of animals and animal products as per the human requirements. The science of animal breeding is concerned with the application of the principles of population genetics to the improvement of domestic animals. Population genetics deals with the forces that influence the genetic composition of biological populations and owes its existence to developments in evolution and population biology and to the global need for improvements in domestic crops and livestock. Livestock breeders, using selection, adapted their stock to meet this need long before animal breeding became a science. With the rediscovery of Mendel in 1900, Wentworth and other animal husbandmen began to explore the art of the breeder in the light of Mendelian genetics. Concurrently, the basic theory of population genetics was formulated by Fisher and Wright. Never before in the history of biology had theory, based on the algebra of ½, so outstripped experimental evidence in any field. This has tended to make population genetics unique among the sciences. Animal breeding used to be in the hands of a few distinguished breeders, individuals who seems to have specific arts and skills to breed good livestock. Now-a-days, animal breeding is much dominated by science and technology. In some livestock species, animal breeding is in the hands of large companies and the role of individual breeders seems to have decreased. There are several reasons for this change. Firstly, the breeding industry has taken up scientific principles. Looking was replaced by measuring and an intuition was partly replaced by calculations and scientific prediction. Other major developments were caused by the introduction of biotechnology. These are roughly the reproductive technologies and the molecular genetic technology. Artificial insemination was introduced in the

1950s in cattle. No doubt that the technology had a major impact on rates on genetic improvement in dairy cattle and just as important, on the structure of animal breeding programs. Nowadays, technologies like ovum pick up, *in vitro* fertilization, embryo transfer, cloning of individuals, cloning of genes and selection with the use of DNA markers are all on the ground. Some of the technologies are already applied, others are further developed or waiting for application. Finally, the rapid development of computer and information technology has greatly influenced data collection and genetic evaluation procedures in livestock populations, now allowing comparison of breeding values across herds, breeds or countries.

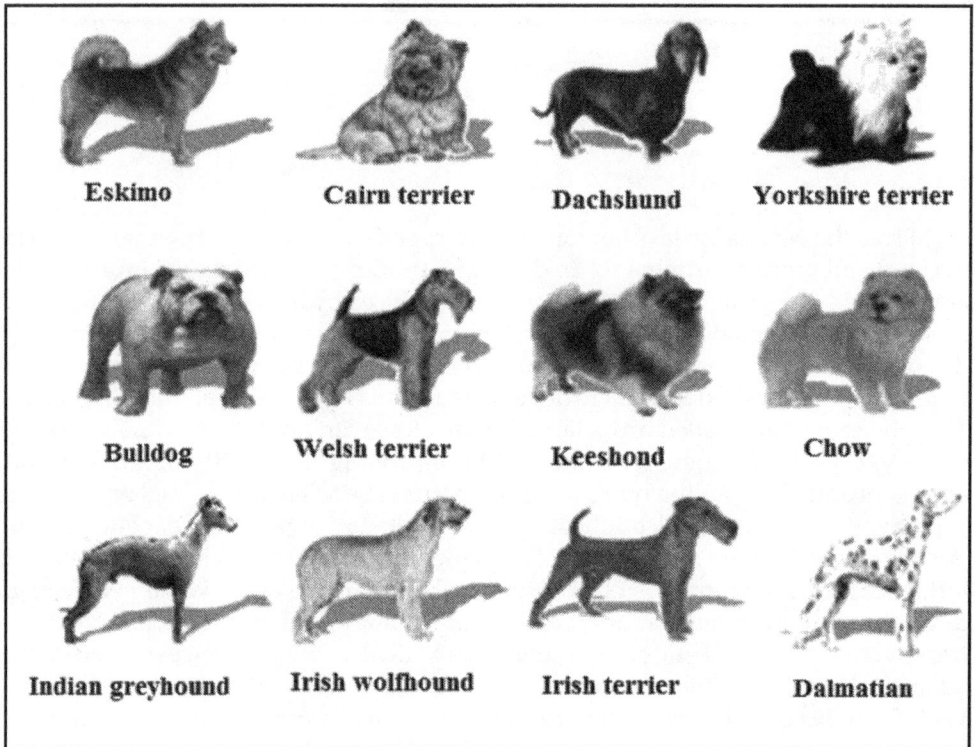

Eskimo	Cairn terrier	Dachshund	Yorkshire terrier
Bulldog	Welsh terrier	Keeshond	Chow
Indian greyhound	Irish wolfhound	Irish terrier	Dalmatian

Figure 3.1: Dog Breeds

3.2 Animals and Human Society

Considering that much of human society is structured through its interaction with non-human animals and since human society relies heavily on the exploitation of animals to serve human needs, human-animal studies has become a rapidly expanding field of research, featuring a number of distinct positions, perspectives and theories that require graded explanation and contextualization. The history of civilization is closely associated with domestic animals. In the early days of human communities, around 10-12,000 years ago, a few large mammalian and bird species were domesticated which have enabled humanity steadily to rise from primitive conditions to life of higher quality. Large domestic animals made possible the move from hunting, gathering and shifting cultivation to more settled life styles. Animals release people from the hard labour of heavy field work; animals make possible the transport of natural resources and farm products to other communities for barter or sale; animals provide animal fat and protein for improved nutrition; animal milk enables infants to survive and grow when quantities of human milk are insufficient; animals provide leather, wool and horn for clothing and shelter; animal fat is used for lighting; dried manure from large animals is fuel for cooking and heating; animal power is used for extracting water from the ground and from rivers for domestic use and for irrigation; animals contribute to improved and integrated farming systems on cropped land; ruminant animals harvest natural vegetation that would otherwise not enter the human food chain; throughout human history, riding animals was the fastest way to travel over land until the invention of the railway in 1829, only 170 years ago. The domestication of animals was the first step to improve the quality of life through science and technology. Now, the majority of people in the world still depend upon animals for these services and, without them life, even in the simplest societies, would disintegrate again into the slavery of food production.

The major advances in European civilization leading to trade, industrialization and the application of science and the development of market economy capitalism were possible because animals had first freed a proportion of the population from the daily routine of food production. Following further applications of science and technology, the majority of people have been set free from work on the land, leaving only 5-10% to farm. This fact can be traced back to the first step of domesticating animals. Freed from the necessity for each family to produce its own food, advanced societies has become immensely creative and modern life has become utterly different.

Influence of domestic animals on human values: For thousands of years everyone was in touch daily with domestic animals. Since animals are a resource of such great value, it is easy to understand why people have held them in high esteem and have sometimes regarded them as sacred. People live in close contact with their animals. Usually each family has a few. Owners give animal's food and care to ensure their health, longevity, ability to serve and to reproduce. Their value is recognized at special celebrations including birth, marriage and death. Animals are wealth and are used both for savings and as currency. The status of a family or community leader is often recorded by numbers of livestock owned. In some parts of Africa today, a bride is given in return for livestock. In India, Hinduism, the major national religion, holds the cow in special honour and sees a link between the life of domestic cattle and human life. In Moslem society, sheep and goats are vital for religious obligations. In early Jewish periods, before AD 70 when Titus destroyed the Temple in Jerusalem, animal sacrifices were a central part of individual and community worship. Domestic animals have greatly influenced community rituals and values in most early societies. We need to distinguish traditions and rituals of life from values. Traditions and rituals are often beautiful and they mark for us the pattern of life, but they are rarely essential and we have dropped many of them from life in the West. In contrast, community and public values in a society, as the name implies, are extremely important. Every society has values. Values determine the direction a society takes. Values enable a society to survive and advance - or they cause its decline. Values lie at the heart of a society and determine the goals people will work to achieve. Values allocate resources in a society and thereby shape its nature. Thus, the values of simpler societies for thousands of years were based upon a holistic view of life. Community embraced all individuals and every-one knew that each component of life is integrated and that life functions as a whole, like an organism with inter-dependent parts which must be sustained for life to continue. In the West, we have lost this world view. We discovered that by focusing upon one component we can make it more productive, but in our enthusiasm we forget the balance of the whole. It is the danger of reductionism. In earlier societies, the intimate dependence upon domestic animals gave more appreciation of the whole environment and helped society to realize that life is knotted with all the natural resources of the world. One cannot take endless quantities of everything without upsetting the balance and eventually precipitating a collapse that will reduce quality of life. The earth is in dynamic equilibrium. In tribes owning large herds of cattle, sheep or goats the dilemma and tension are well known. The attractions of larger numbers of animals to ensure that some survive periods of drought have to be balanced against overgrazing and poorer quality animals.

3.3 Animal Breeding

Breeding is inherent in the keeping of animals, because it is the animal keeper who determines which animals will produce offspring. Breeding is the selection and mating of animals for the purpose of changing the characteristics of the next generation to better correspond to a breeding goal formulated by humans. Therefore, breeding is beneficial to people, but it is not always in the interest of the involved animals. Breeding raises ethical concerns. Breeding require interest to be weighed such as interest of human and animal welfare, interest of climate, biodiversity and food supply and sustainability. Animal breeding controlled propagation of domestic animals in order to improve desirable qualities. Humanity has been modifying domesticated animals to better suit human needs for centuries. Selective breeding involves using knowledge from several branches of science. These include genetics, statistics, reproductive physiology, computer science and molecular genetics.

Animal breeding, as an applied field of population genetics, has a well-developed mathematical foundation that was laid early in its development. Facets of major emphasis in current animal breeding include the utilization of new estimation procedures for random effects, the incorporation of economics in the development of breeding programmes designed for the livestock industry, the verification of theory and testing of breeding schemes using laboratory organisms, the evaluation of new germplasm available in livestock populations and the application of breeding principles to the livestock industry. There are real opportunities in animal breeding to serve the current livestock industry. The animal breeder faces many complex problems during hybridization experiments because many traits of animals are dependent on the interaction of multiple genes. When the attempts are made only to increase the size of eggs in fowls, it was observed that the progeny produced yielded few number of eggs or even they die sometimes. That is if only one character is taken for improvement of the animals; the other characters will degenerate or result in harmful effects. Hence, at the time of selection all the desirable characters are to be taken into consideration. The techniques for the improvement of animals involve principles of selection based on quantitative variations. It is not possible for all of the desirable traits to be obtained in one individual. The successful product must contain maximum number of desirable traits and a minimum number of undesirable traits.

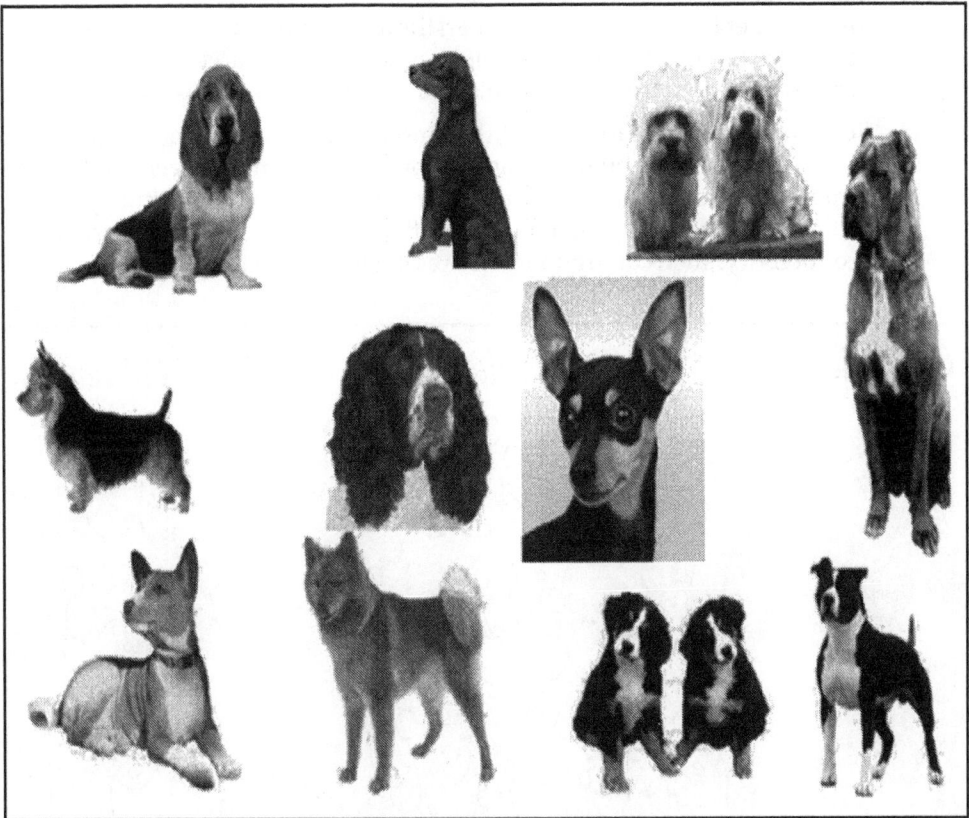

Figure 3.2: Selection of Phenotype

i.   **Body form:** It is an important factor in selecting racially improved variety of animals. A certain body form in cattle and broilers will be having high market value. They yield delicious mutton if they are having well built body form.

ii. **Productivity:** This is of great significance to the breeder. Sometimes it has first priority over other traits. For example the number of eggs, quantity of milk or wool per animal is an important criterion in any programme of improvement of animals.

iii. **Quality of product:** In addition to the quantity, the quality of the productivity is also to be taken into consideration during breeding experiments. The cattle which yield low quantity of milk but having high percentage of fat content are more prominent than those which yield high quantity of milk but with low percentage of fat content. Similarly the quality of wool in a sheep is more important than the quantity of wool.

iv. **Resistance to diseases:** The ability of the animal to resist diseases, to withstand adverse environmental conditions are also important in the animals produced by hybridization experiments.

v. **Early maturity:** It is another trait that the animal breeders look into for improvement of animals. The earlier, the animals mature to the productive age, lesser is the cost of maintaining them. If a hen matures early and begins egg production, it is more valuable than that which matures later.

vi. **Economy in the use of food:** If the amount of food required producing a certain quantity and quality of animal product is comparatively higher, the commercial value of such an animal is said to be very low. In milk yielding cattle and egg yielding fowls if most of their food material is converted into productivity, such cattle and fowls are considered as more valuable.

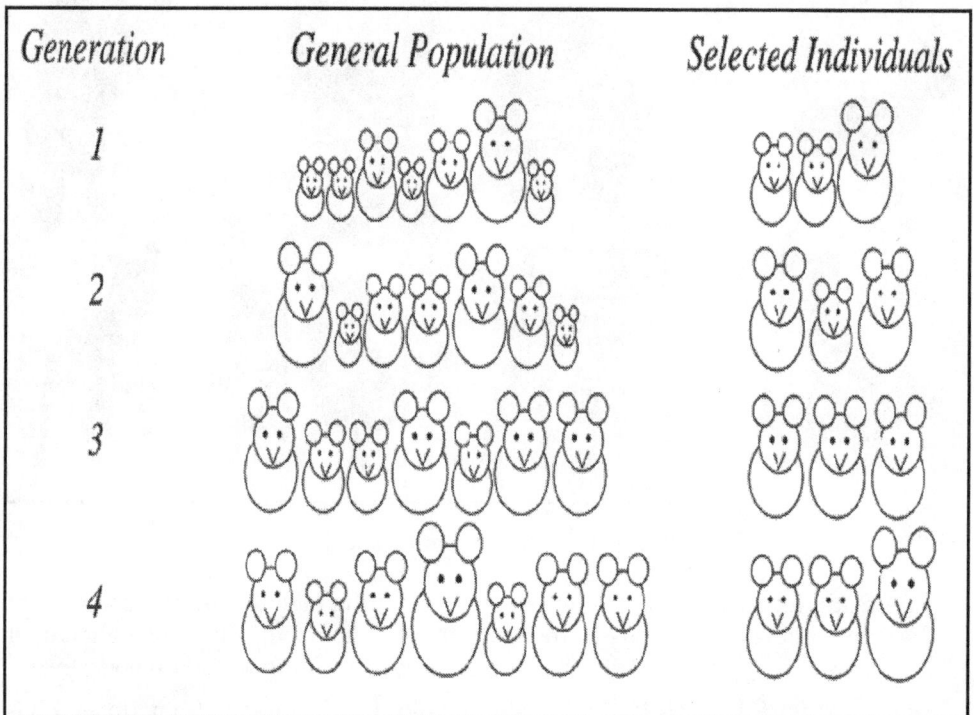

Figure 3.3: Illustration of phenotypic selection for increased body size in mice

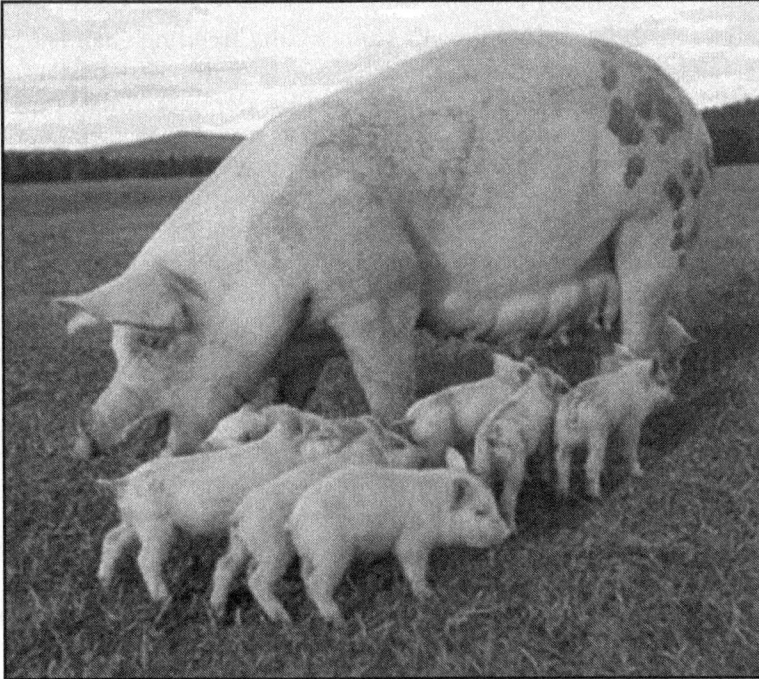

Figure 3.4: Pig and its breed

BOX 3.1

BREEDERS AND ASSOCIATIONS

A breeder is an individual animal keeper who selects animals and mates them for the purpose of producing offspring. Generally, Breeders are private animal owners with just a few animals, as is typically the case in the breeding of dogs and horses. However, breeders may also be large, multinational enterprises. In most cases the breeder owns the female animals, but not generally the male animals. The breeder selects from male animals belonging to others (when natural mating is used) or from sperm (when artificial insemination is used) derived from males owned by another breeder or breeding organization. Breeders seek to improve their own animals through selection and targeted mating of female animals. To modify a population, breeders have to work together. Breeders are typically organized in associations, such as breed registries, studbooks, breeding organizations and breed clubs. These partnerships are essential for making and implementing breeding programme. Within these associations, members agree on the desired direction of population development, the role of individual breeders and the sharing of genetic material. In dairy cattle breeding organizations play a major role in bull selection and therefore in determining the genetic make-up of the population. The breeding organization selects from the population bulls with a high breeding value or genetic value for the breeding goal. The breeding value is determined based on progeny testing. Only the very best animals are selected as breeding bulls. Livestock farmers (breeders) can utilize the semen of breeding bulls from various breeding organizations on their farm. In doing so, they can modify the genetic make-up of their own group. In addition, a breeder can contribute to the improvement of the entire population by selling female animals and even more so, by producing a breeding bull. In laying hens the breeding organization owns both female and male animals in the purebred lines. These organizations' breeding programmes are aimed at genetic improvement of the purebred lines. In this case, the breeding organization is also the breeder. The breeding organization sells crossbred hens and roosters to poultry farmers (multipliers). Poultry farmers mate these animals to produce offspring, which they use for egg or meat production. According to the definition, these poultry farmers are breeders too, since they produce offspring. But the animals produced by these breeders do not contribute to the genetic improvement of the population as a whole, because that is dependent on the selection done in the purebred lines. Only breeders who exchange no genetic material with other breeders such as the large poultry breeding companies can implement a breeding programme entirely on their own. All other breeders are dependent to some extent on other breeders to implement their breeding programme. Dairy farmers can decide for themselves which bulls to use to fertilize their cows, but their choice is limited by the assortment of bulls on offer by the AI organizations. Another example is that of dog breeders. While they can choose for themselves which male to mate with their females, they are nonetheless strongly dependent on which stud dogs are being offered by other breeders and on the information that these breeders provide.

Inbreeding

Inbreeding is the mating of related individuals. A more technically correct definition of inbreeding is the mating of individuals more closely related than average for the population. Inbreeding has a number of effects, but the chief one and the one from which all the others stem is an increase in homozygosity, an increase in the number of homozygous loci in inbred animals and an increase in the frequency of homozygote genotypes in an inbred population. Because inbred individuals have fewer heterozygous loci than non-inbreds, they cannot produce as many different kinds of gametes. The result is fewer different kinds of zygotes and less variation in the offspring. A second consequence of inbreeding is the expression of deleterious recessive alleles with major effects and it is this aspect of inbreeding, more than any other that gives inbreeding a bad reputation. People associate inbreeding with genetic defects. It is true that defects caused by recessive alleles often surface in inbred populations. But inbreeding does not create deleterious recessive alleles; they must already have been present in a population. Inbreeding by itself simply increases homozygosity and it does so without regard to whether the newly formed homozygous combinations contain dominant or recessive alleles. It increases the chance of deleterious alleles becoming homozygous and expressing themselves. Expression of deleterious recessive alleles with major effects, particularly lethal genes, is a very visible consequence of inbreeding. It is an example of the effect of inbreeding can have on certain simply-inherited traits. Less obvious is the expression of unfavorable recessive alleles influencing polygenic traits. The individual effects of these genes are small but, taken together, can significantly decrease performance- a phenomenon known as inbreeding depression.

3.4 Genetic engineering applications in Animal Breeding

Genetic engineering is the name of a group of techniques used for direct genetic modification of organisms or population of organisms using recombination of DNA. These procedures are of use to identify, replicate, modify and transfer the genetic material of cells, tissues or complete organisms. Most techniques are related to the direct manipulation of DNA oriented to the expression of particular genes. In a broader sense, genetic engineering involves the incorporation of DNA markers for selection (marker-assisted selection, MAS), to increase the efficiency of the so called traditional methods of breeding based on phenotypic information. The most accepted purpose of genetic engineering is focused on the direct manipulation of DNA sequences. These techniques involve the capacity to isolate, cut and transfer specific DNA pieces, corresponding to specific genes. The mammalian genome has a larger size and has a more complex organization than in viruses, bacteria and plants. Consequently, genetic modification of animals, using molecular genetics and recombinant DNA technology is more difficult and costly than in simpler organisms. In mammals, techniques for reproductive manipulation of gametes and embryos such as obtaining of a complete new organism from adult differentiated cells (cloning) and procedures for artificial reproduction such as *in vitro* fertilization, embryo transfer and artificial insemination, are frequently an important part of these processes.

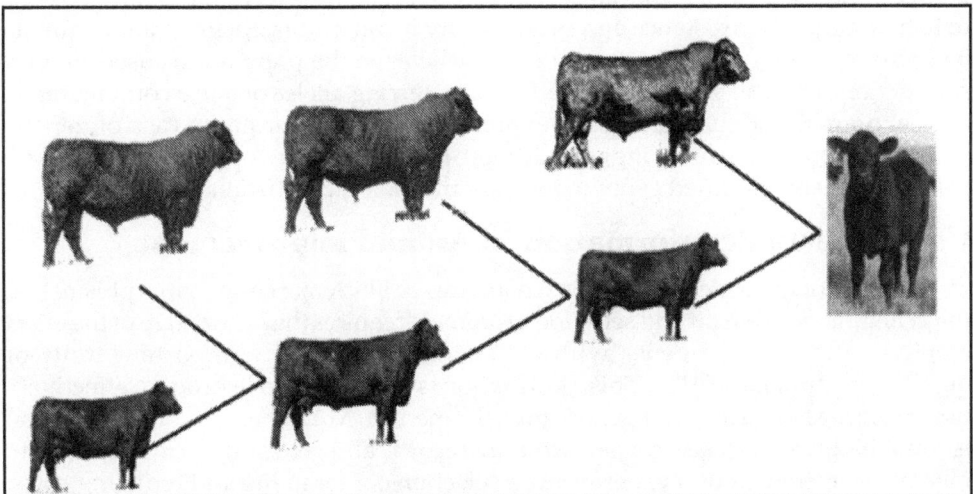

Figure 3.5a: Pedigree information

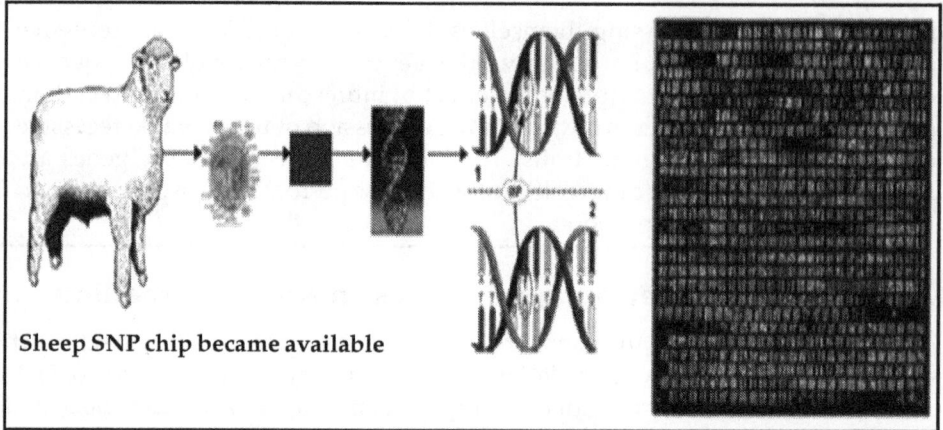

Sheep SNP chip became available

Figure 3.5b: Genetic revolution

Current research in genetic engineering of animals is oriented toward a variety of possible medical, pharmaceutical and agricultural applications. Also, there is an interest to increase basic knowledge about mammalian genetics and physiology, including complex traits controlled by many genes such as many human and animal diseases. The interest in genetic engineering of mammalian cells is based in the idea of use gene therapy to cure genetic diseases such as cystic fibrosis by replacing the damaged copies of the gene by normal ones in fetuses or infants (gene therapy). Genetically engineered animals such as the knockout mouse, in which one specific gene is turned off, are used to model genetic diseases in humans and to discover the function of specific sites of the genome. Genetically modified animals such as pigs will probably be used to produce organs for transplant to humans (xeno-transplantation). Other applications include production of specific therapeutic human proteins such as insulin in the mammary gland of genetically modified milking animals like goats (transgenic animals, bioreactors). These techniques may be used to increase disease resistance and productivity in agriculturally important animals by increasing the frequency of the desired alleles in the populations used in food production. This can be accomplished by transferring alleles or allele combinations, over expressing or eliminating the expression of particular genes (use of genetic engineering in animal breeding). In addition, these techniques open the possibility of using artificially modified genes to increase the biological efficiency of proteins.

Use of Genomic information in Animal improvement

The use of genomic information (sequences or DNA marker polymorphisms) for the genetic improvement and selection of animals requires the knowledge of the effect of physically mapped genes with effects on economically important traits or quantitative trait loci (QTL). This information is also required in order to effectively use transgenesis and MAS for genetic improvement. In MAS, the genomic information is combined with the classical performance records and genealogical information to increase selection accuracy, performing selection earlier in life and reducing costs. The traits, on which the application of marker-assisted selection can be more effective, are those that are expressed late in the life of the animal, have low heritability, sex limited, expensive to measure or controlled by a few genes. Examples are longevity, carcass traits in meat producing animals and diseases or defects of simple inheritance. Expected increments in selection response from MAS for a single complex trait, using known QTL genotypes plus linear model predictions (BLUP; B= Best, L= Linear, U=Unbiased, P=Prediction), compared to selection on BLUP alone, ranges from 0.7 to 64%. In practice, results will depend on many parameters which are likely to be very different for each trait combination and population. The statistical properties of genetic evaluations (predictions) of animals for quantitative traits obtained through mixed model methodology using phenotypic records and genealogical information as inputs are known as BLUP. Best means minimum variance of prediction, Linear; because predictions are linear functions of observations, Unbiased means that the expected value of predictors obtained with linear model have an expected value equal to the expected value of the mean of the breeding values, conditional to data and Prediction; because involves prediction of random breeding value.

Most experiments on QTL detection in animals allow only the estimation of wide chromosomal regions (practical maximum resolution is of about 1 cM, but usual resolution is about 30 cM) that harbour a QTL in a statistical sense, estimated from the effects of some marker haplotypes on quantitative traits. Thus, further confirmation is required in order to assure the use of the causative gene. Identification of the causative gene has proven to be difficult. The process to identify the gene responsible for the effect is known either as fine mapping studies (targeting mapping smaller genomic regions) or candidate gene studies (targeting individual genes based on their probable function). In practice, MAS is useful to select genes with effects well identified and precisely located in the genome such as those controlling monogenic recessive diseases such as the pig stress syndrome gene. However, for most recessive alleles with lethal or semi-lethal effects, natural selection will maintain their frequencies very low making MAS unnecessary.

Unless the additive and non-additive effects for most genes involved in the phenotypic expression of complex, economically important traits are determined, MAS should be regarded just as a tool to increase the rates of genetic gains and not a method to fully open the black box of the genetic control of complex traits that would render phenotypic selection obsolete. Therefore, the perspectives on the optimum use of DNA marker information in the framework of a genetic program is still a matter of debate. Quantitative trait loci experiments using crosses between breeds or lines with extreme genotypes for a trait, increases the power of detecting QTLs for that trait, compared to within family designs. These across population's polymorphisms are not necessarily useful to perform MAS for within population selection. The favorable allele could be fixed in parental populations and crosses may be commercially irrelevant. Wide genome scans for positioning a QTL using crosses or within family experiments, are only the initial phase of the search for a true mayor gene involved in a complex trait. Another source of complexity for detection and use of QTL for selection is genetic heterogeneity, where DNA mutations in several sites produce the same phenotype. Major single gene effects can be sometimes compensated in the organism using alternative metabolic pathways.

Problems related to false positive detection of candidate genes are also common. Using crosses between two pig breeds, a polymorphism on the estrogen receptor locus (ESR) was associated to litter size in pigs with 1.5 piglet advantage for homozygous sows for the beneficial allele and where followed by immediate recommendations for commercial use and patenting. Further research did not confirm the effect. Different phases of linkage between the markers and the QTL could explain the fact that the effect of the ESR locus varied widely between populations. Thus, very probably, despite the ESR gene is probably a plausible candidate from their inferred physiological functions the gene involved seems to be another one, still unknown or the effect initially observed was the product of several, interacting genes (epistasis). Main problems related to the use of molecular genetics in the improvement of agricultural populations are:

i.   Direct use of a discovered QTL effect for selection across families is not possible.

ii. By the time the information about the inferred genotypes is known, frequently the animals involved in the study are not available as candidates for selection, because they will be too old.

iii. Advantage from within family selection for a QTL bracketed by markers over BLUP or phenotypic selection alone is frequently low and the methodology to exploit this information for selection is complex and relatively inefficient.

iv. There are statistical estimation errors, causing both false positive and false negative effects, particularly when the effect of QTL is small.

v.   There is a lack of consistency of the effect of the same QTL between studies, caused by QTL by genetic background (epistasis) of QTL by environment interactions.

vi. The net economic effect of the QTL may be lower than the effect on single traits, because unfavorable effects on other traits.

vii. Selection using QTL is more complex than phenotypic selection alone. QTL information (whether the information on QTL is direct or indirect), adds to the list of traits used as selection criteria. Issues such as reduction of selection intensities and relative emphasis given to each trait, make optimal selection more difficult, with a need for adequate relative weights for the QTL and the polygenic portions of the genetic variation for each trait at each generation (year).

viii.Short term gains due to MAS may be at the expense of medium to long-term polygenic responses for important traits.

Theoretically, it is possible to predict accurately the breeding values of animals using many markers. From this knowledge, it is possible to develop a model for *in vitro* genetic improvement of animals. This is known as velogenetics. The model involves *in vitro* selection of cells containing the desired genes the use of totipotent embryonic stem cells (ES). The procedure uses transfection of the desired genes, selection *in vitro* of the cells and nuclear transfer of the desired genotypes into receptor oocytes. This approach is supposed to increase the rate of genetic improvement by obtaining many generations in a short time by avoiding rearing, reproduction and selection of real animals. Selection on the basis of genomic information only, such in this *in vitro* system, even with major genes with known effects well localized, may be dangerous, because in these artificial populations, unlike in real populations, natural selection would not be allowed to act at each generation on fitness traits under real, perhaps changing, environmental conditions. Changes on economically important traits will not be evaluated directly. This may potentially reduce the responses on selected traits because of genotype x environment interactions. This is because selection is performed in artificial conditions that may deteriorate the fitness of the population and economic response.

Using MAS for improving health in animals by reducing disease prevalence (increasing disease resistance) or increasing resilience (ability to withstand the disease without harmful effects), for infectious or parasitic diseases has been difficult. In most cases, excepting some rare examples such as Scrapie in sheep, complete resistance could not be obtained with the manipulation of a small number of genes. For most diseases, single-gene approaches are expected to have only a partial contribution. Gene interactions are common. For many diseases, heritabilities are often low. That indicates the existence of many environmental factors affecting both the probability of infection and the response of the host. In spite of responses attained using conventional selection for some traits that are used as indicators of disease, the result is not well known. The existence of contradictory results regarding associations between production and disease resistance, the complexities of immune and resistance mechanisms and the interaction with other methods of control such as vaccination, sanitation, management and chemotherapy, makes the whole issue of selecting for disease resistance more difficult, in principle, that selecting for production traits. Moreover, we know that heritable resistance or resilience to more virulent form of pathogens would be increased by natural selection. As heritability for survival are generally low, we know that the genetic control of disease may be very complex, making difficult to change the outcome by manipulating single genes. Other very important applications of genetic markers in animal improvement include the optimization of mating strategies for non-additive genetic effects (estimation and managing of inbreeding and heterosis), parentage determination, genetic characterization of diverse animal breeds and populations using studies of between and within population (breeds) diversity and marker-assisted introgression of particular alleles.

Cloning Adult Mammals

Cloning an animal is the production of a genetically identical individual, by transferring the nucleus of differentiated adult cells into an oocyte from which the nucleus has been removed. This is known as Nuclear Transfer and is how the Dolly sheep was produced. There are several other reports on adult cloned animals involving mice, cattle, cats, goats, pigs, sheep and rabbits involving the same and other cloning techniques.

Cloning Methods: In the case of Dolly, mammary gland cells in culture from a 6-year old donor ewe, where subjected to a reduction in the concentration of serum and thus obliged to enter in a quiescent state of the cell cycle (G_0). Nuclear transfers to enucleated oocytes, was followed by electrical pulses for fusion of the donor cell nucleus and oocyte membranes and activate division.

Problems: Currently, there is no doubts regarding the genetic similarity of the donor and the clone in the case of Dolly, besides low success rates, several health problems related to the technique have been described. Normal development of an embryo is dependent on the methylation state of DNA contributed by the sperm and egg and on the appropriate reconfiguration of the chromatin structure after fertilization. Somatic cells have very different chromatin structure to sperm and reprogramming of the transferred nuclei must occur within a few hours of activation of reconstructed embryos. Incomplete or inappropriate reprogramming will lead to de-regulation of gene expression and failure of the embryo or foetus to develop normally or to non-fatal developmental abnormalities in those that survive. These facts indicate that there is a need for studies to determine further biological consequences of cloning. Cloning has important potential applications in gene transfer procedures.

Use of Cloning in Animal Breeding

Use of cloning in animal genetic improvement may increase the rates of selection progress in certain cases, particularly in situations where artificial insemination is not possible, such as in pastoral systems with ruminants. Currently, high costs of cloning are one of the main factors limiting their use as a technique in practical animal breeding. However, clonal groups more uniform than full sibs will have all differences caused by the environmental fraction of variation for measured traits, which is usually more than 50% of total variation. Selection among many cloned germlines allows the use of the non-additive genetic effects. These effects are not exploited when traditional selection methods involving sexual reproduction are used in animal improvement, but most of the observed genetic variation between animals is additive. Advantages in terms of additional genetic progress however, seems to be only marginal from clone evaluation in selection nucleus herds. Production based on clones of the best animals of the population, may allow for a one time large jump in breeding value, so the commercial animals might be very close to those in the nucleus. However, further genetic improvement must be based in the continued use of the genetic variation by selection programs.

Transgenic Animals

Transgenesis is a procedure in which a gene or part of a gene from one individual is incorporated in the genome of another one. Transgenic animals have any of these genetic modifications with potential use in studying mechanisms of gene function, changing attributes of the animal in order to synthesize proteins of high value, create models for human disease or to improve productivity or disease resistance in animals. In the early 1980s, several research groups reported success in gene transfer and the development of transgenic mice. The definition of transgenic animal has been extended to include animals that result from the molecular manipulation of endogenous genomic DNA, including all techniques from DNA microinjection to embryonic stem (ES) cell transfer and knockout mouse production. Since the early 1980s, the production of transgenic mice by microinjection of DNA into the pronucleus of zygotes has been the most productive and widely used technique. Using transgenic technology in the mouse, such as antisense RNA encoding transgenesis, it is now possible to add a new gene to the genome, increase the level of expression or change the tissue specificity of expression of a gene and decrease the level of synthesis of a specific protein. Removal or alteration of an existing gene via homologous recombination required the use of ES cells and was limited to the mouse until the advent of nuclear transfer cloning procedures.

Transgenic Methods

Microinjection of DNA and now nuclear transfer, are two methods used to produce transgenic livestock successfully. The steps in the development of transgenic models are relatively straightforward. Once a specific fusion gene containing a promoter and the gene to be expressed has been cloned and characterized, sufficient quantities are isolated, purified and tested in cell culture if possible and readied for preliminary mammalian gene transfer experiments. In contrast with nuclear transfer studies, DNA microinjection experiments were first performed in the mouse. While the transgenic mouse model will not always identify likely phenotypic expression patterns in domestic animals, there have not been a single construct that would function in a pig when there was no evidence of transgene expression in mice. Preliminary experimentation in mice has been a crucial component of any gene transfer experiment in domestic animals. While nuclear transfer might be considered inefficient in its current form, major advances in experimental protocols, can be anticipated. The added possibility of gene targeting through nuclear transplantation opens up a host of applications, particularly with regard to the use of transgenic animals to produce human pharmaceuticals. The only major technological advance since the initial production of transgenic farm animals has been the development of methods for the *in vitro* maturation of oocytes (IVM), *in vitro* fertilization (IVF) and subsequent culture of injected embryos prior to transfer to recipient females. Another highly efficient technique for transgenesis has been recently developed based on the use of lentiviral vectors to transform cow and pig oocytes. These vectors are more efficient than microinjection in terms of transformation and expression rates. One limitation is that the size of the transgene and the internal promoter has to be less than 8.5 kb in size.

Transgenesis in Improvement of Production Traits

The technology of transgenesis is potentially useful to modify characters of economic importance in a rapid and precise way. Contrary to the classical selection programs, it is necessary a knowledge of the genes that control these characters and their regulation.

(a) **Growth and meat traits:** In most of the earlier work in domestic species (pig, sheep, rabbit) growth hormone was enhanced by the metallotionein promoter to control its expression. Subsequent efforts to genetically alter growth rates and patterns have included production of transgenic swine and cattle expressing a foreign c-ski oncogene, which targets skeletal muscle and studies of growth in lines of mice and sheep that separately express transgenes encoding growth hormone-releasing factor (GRF) or insulin-like growth factor I (IGF-I). Transgenic pigs and sheep with high levels of serum growth hormone were obtained, but an increment of its rate of growth was not observed and only in some lines average daily gain increased with the supplement of the diet with high levels of protein. The highest effects were observed in the reduction of body fat. There is evidence for the use of transgenesis allowing to important reductions in body fat and increased diameter of muscle fiber by increased IGF-I levels and growth hormone without serious pathological side effects in 1998. Frequently the used promoters have not allowed an efficient control of the expression of the transgene. It was assessed that it is necessary to develop more complex constructions that activate or repress the expression of the transgene more precisely. Adams in 2002, found inconsistent results regarding the effect of a growth hormone construct in sheep on growth and meat quality.

(b) **Wool production:** The major objective in wool productions is to improve production of sheep wool and to modify the properties of the fiber. Because cystein seems to be the limiting amino acid for wool synthesis, the first approach is to increase its production through transfer of cystein biosynthesis from bacterial genes to sheep genome. This approach cannot achieve the efficient expression of these enzymes in the rumen of transgenic sheep.

(c) **Milk Composition:** Milk proteins are coded by unique copy genes that can be altered to modify milk composition and properties. Among the different applications of milk modification in transgenic animals, the following can be highlighted:

i.   To modify bovine milk to make it more appropriate to the consumption of infants. Human milk lacks â-lactoglobulin, has a higher relationship of serum proteins to caseins and has a higher content in lactoferrin and lysozyme when compared to bovine milk. Lactoferrin is responsible for the iron transport and inhibits the bacterial growth. To introduce the human lactoferrin into the bovine milk, transgenic cows have been obtained. The elimination of the â-lactoglobulin in the cow milk would be another interesting objective because is one of the major allergens of cow's milk.

ii. To reduce the content of lactose in the milk to allow their consumption to people with intolerance to lactose. It is considered that 70 per cent of the world population is lacking the intestinal lactase, the enzyme required to digest the lactose. The reduction in lactose may be obtained by expressing â-galactosidase in the milk or diminishing the content of α-lactalbumin. Transgenic mouse with inactivated α-lactalbumin gene produce milk without lactose. However, a serious practical drawback of this method is that this milk is very viscous and it is not secreted to the exterior of the mammary gland, due to the importance of the lactose in the osmoregulation of the milk.

iii. To alter the content of caseins of the milk to increase their nutritive value, cheese yield and processing properties. Research has intended to increase the number of copies of the gene of the ê-casein, to reduce the size of the micelles and modificating the ê-casein to make it more susceptible to the digestion with chymosin. This has only been done using the mouse as a model. Brophy in 2003 engineered female bovine foetal fibroblasts to express additional copies of transgenes encoding two types of casein; bovine α-casein and ê-casein. The modified cell lines of fibroblasts were used to create eleven cloned calves. Milk from the cloned animals was enriched for α and-β casein, resulting in a 30 per centincrease in the total milk casein or a 13 per cent increase in total milk protein, demonstrating the potential of this technology to make modified milk.

iv. To express antibacterial substances in the milk, such as proteases to increase mastitis resistance. The objective is to alter the concentrations of antibacterial proteins such as lyzozyme or transferrin in the milk.

Future Perspectives of Transgenesis

The techniques for obtaining transgenic animals in species of agricultural interest are still inefficient. Some approaches that may overcome this problem are based on cloning strategies. Using these techniques it is feasible to reduce to less than 50% the number of embryo receptor females, which is one of the most important economic limiting factor in domestic species. It would also facilitate the further proliferation of transgenic animals. Recent results relate these techniques with still low success rates, high rates of perinatal mortality and variable transgenic expression that requires to be evaluated before generalizing their application. Considerable effort and time is required to propagate the transgenic animal genetics into commercial dairy herds. Rapid dissemination of the genetics of the parental animals by nuclear transfer could result in the generation of mini-herds in two to three years. However, the existing inefficiencies in nuclear transfer make this a difficult undertaking. It is noteworthy that the genetic merit of the cloned animals will be fixed, while continuous genetic improvements will be introduced in commercial herds by using artificial insemination breeding programs. Detecting genes related to disease and their expression in humans from studies on the genome, could lead to the development of therapies and the development of drugs for specific individuals and enhanced early diagnosis of individuals with high-risk genotypes, allowing for preventive or remedial actions, even gene therapy. In animals, this knowledge could lead to select against defective genes. In livestock, knowledge of effects of specific genes and gene combinations on important traits could lead to their enhanced control to create new, more useful populations. The use of specific gene information is not a panacea, but could help to increase rates of genetic improvement and open opportunities for using additive and non-additive genetic effects of domestic species, provided wise improvement goals are used and this new technology is optimally used together with the so called traditional or conventional methods based on phenotypic and genealogical information.

These methods will help to increase our knowledge about the genetic architecture of complex quantitative traits in domestic animal populations and to estimate the distribution of the genetic variation across and within breeds and population. It will also aid in ascertaining the genetic merit of local, less known populations. Studies for using genetic diversity in structured populations using DNA markers are very useful in order to set priorities for conservation of distant or unique populations as reservoirs of potentially unique genes, because their contribution to biodiversity would be greater. Currently, the main practical application of DNA markers is for parenting determination and to trace products such as meat.

One promising applications of transgenesis is the synthesis of biomedical products of high commercial interest. Transgenic bioreactors and the use of exogenous or artificial genes interfering with particular cell mechanisms or with pathogens but not or only marginally, with the physiology of the animals are potential applications. A greater knowledge on the mechanisms that determine the integration of the transgenes and genic regulation will allow a more precise control of the expression of the transgenes and it will probably facilitate a larger number of applications in the domestic species, including modifications beyond normal limits, such as to increase the number of copies of the gene and their expression. These transformations could be regarded as a form of mutation. The expressions of complex traits are the result of several mechanisms involving both regulatory and structural portions of the genome. Advances in molecular genetics, genomics, proteomics and transcriptomics might perhaps help to shorten the gap between the more holistic approaches of quantitative genetics with the more reductionistic approach of molecular genetics. The release of genome sequence information in cattle and pig, may allow for a more efficient use of MAS and also to address some consumers concerns regarding product quality and safety. Cloning is another technique that raises concerns both from the ethical and practical point of view. Whether it is acceptable to clone humans is a very difficult issue. In animals, besides the very low success rates, some abnormalities should suggest that more information is required on the consequences of such practices in humans but also in animals, before its routine use. Advantages for animal breeding programs derived from cloning with no use of transgenesis are like to be small. A reasonable degree of regulation, open information on the issues of genetic engineering technologies from the academic world and an involvement of the whole society in the developments of the laws concerning these issues, seems to be the best way to circumvent an exaggerated or negative reactions to some of these knowledge and to avoid or reduce unethical or abusive use of these techniques. A specific set of conclusions regarding safety of food from genetically modified animals is available from a FAO/WHO expert consultation panel. Most of the important potential technical advances offered by genetic engineering technology in animal breeding are still ahead. Their use has both advantages and problems. Advantages are related to a more complete control over the animal genome. Problems are related to technical complexity, high costs, in some cases, public acceptance and ethical dilemmas.

BOX 3.2

ENHANCING LIVESTOCK PRODUCTIVITY

Farmers in developing countries, due to the pressure for higher animal output and the trend to promote the advantages of a small number of highly specialized breeds from the developed world, have been replacing or crossbreeding their local breeds with exotic animals for many years. The genetic improvement has been quite successful in many instances; selective inbreeding and use of highly productive genetic lines and breeds while neglecting or blanket upgrading indigenous animals with exotic breeds is leading to deterioration in genetic diversity. Genetic biodiversity allows the expression of advantageous traits influencing adaptability to harsh environments, productivity or disease resistance. There are indigenous breeds with some degree of enhanced resistance compared to exotic ones reared in the same environment, especially for gastro-intestinal nematode infections. Similar resistance occurs for diseases due to mycotoxins, bacterial diseases including foot rot and mastitis, ectoparasites such as flies and lice and scrapie. However, indigenous animals are underutilized in conventional breeding programmes, due to misconceptions over their value and failure to identify breeds and animals carrying advantageous traits. The Subprogramme is conducting several studies to genetically characterize local breeds to identify beneficial traits that can be used for breed selection and therefore, supporting genetic conservation. In an on-going project, characterization and mapping of genes that control such traits, through genomic studies using radiolabelled nucleotides in DNA hybridization, DNA characterization and hybrid mapping procedures, along with the phenotypic evaluation of the resistance to gastrointestinal parasites of sheep and goat breeds will allow the identification of single-nucleotide polymorphism (SNP) markers that would be suitable for selecting resistant breeding stock. The hybrid map will be a fundamental tool for member states working on the genetic characterization of small ruminants and for comparative genomic analyses.

Efficient reproduction is of the utmost importance for the sustainable improvement of animal productivity and is a critical factor influencing the economic viability of livestock farmers. Low fertility is identified as one of the primary constraints hindering the effectiveness of livestock production systems in developing countries. Decreasing the age at first parturition, the interval from parturition to conception, interval between parturitions and peripartal mortality and increasing conception rate, litter size and productive life are the key targets and crucial factors in improving livestock productivity. Increased numbers of animals also enables more intense selection of animals of superior quality to serve as parents of the next generation. Individual or corporate farmers, by using simple but well established and validated field and laboratory protocols, can monitor and evaluate the performance of both individual animals and whole herds. This will allow them to run a programme where animals can reach sexual maturity and first parturition at an earlier age, produce offspring at a higher frequency and in consequence, farmers can obtain higher and sustainable economic returns. The monitoring of reproductive hormones, through radio-isotopic techniques such as radioimmunoassay (RIA), in conjunction with field protocols for sampling, collection of behavioural and biological data and the use of computer software applications, developed by the IAEA such as AIDA Asia, AIDA Africa, LIMA and SPeRM has proved of enormous benefits to livestock producers and extension workers. This has included obtaining a better understanding of the reproductive physiology of livestock species, identification and amelioration of limiting factors affecting reproductive efficiency and provision of diagnostic tools to ensure proper AI timing, to monitor ovarian cyclicity and to identify anoestrus and non-pregnant females. It has also assisted

AI centres and AI service providers on identifying management and human errors on AI, efficiency of inseminators, failures in heat detection and fertility of sires. RIA is a mature, sound and unbeatable nuclear technique that can be established in decentralized laboratories and only requires a basic set of equipment and consumables. The technique provides tremendous support to research and extension laboratories by assisting farmers to improve livestock productivity and income. IAEA Member States, through Technical Cooperation (TC) Projects and Coordinated Research Projects (CRP) are assisted in its application, quality control and data interpretation. Healthy and well-fed animals, properly reared and genetically selected will grow faster and produce more and better quality yields. Based on this simple but important principle, actions should be focused on integrated programmes that address the efficient use of locally available feed resources for feeding the animals in a sustainable manner, the selection of superior animals for improved reproductive and productive efficiency, the alleviation of fertility constraints, the implementation of artificial insemination (AI) programmes and the prevention and control of infectious diseases, with emphasis in transboundary diseases.

3.5 Breeding and Variation

Selective breeding utilizes the natural variations in traits that exist among members of any population. Breeding progress requires understanding the two sources of variation; genetics and environment. For some traits there is an interaction of genetics and the environment. Differences in the animal's environment, such as amount of feed, care and even the weather, may have an impact on their growth, reproduction and productivity. Such variations in performance because of the environment are not transmitted to the next generation. For most traits measured in domestic animals, the environment has a larger impact on variation than do genetic differences. For example, only about 30 per cent of the variation in milk production in dairy cattle can be attributed to genetic effects; the remainder of the variation is due to environmental effects. Thus, environmental factors must be considered and controlled in selecting breeding stock. Genetic variation is necessary in order to make progress in breeding successive generations. Each gene, which is the basic unit of heredity, occupies a specific location or locus, on a chromosome. Two or more genes may be associated with a specific locus and therefore with a specific trait. Traits that can be observed directly, such as size, colour, shape and so forth, make up an organism's phenotype. These genes are known as alleles. If paired alleles are the same, the organism is called homozygous for that trait; if they are different, the organism is heterozygous. Typically, one of the alleles will be expressed to the exclusion of the other allele, in which case the two alleles are referred to as dominant and recessive, respectively. However, sometimes neither dominates, in which case the two alleles are called codominant.

Although no complete knowledge of the genetic makeup of any breed of livestock exists yet, genetic variations can be used for improving stock. Researchers partition total genetic variation into additive, dominance and epistatic types of gene action, which are defined in the following paragraphs. Additive variation is easiest to use in breeding because it is common and the effect of each allele at a locus just adds to the effect of other alleles at that same locus. Genetic gains made using additive genetic effects are permanent and cumulate from one generation to the next. Although dominance variation is not more complex in theory, it is more difficult to control in practice because of how one allele masks the effect of another. For example, let a indicate a locus, with a_1 and a_2 representing two possible alleles at that location. Then a_1a_1, a_1a_2 (which is identical to a_2a_1) and a_2a_2 are the three possible genotypes. If a_1 dominates a_2, the genotypes a_1a_2 and a_1a_1 cannot be outwardly distinguished. Thus, the inability to observe differences between a_1a_2 and a_1a_1 presents a major difficulty in using dominance variance in selective breeding. Additive and dominance variations are caused by genes at one locus. Epistatic variation is caused by the joint effects of genes at two or more loci. There has been little deliberate use of this type of genetic variation in breeding because of the complex nature of identifying and controlling the relevant genes.

Breeding can be discussed in terms of changing the genetic makeup of a population of animals, where population is defined as a recognized breed. Choice of breeding goals and design of an effective breeding program is usually not an easy task. Complicating the implementation of a breeding program is the number of generations needed to reach the initial goals. Ultimately, breeding goals are dictated by market demand; it is not easy to predict what consumers will want several years in advance. Sometimes the marketplace demands a different product than was defined as desirable in the original breeding objective. When this happens, breeders have to adjust their program, which results in less efficient selection than if the new breeding goal had been used from the beginning. For example, consumers want leaner beef that is tender. Thus, ranchers have changed their cattle breeding programs to meet this new demand. These trends have gradually changed over the last few decades; Angus cattle are particularly noted for the quality of beef produced. The use of ultrasound is now widespread in determining the fat and lean content of live animals, which will hasten the changing of carcass quality to meet consumer demands. Additional complications arise from simultaneously trying to improve multiple traits and the difficulty of determining what part of the variation for each trait is under genetic control. In addition, some traits are genetically correlated and this correlation may be positive or negative the traits may be complementary or antagonistic. Breeding methods depend on heritability and genetic correlations for desirable traits.

Heritability and Genetic correlations in Breeding

Heritability is the proportion of the additive genetic variation to the total variation. Heritability is important because without genetic variation there can be no genetic change in the population. Alternatively, if heritability is high, genetic change can be quite rapid and simple means of selection are all that is needed. Using an increasing scale from 0 to 1, a heritability of 0.75 means that 75 per cent of the total variance in a trait is controlled by additive gene action. With heritabilities this high, just the record of a single individual's traits can easily be used to create an effective breeding program. Some general statements can be made about heritability, keeping in mind that exceptions exist. Traits related to fertility have low heritabilities. Examples include the average number of times that a cow must be bred before she conceives and the average number of pigs in a litter. Traits related to production have intermediate heritabilities. Examples include the amount of milk a cow produces, the rates of weight gain in steers and pigs and the number of eggs laid by chickens. So-called quality traits tend to have higher heritabilities. Examples include the amount of fat a pig has over its back and the amount of protein in a cow's milk. The magnitude of heritability is one of the primary considerations in designing breeding programs. Genetic correlation occurs when a single gene affects two traits. There may be many such genes that affect two or more traits. Genetic correlations can be positive or negative, which is indicated by assigning a number in the range from +1 to -1, with 0 indicating no genetic correlation. A correlation of +1 means that the traits always occur together, while a correlation of -1 means that having either trait always excludes having the other trait. Thus, the greater the displacement of the value from 0, the greater the correlation (positive or negative) between traits. The practical breeding consequence is that selection for one trait will pull along any positively correlated traits, even though there is no deliberate selection for them. For example, selecting for increased milk production also increases protein production. Another example is the selection for increased weight gain in broiler chickens, which also increases the fat content of the birds. When traits have a negative genetic correlation, it is difficult to select simultaneously for both traits. For example, as milk production is increased in dairy cows through genetic selection, it is slightly more difficult for the high-producing cows to conceive. This negative correlation is partly due to the partitioning of the cows' nutrients between production and reproduction, with production being prioritized in early lactation. In the case of dairy cattle, milk production is on the order of about 10,000 liters per year and is increasing. This is a large metabolic demand, so nutrient demand is large to meet this need. Thus, selecting for improved fertility may result in a reduction in milk production or its rate of gain.

Methods of selection: Types of selection are individual or mass selection, within and between family selection, sibling selection and progeny testing, with many variations. Within family selection uses the best individual from each family for breeding. Between family selection uses the whole family for selection. Mass selection uses records of only the candidates for selection. Mass selection is most effective when heritability is high and the trait is expressed early in life, in which case all that is required is observation and selection based on phenotypes. When mass selection is not appropriate, other methods of selection, which make use of relatives or progeny, can be used singularly or in combination. Modern technologies allow use of all these types of selection at the same time, which results in greater accuracy.

Elements needed to make genetic progress: Genetic gain per year (Δ) depends on balancing several factors, as expressed in the equation $\Delta G=(A\sigma g i)/1$, where A is the accuracy of selection, $\acute{o}g$ is the standard deviation of the additive genetic variation in the population, i is the selection intensity (proportion selected for further breeding) and I is the generation interval (age of breeding). The αg factor cannot be easily changed within a breed, though it can be changed by crossbreeding. The other quantities in the equation can be changed. More complete pedigree records on candidates for breeding can increase the accuracy of selection, but waiting for candidates to reach full maturity in order to have better genetic data will increase the generation interval. Whether an increase in generation interval is justified by a more accurate selection process depends on individual circumstances. Selection intensity can also be increased, by narrowing the proportion of the population used in breeding, but it should be done without increasing the generation interval. Because generation interval is the divisor in the genetic gain equation, anything that increases the generation interval has an unfavorable impact on genetic progress, all else being equal.

Evaluation of animals: Methods of ranking animals for breeding purposes have changed as statistical and genetic knowledge has increased. Along with increases in breeding knowledge, advancements in computing have enabled breeders to quickly and easily process routine breeding evaluations, as well as to develop research needed to rank large populations of animals. Evaluating and ranking candidates for selection depends on equating their performance record to a statistical model. A performance record (y) can be expressed as $y = g + e + å$, where g stands for genetic effects, e indicates known (categorized) environmental effects and $å$ indicates random environmental effects. The first task in estimating g is to statistically eliminate environmental effects, a process that involves setting up a system of equations to simultaneously solve for all of the genetic effects for the sires and cows. Information from relatives is included in g and increases the accuracy of evaluation of the candidates for selection. All relatives that are available can be incorporated in this type of evaluation. This model is called the animal model.

The animal model is used extensively in evaluating beef and dairy cattle, chickens and pigs. To apply this model for evaluating large populations requires use of high speed computers and extensive use of advanced mathematical techniques from numerical analysis.

Accuracy of selection: In some cases the accuracy of selection for a trait can be measured using a calibrated tool or a scale. Thus, measurements of such traits can be replicated with high reliability. Alternatively, some traits are difficult to measure on an objective scale, in which case a well designed subjective scoring method can be effective. An excellent example is hip dysplasia, a degenerative disease of the hip joints that is common in many large dog breeds. Apparently, hip dysplasia is not associated with a single allele, making its incidence very difficult to control. However, an index has been developed by radiologists that allow young dogs to be assigned a score indicating their likelihood of developing the disease as they age. In 1997, American animal geneticist E.A. Leighton reported that, in fewer than five generations of selection in a breeding experiment using these scores, the incidence of canine hip dysplasia in German shepherd dogs measured at 12 to 16 months of age had decreased from the breed average of 55 per cent to 24 per cent among the experimental population; in Labrador retrievers the incidence dropped from 30 to 10 per cent.

Because close relatives share many genes, an examination of the relatives of a candidate for breeding can improve accuracy of selection. The more complete the genealogical record or pedigree, the more effective the selection process. A pedigree is most useful when the heritability of a trait is relatively low, especially for traits that are expressed later in life or in only one sex.

Reproductive techniques can be used to increase the rate of genetic progress. In particular, for species that are mostly bred by artificial insemination, the best dams can be chosen and induced to super ovulate or release multiple eggs from their ovaries. These eggs are fertilized in the uterus and then flushed out in a nonsurgical procedure that does not impair future conception of the donor female. Using this procedure, valuable females can produce more than one calf per year. Each embryo is implanted in a less-valuable host female to be carried through gestation. The sex of the embryos can be determined in utero at about 50 days of gestation. The normal gestation for Holstein-Friesian cattle is about 280 days, so this early determination of sex saves many days and allows the breeding program to be adjusted. The donor cow could be collected again or another superior cow could be bred to produce males. Thus, these reproductive technologies reduce the generation interval and increase selection intensity by getting more than one male calf from superior females. Both super ovulation and sex determination are now commonly used procedures. Super ovulation is also used when breeders want to increase the number of female calves from a valuable cow.

Progeny testing: Progeny testing is used extensively in the beef and dairy cattle industry to aid in evaluating and selecting stock to be bred. Progeny testing is most useful when a high level of accuracy is needed for selecting a sire to be used extensively in artificial insemination. Progeny testing programs consist of choosing the best sires and dams in the population based on an animal model evaluation. The best 1 to 2 per cent of the cows from the population are chosen as bull mothers and the best progeny-tested bulls are chosen to produce another generation of sires. The parents are mated to complement any individual deficiencies. The accuracy of evaluation of bull mothers is typically about 40 per cent and of sires that produce young bulls the accuracy is more than 80 per cent. This is not as high as the industry wants for bulls to be used in artificial insemination. To reach greater accuracy, the next generation of sires is mated to enough cows in the population for each sire to produce 60 to 80 progeny. After the daughters of the young sires have a production record, the young sires are evaluated and about the best 10 per cent are used extensively to produce commercial cows. Some of the progeny-tested sires will have thousands of daughters before a superior sire is found to replace them. About 70 per cent of dairy cattle are bred by artificial insemination, so these sires control the genetic destiny of dairy cattle. Consistently applying this selection procedure has been very successful. The genetic gain has been consistent over the years. The actual first-lactation milk production varies more than the sire breeding value because differences in environmental conditions affect first-lactation production, but these environmental effects have been adjusted out of the breeding value calculations. There is no indication that the rate of gain in the sire breeding values is about to reduce. This level of achievement can only be realized if artificial insemination organizations and producers work together.

Crossbreeding: Crossbreeding involves the mating of animals from two breeds. Normally, breeds are chosen that have complementary traits that will enhance the offsprings' economic value. An example is the crossbreeding of Yorkshire and Duroc breeds of pigs. Yorkshires have acceptable rates of gain in muscle mass and produce large litters and Durocs are very muscular and have other acceptable traits, so these breeds are complementary. Another example is Angus and Charolais beef cattle. Angus produce high quality beef and Charolais are especially large, so crossbreeding produces an animal with acceptable quality and size. The other consideration in crossbreeding is heterosis or hybrid vigour, which is displayed when the offspring performance exceeds the average performance of the parent breeds. This is a common phenomenon in which increased size, growth rate and fertility are displayed by crossbred offspring, especially when the breeds are more genetically dissimilar. Such increases generally do not increase in successive generations of crossbred stock, so purebred lines must be retained for crossbreeding and for continual improvement in the parent breeds. In general, there is more heterosis for traits with low heritability. In particular, heterosis is thought to be associated with the collective action of many genes having small effects individually but large effects cumulatively. Because of hybrid vigour, a high proportion of commercial pork and beef come from crossbred animals.

Inbreeding: Mating animals that are related causes inbreeding. Inbreeding is often described as narrowing the genetic base because the mating of related animals results in offspring that have more genes in common. Inbreeding is used to concentrate desirable traits. Mild inbreeding has been used in some breeds of dogs and has been extensively used in laboratory mice and rats. For example, mice have been bred to be highly sensitive to compounds that might be detrimental or useful to humans. These mice are highly inbred so that researchers can obtain the same response with replicated treatments. Inbreeding is generally detrimental in domestic animals. Increased inbreeding is accompanied by reduced fertility, slower growth rates, greater susceptibility to disease and higher mortality rates. As a result, producers try to avoid mating related animals. This is not always possible, though, when long-continued selection for the same traits is practiced within a small population, because parents of future generations are the best candidates from the last generation and some inbreeding tends to accumulate. The rate of inbreeding can be reduced, but, if inbreeding depression becomes evident, some method of introducing more diverse genes will be needed. The most common method is some form of crossbreeding.

DNA: Deoxyribonucleic acid (DNA) is the genetic material that contains the instructions in each cell of organisms. DNA determines the genome and thus the genetic code, which is a blueprint for development of all body organs and structures. The structure of DNA can be visualized as a spiral staircase. The handrails are made up of sugar and phosphate molecules and the steps are composed of four nitrogenous bases; adenine, thymine, cytosine and guanine. These bases are paired; adenine is paired with thymine and cytosine is paired with guanine. The order of these four base pairs is the genetic code that determines the genotype of an individual. The DNA is arranged on chromosomes inside cells, with cells having two methods of dividing and replicating. In mitosis, a cell divides into two daughter cells such that each contains an exact copy of the original cell's chromosomes. In meiosis, a germ cell's chromosomes are duplicated before the cell undergoes two divisions to produce four gametes or sex cells, each with half (male or female) of the original cell's chromosomes. During the process of fertilization, male and female gametes from different organisms pair their chromosomes to form a zygote, which eventually becomes an adult. Genetic progress in domestic animals has been made using quantitative methods to date. It would be very desirable to know the genes that control the many traits that have economic significance in domestic animals. This should make selection more accurate. Information from sequencing human genes, as well as those of other species, is being used to find chromosomal segments with high probabilities of coding genes in livestock. Another approach is to scan a chromosome segment and look for associations with economic traits. Several quantitative trait loci have been discovered that are or promise to be useful in livestock breeding. For example, an estrogen receptor in pigs is associated with increased litter size, on average, an increase of 0.6 to 2.0 pigs per litter, depending on the genetic background in which the gene is expressed. Other genes have been found that control the secretion of casein in cow's milk. Genes are also known for growth hormone and many others could be enumerated. With improvements in sequencing DNA, more genes will be discovered that affect economic traits, genes that will need to be tested in different genetic backgrounds and environments before they can be commercialized. It is now much less expensive to sequence DNA, which has led to new methods of evaluating animals using large segments of 30,000–50,000 bases. With the use of these large segments of DNA, animals are evaluated without looking for markers for individual traits. This is intuitively an appealing approach because much more of the DNA can be evaluated; perhaps in the future the entire genome can be used to evaluate animals. This method of selection, called genomic selection, is now being applied to dairy cattle.

Immunogenetics: The connection between an organism's genetic makeup and its immune system, as well as applications of that knowledge, forms the young science of immunogenetics. The producers must control diseases in their livestock if they are going to be profitable. While vaccines, hygiene and other therapeutic methods control most diseases, vaccines are expensive and none of these methods is completely effective. However, there is evidence from experiments and field data of some degree of genetic control over the immune system in humans and animals. For example, bovine leukocyte adhesion deficiency (BLAD) is a hereditary disease that was discovered in Holstein calves in the 1980s. The presence of the BLAD gene leads to high rates of bacterial infections, pneumonia, diarrhea and typically death by age four months in cattle and those that survive their youth have stunted growth and continued susceptibility to infections. It was soon found that these calves carried two copies of a recessive gene that was present in nearly 25 per cent of Holstein bulls. Cattle with only one copy of the gene or carriers, had normal growth patterns and immune systems. Holstein bulls are now routinely tested for the BLAD gene before being used for artificial insemination. With a high percentage of Holsteins being bred artificially, a potentially major problem has been avoided.

Genetic control of the immune system is based on the DNA of the individuals. Histocompatibility genes that serve several functions are on one area of a chromosome, called the major histocompatibility complex (MHC), which exists in all higher vertebrates. There are large numbers of genes involved in the MHCs of different species. There are more than 60 different alleles at one locus and other loci are multi-allelic. There are also differences among species in the number of genes known. In addition, selection experiments have demonstrated genetic variation between lines selected for high and low response to different antigens. Some vaccinations are more efficacious when the animals have been selected for resistance to the antigen for which they are vaccinated. Substantial progress has been made in the field of immunogenetics, but limited use has been made of this knowledge. One reason for this is that immune systems have evolved to be generally robust. Changing the frequency of some genes that control immune function may inadvertently change the function of other genes and result in adverse effects. Experiments are now under way to determine whether sires' immune responses can be used to predict the health of their daughters under field conditions. The results indicate that there are differences among sires' daughter groups, but the differences are not large enough to control a high proportion of the variability. The tests used were based primarily on leukocytes, which are the first line of defense when an antigen invades an animal. Application of knowledge in the area of immunogenetics must be used with caution. It might seem that integrating molecular markers and quantitative methods would be a trivial task. However, the effect of some genes depends on the presence of others and these interactions need to be considered along with the particular breeding scheme. Furthermore, there are nongenetic influences that may turn genes on and off. Thus, some genes act individually, some genes interact and the environment has a further impact. Finding how these all affect the phenotypic expression of an organism is complicated. However, this challenge presents an opportunity for future research and for producers. Many advances in reproductive technologies have been made, though many are too expensive for everyday use. Most of the advanced techniques use artificial insemination, which was developed decades ago, though refinements continue.

Cloning: Cloning, an asexual method of reproduction produces an individual with the same genetic material (DNA) as another individual. Probably the best-known examples of clones are identical twins, which result when cells in the early development stage separate and develop into different individuals. Though the DNA in cloned individuals is the same, environmental influences may make them differ in phenotype. Thus far, the commercial use of clones has been limited. Cloning can be used to produce clones from a highly productive individual, but the cost would have to be low enough to recover the expense quickly. Animals have been cloned by three processes: embryo splitting, blastomere dispersal and nuclear transfer. Nuclear transfer is most common and involves enucleating an ovum or egg, with all the genetic material removed. This material is replaced with a full set of chromosomes from a suitable donor cell, which is microinjected into the enucleated cell. Then the enucleated cell, with the transplanted chromosome, is placed into a recipient female to be carried through gestation.

Determining sex from sperm: There is a commercial demand for the ability to predetermine the sex of livestock. For example, a producer may want female calves from the best cows for replacements and male calves for beef production. Dairy producers may want more females for replacing cows or for expansion of their herds. The sex of mammals is determined by the sex chromosomes or X and Y chromosomes. Animals with two X chromosomes develop into females; animals with an X and a Y chromosome develop into males. Thus, the detection of X and Y chromosomes on sperm has been the focus of research to predetermine the sex of domestic animals. In one process, sperm is pretreated with a dye that fluoresces when exposed to short wavelength light. The fluorescence is brighter from a sperm bearing X chromosomes, which contain about 4 per cent more DNA than the Y chromosome. A stream of dyed sperm is passed through a flow cytometer, a computer determines the degree of fluorescence and the sperm is separated into different containers. The success rate can be as high as 40 per cent. When sexed sperm has been used on a commercial basis, though, it has had limited success. The conception rate using sexed sperm is lower in cows, though it is higher in primiparous cows. In addition, sperm are killed in the typing process and the rate of sexing the sperm is slower than desired. While economical processing of sperm is just getting started, it is expected to become another useful tool in animal agriculture.

BOX 3.3

NEW TECHNOLOGIES IN ANIMAL BREEDING

Swine breeders and livestock breeders in general, are continuously challenged by the need to evaluate new developments and new technologies; breeding is a business and just like any other business, only breeding organizations that stay up-to-date with new developments, can recognize developments and innovations that can aid their business and able to implement such developments in an effective and rapid manner will be successful in tomorrow's increasingly competitive market for supplying superior germplasm. Examples of important technologies that have impacted swine breeding programs over the past decade are the selection index, Best Linear Unbiased Prediction (BLUP) of breeding values, the halothane test and Ryanodine Receptor test, as well as artificial insemination and ultra-sound technology. With advances in reproductive and molecular genetic technology, the number of new developments that have the potential to impact swine breeding programs is increasing rapidly.

Role of Molecular Genetics

To date, most genetic progress for quantitative traits in livestock has been made by selection on phenotype or on estimated breeding values (EBV) derived from phenotype, without knowledge of the number of genes that affect the trait or the effects of each gene. In this quantitative genetic approach to genetic improvement, the genetic architecture of traits has essentially been treated as a black box. Despite this, the substantial rate of improvement that has been and continues to be achieved in commercial populations is clear evidence of the power of these approaches. However, genetic progress may be further enhanced if we could gain insight into the black box of quantitative traits. Molecular genetics allows for the study the genetic make-up of individuals at the DNA level and may provide the tools to make those opportunities a reality, either by direct selection on genes that affect traits of interest, major genes or quantitative trait loci (QTL) - or through selection on genetic markers linked to QTL. The main reasons why molecular genetic information can result in greater genetic gain than phenotypic information are:

a. Assuming no genotyping errors, molecular genetic information is not affected by environmental effects and has heritability equal to 1.

b. Molecular genetic information can be available at an early age, in principle at the embryo stage, thereby allowing early selection and reduction of generation intervals.

c. Molecular genetic information can be obtained on all selection candidates, which is especially beneficial for sex-limited traits, traits that are expensive or difficult to record or traits that require slaughter of the animal (carcass traits).

The eventual application of molecular genetics in breeding programs depends on developments in the following four key areas:

(i) *Molecular genetics*: identification and mapping of genes and genetic polymorphisms

(ii) *QTL detection*: detection and estimation of associations of identified genes and genetic markers with economic traits

(iii) *Genetic evaluation*: integration of phenotypic and genotypic data in statistical methods to estimate breeding values of individual animals in a breeding population

(iv) *Marker-assisted selection*: development of breeding strategies and programs for the use of molecular genetic information in selection and mating programs.

Molecular Genetics: Through advances in molecular genetic technologies, the number of genes that has been mapped in the pig and other livestock species has increased exponentially during the past decade. The majority of mapped genes are so-called anonymous marker genes. These genes are not directly responsible for differences in economic traits but they may be linked to QTL. As such, they can be used to find QTL and to select for QTL through marker-assisted selection.

QTL Detection: Two approaches have been used to identify genes affecting traits of interest: the candidate gene approach and the genome scan approach. In the candidate gene approach, knowledge from species that are rich in genome information *e.g.* human, mouse and/or knowledge of the physiological basis of traits is used to identify genes that are thought to play a role in physiological mechanisms underlying economic traits. Using this information, candidate genes are identified in the species of interest and polymorphisms in the coding, but usually non-coding, regions of the gene are detected. Associations of these polymorphisms with the trait of interest are then identified using statistical analysis of phenotypic records of a sample of individuals from the population of interest. Using this approach, several genes with major effect have been identified, a prime example being the estrogen receptor gene (ESR) affecting litter size in pigs. The genome scan approach to QTL detection uses anonymous genetic markers spread over the genome to identify QTL. Unless marker density is high, these studies cannot rely on population-wide linkage disequilibrium between markers and QTL. Instead, they rely on the linkage disequilibrium that exists within families in outbred populations or that is created in crosses between breeds or lines. Using statistical methods QTL can be identified and their position and effect estimated by associating marker data to phenotypic records. The precision of estimates of QTL position that can be obtained from these approaches is limited and large population sizes are needed. Although the candidate gene and the genome scan approach are often viewed as alternate approaches for identifying genes of interest, it is clear that they can be complementary, with a genome scan identifying regions of the genome that harbor potential QTL, followed by further investigation of genes known to be located in that region using the candidate gene approach.

Use of Gene Marker Information in Genetic Evaluation: Although candidate gene and QTL mapping experiments can result in identification of genes of interest, the use of these genes in genetic improvement programs requires estimation of the effects of these genes in commercial breeding populations. In particular with the use of anonymous markers, marker and QTL effects must be estimated and re-estimated on a within-family basis. This requires routine systems for DNA collection and marker genotyping. Even when the actual gene has been identified, there will be a need to re-estimate gene effects on a regular basis to improve accuracy and to guard against unfavorable associations with other traits and against interactions with the background genome or environment.

Use of Gene or Marker Information in Within-Breed Selection: Once a QTL or a marker closely linked to it has been identified, the important question that remains is how to use this information in selection. In this regard it is important to recognize that, although an identified QTL provides (accurate) information on the animal's genetic value for one of the genes that affect the trait, there are many other genes that affect performance. An individual's phenotypic performance can be used to estimate an animal's breeding value for the collective effect of all other genes, like animal breeders have always used phenotypic data. Although the estimate of this polygenic breeding value may not be as accurate as the estimate of the breeding value for the QTL, maximum genetic progress will be made by using both estimates, rather than basing selection on only one of them. Then question becomes how we can best combine the effect of the QTL with the EBV for the polygenes into a selection criterion.

For selection on a known QTL, the following strategies can be distinguished:

  (i) Two-stage selection, with selection on the QTL in the first stage, followed by selection on polygenic EBV among selected animals with the poorest QTL genotype.

  (ii) Standard QTL index selection, with selection on $I = g + EBV$, where g is the breeding value for the QTL and EBV refers to the polygenic EBV.

(iii) Although the index in strategy provides the best estimate of the animal's total breeding value, several studies have shown that selection on this index may not maximize response to selection over multiple generations.

(iv) Optimal QTL index selection, with selection on I = b g + EBV, where b is an index weight on the QTL breeding value, which can be optimized following procedures outlined by Dekkers and van Arendonk (1998), with the aim to maximize cumulative response after a given number of generations.

With standard QTL index selection, the frequency of ESR also increased rapidly, with fixation in generation 4. For the optimal selection strategies, ESR also reached near fixation by the end of the planning horizon (2, 3, 4, 5 or 10 generations) but the increase in gene frequency was almost linear. This in contrast to standard QTL index selection, which resulted in a very rapid increase in frequency in the first two generations, followed by much smaller increases to reach fixation. Thus, optimal selection resulted in a much more balanced increase in gene frequency than standard index selection and it achieved that by reducing the index weight on the QTL (b<1). Standard index selection was superior to phenotypic BLUP selection for the first 5 generations. After 6 generations, cumulative response with selection ignoring ESR was greater than response from standard index selection due to the reduced selection emphasis on other genes that affect litter size when selection emphasis is placed on the QTL. Standard index selection was, however, superior to two-stage QTL selection for all generations. The reason for this is that two-stage selection on ESR allowed selection of individuals with inferior polygenic EBV which, although they had the favorable ESR genotype, did not have superior overall breeding values for litter size because of their inferior polygenic EBV. Index selection results in a balance between selection on ESR and polygenic EBV, which allows selection of individuals with the unfavorable ESR genotype if the superiority of their polygenic EBV compensates for the unfavorable ESR genotype. This result clearly demonstrates the importance of balancing selection on a QTL with selection on polygenic EBV. An even better balance between the QTL and polygenic EBV is achieved by the optimal selection strategies. Although the optimal strategies resulted in less response in initial generations than standard index selection, responses were 3 to 5% greater in the final generation of the respective planning horizons. Optimal selection over 10 generations also resulted in slightly greater response to selection than phenotypic BLUP selection.

Integrating Molecular and Reproductive Technologies: The main challenges for the use of molecular genetic information in selection is that it reduces selection on polygenes and, unless selection on the QTL is properly balanced against lost response in polygenes, QTL selection can be detrimental in the long-term and suboptimal in the short term. QTL selection is incorporated into traditional selection stages, where QTL selection competes with polygenic selection. The most effective manner to capitalize on QTL information is by incorporating it at stages, where selection is not possible previously and prior to availability of phenotypic information.

Use of Molecular Information in Crossbreeding Programmes: Although breeding programs primarily rely on selection within purebred populations, in many cases the objective is to improve crossbred performance. This raises important additional questions on how to incorporate molecular genetic information in selection programs within pure breeds that contribute to crossbreeding programs, in particular for QTL that exhibit non-additive effects. The QTL may not be the same for sire and dam breeds and that there will be a need to simultaneously optimize selection on identified QTL within both breeds in order to maximize both the rate of improvement within the pure breeds and the level of performance in the crossbreds. The design of selection criteria and strategies will be further complicated when multiple QTL are available, each with their own mode of action and epistatic interactions.

Possible directions for Selection within Sire and Dam breed (2-way cross on QTL)

Mode of geneaction at QTL	Direction for QTL selection on favorable allele in	
	Sire breed	*Dam breed*
Additive	Increase	Increase
Partial dominance	Increase	Increase but at slower rate
Negative dominance	Increase	Increase
Over dominance	Increase	Decrease

3.6 Aquaculture

3.6.1 Prefixture

Aquaculture on the other hand is a branch of animal husbandry involving raising or breeding of aquatic living things either plants *e.g.* seaweed, plankton and algae or animals *e.g.* fin-fish, shell-fish, oyster shell, clams, cockles, shrimps, crayfish, periwinkles, turtles in a controlled water body to marketable size. Aquaculture has been around for centuries in small, rural settings, but it has exploded worldwide in the past few decades into a commercial activity for the global market. Today, farmed fish make up more than one-fourth of the fish we eat and fish production from the aquaculture industry is an attractive means to relieve the stress on the ocean's fisheries. Unfortunately, if it is mismanaged or done without consideration for its external impacts, aquaculture also has the potential to damage the environment and to contribute to the collapse of global fisheries. The heterogeneity of aquaculture systems, in size, location and contribution to the local economy, makes it difficult to characterize the industry as good or bad. Each type of aquaculture has legitimate benefits as well as serious costs and because aquaculture products are traded on an international market, there is a global responsibility to promote sustainable aquaculture. For effective aquaculture, one has to gain familiarity and control water quality to enhance its biological productivity; one has to understand fish nutrition so as to be able to formulate nutritionally balanced fish diet; one has to delve deep into fish genetics so as to be able to evolve new varieties and strains which bestow commercial advantages to the product in terms of superior growth rate, nutritive value, bonelessness, taste, odour etc. one has to prevent incidence of fish infections and diseases through prophylatics and therapeutics. Aquaculture also known as fish or shellfish farming refers to the breeding, rearing and harvesting of plants and animals in all types of water environments including ponds, rivers, lakes and the ocean. Researchers and aquaculture producers are farming all kinds of freshwater and marine species of fish, shellfish and plants. Aquaculture produces food fish, sport fish, bait fish ornamental fish, crustaceans, mollusks, algae, sea vegetables and fish eggs. Aquaculture includes the production of seafood from hatchery fish and shellfish which are grown to market size in ponds, tanks, cages or raceways. Stock restoration or enhancement is a form of aquaculture in which hatchery fish and shellfish are released into the wild to rebuild wild populations or coastal habitats such as oyster reefs. Aquaculture also includes the production of ornamental fish for the aquarium trade and growing plant species used in a range of food, pharmaceutical, nutritional and biotechnology products.

Branches of Aquaculture

Fish farming: Fish farming is the primary form of aquaculture. Fish farming is cultivation of fish for commercial purposes in man-made tanks and other enclosures. The most common types of farmed fish are catfish, tilapia, salmon, carp, cod and trout. With the increase in over-fishing and the demand on wild fisheries, the fish-farming industry has grown in order to meet the demand for fish products.

Mariculture: Mariculture is the branch of aquaculture that cultivates marine organisms either in the open ocean, an enclosed portion of the ocean or tanks or ponds filled with seawater. Finfish such as flounder and whiting, shellfish like prawns and oysters and sea plants like kelp and seaweed are cultured in saltwater. Mariculture products are also used for cosmetics, jewelry such as cultured pearls and fish meal.

Algaculture: Algaculture is the type of aquaculture that cultivates algae. Most algae harvested are either microalgae (phytoplankton, microphytes or planktonic algae) or macroalgae, commonly known as seaweed. Although macroalgae is used for a variety of commercial purposes, its size and cultivation needs make it hard to grow. Microalgae are easier to harvest on a large scale. To successfully harvest algae, an algae farm needs the right temperature range, light source and nutritional characteristics in the water source. Algae are most commonly cultivated in open-pond systems, such as ponds, pools and lakes. However, these systems do not allow for control of light or temperature. Yet, they are the most popular type of pond system, since they are cheaper to build and produce the highest yield of algae. On the other hand, closed-pond systems remedy some of the problems with the open-pond systems. Closed-pond systems are pools or ponds that are covered. Even though the closed-pond system allows more species to grow, it tends to be smaller in scale, so it produces a smaller crop. One variation of the closed-pond system is the photobioreactor, a system that incorporates a light source. For example, placing a greenhouse cover over a pond or pool creates a photobioreactor. Although nutrients must be brought into this type of system, it can produce high-yield crops. In fact, it can even produce excess crops, which could end up destroying the system. However, with proper care, photobioreactor systems produce successful results.

Integrated multitrophic aquaculture: Integrated multitrophic aquaculture (IMTA) is a more advanced system of aquaculture. In a multitrophic system, different species with various nutritional needs are combined into one system. IMTA uses the waste products of one species as feed or fertilizer for another species. For example, seaweed grows from the phosphorus and ammonia that fish and shrimp excrete. Shellfish feed on the solids that fish and shrimp produce. Although there are many different types and degrees of IMTA, the main principle behind the system is balance.

3.6.2 History of Aquaculture

In the historical past, aquaculture remained multilocational and isolated, each location having evolved its own pattern, until in recent times, when with the development of fast means of communication and travel bridging distances in progressively decreasing time, species are being cultured adopting a measure of standardised practices and sites when they are most suited. The evidence that Egyptians were probably the first in the world to culture fish as far back as 2500 B.C. come from pictorial engravings of an ancient Egyptian tomb showing tilapia being fished out from an artificial pond. The Romans are believed to have reared fish in circular ponds divided into breeding areas. Culture of Chinese carps was sidespread in China in 2000 B.C. Writings in India made in 300 B.C. suggest means of rendering fish poisonous in the Indian sub-continent in times of war. This implies that fish culture prevailed in some Indian reservoirs. Some historical documents compiled in 1127 A.D. describe methods of fattening fish in ponds in India. Culture of Gangetic carps in Bengal in the Indian Sub-continent is of historical origin. The Chinese carried with them their traditional knowledge of carp culture to the countries they emigrated like Malaysia, Taiwan, Indonesia, Thailand, Cambodia, Vietnam etc. In the Philippines, fish culture has been done in brackishwater ponds for centuries. Eel culture in Japan is also very old. In Central and occidental Europe, common carp culture developed along with monasteries in the Middle Ages. Later, with the development of pond fertilization and artificial feeding, carp culture got a new lease of life especially in Central and Oriental Europe. Simultaneously in Europe, salmonid culture began, fillip having been provided by salmon breeding and rearing techniques which were developed by them. Pollution in the aftermath of industrialisation and hydro-electric development, led to restocking of open waters in Europe. This gave a new texture to development of aquaculture in Europe. In North America, fish culture has developed from the turn of the century emphasis having been laid on trout for stocking in coldwater and black bass in warm waters. Except for the referred culture of tilapia in Egypt, the origin of fish culture in Africa is recent. It was only at the end of II world war that efforts were made to introduce and develop fish cultivation. The prize species in Africa is tilapia, which, in recent years, has been extensively transplanted into many warm countries almost round the equator. Tilapia has been referred to as the wonder fish of Africa and several attempts to popularize tilapia culture in various African countries did not achieve so much success as expected. In some countries mixed culture of tilapia and catfish (*Clarias gariepinus*) have achieved some success lately; aquaculture prospects and priorities for Africa are now subject to a fresh scrutiny in attempts to make it a successful venture, especially in view of its role in rural development. Fish culture is only beginning in Latin America and most of the Middle-East. In Israel, it has made phenominal progress. Since World War II, four factors have contributed to rapid development of aquaculture. These are:

a.   Facilities of fish transport by modern forms of communication bridging distances by quick transport.

b.   Use of polythene bags and fish transported therein under oxygen with addition, when necessary, of transquilizer to water.

c.   Artificial propagation of farmed fish by hypophysation and its application to difficult-to-breed fish *e.g.* Chinese and Indian carps and development of hatching techniques to rear eggs and larvae.

d.   Availability of feed concentrates and their distribution in pellet form.

The fish which have figured most in inter-regional transplantation are rainbow trout, carp, certain species of tilapia (*T. mossambica* and *T. nilotica*) and Chinese carps (*Ctenopharyngodon idella* and *Hypophthalmichthys mollitrix*). Fish culture using some standard methods has got itself extended to many parts of the world. Fish breeding, artificial fertilization and pellet feeding, which at one time were applied to selected species, are now made applicable to many cultured species and, as time advances, more and more species are falling in line, though details vary. With further research in aquaculture, especially on production of fish seed and fish feed technologies, aquaculture in heading towards a quantum jump in years to come. Despite the fact that fish culture is an age-old practice in some regions of the world, it is relatively new as a significant industry in most countries. Aquaculture is considered to be a labour-intensive, but a high-risk bio-industry. An important characteristic feature of aquaculture is that, depending on its intensification, it can be organized as systems which may be termed as:

(a)   **Extensive :** Adoption of traditional techniques of aquaculture *e.g.* dependence on natural productivity and little control over the stocks.

(b)   **Intensive :** Adoption of full complement of culture techniques including scientific pond design, fertilization, supplemental feeding or only feeding without fertilization; full measure of stock manipulation, disease control, scientific harvesting, high level inputs and high rate of production.

(c)   **Semi-intensive :** Adoption of mid-level technology, partial dependence on natural productivity, fertilization, supplementary feeding, with stock manipulation, medium level inputs and medium rate of production.

Another characteristic of aquaculture is that it can be organized on the basis of:

a.   Small scale rural aquaculture (even as one-family-unit).

b.   Large-scale vertically integrated aquaculture (VIA) which is defined as a centrally mamaged comprehensive system such that all components from input of energy to final level of produce in the market are coordinated and kept in harmony.

3.6.3 Types of Aquaculture

Aquaculture is most commonly known for the production of food organisms such as fish, prawns and shellfish. However aquaculture is also used in producing aquatic organisms for bait, aquaria, fee-fishing, lake stockings, biological supply houses, chemicals and pharmaceuticals. Aquaculture species can be produced in marine or freshwater environments using various production systems. Some systems, such as those containing animals in ponds, tanks, aquaria or raceways, can incorporate water-recirculating systems that reduce the reliance on large quantities of water to maintain water quality and the health of cultured organisms. As habitats of aquaculture, there are three categories of waters, *viz.* fresh, salt and brackish. Fresh waters, generally abounding in the inland areas of a country and the salt water of the seas and oceans are characterized by a wide difference in their salinities ranging from nil in the former to nearly 35 ppt (parts per trillion) in the latter.

The difference in salinity within each category of water, fresh and sea is restricted to rather narrow limits. The salt content of fresh and sea water exercises a very selective influence on the fauna and flora that live in each type of water. In as far as finfish and shellfish are concerned, the normal residents of each type of water are said to be stenohaline *i.e.* they can withstand only a narrow variation in the salinities of their surrounding medium. A carp is an example of stenohaline freshwater fish and a sardine or a mackerel may be cited as examples of stenohaline saltwater fish. Brackish water normally naturally occurs in estuaries, deltas of rivers, lagoons and backwaters, which everywhere in the world are under tidal regime. In such habitats the salinity of the water fluctuates widely between negligible to 35 ppt, depending on the phase of the tide and volume of fresh water discharged through the river into the sea. The finfish and shellfish that inhabit brackish waters are invariably euryhaline *i.e.* they form a group of organisms which physiologically withstands wide changes in salinity of the surrounding medium. Stenohaline organisms are devoid of physiological mechanisms to tolerate wide changes of salinity. So, a special type of fauna inhabits the estuarine habitat beyond the sea-end of which live the stenohaline and saltwater forms.

Examples of euryhaline fish are a mullet (*Mugil cephalus*) and mud-skipper, *Periophthalmus* and those of crustaceans are several species of penaeids *e.g. Penaeus monodon* and crab *e.g. Scylla serrata*. The capacity of the residents of an estuary to tolerate a wide range of salinity that prevails there is by virtue of a dynamic physiological process of osmoregulation in which the gills, the kidneys, the skin and the buccal cavity lining play significant roles. *Periophthalmus koelereuteri*, *Penaeus notialis* and the crab, *Callinectes* are corresponding species which we encounter in ARAC fish farm at Buguma.

There are finfish and shellfish which spend different phases of their lives in sea, estuaries and freshwater streams. These forms transcend the salinity barrier by their osmoregulation. Such animals are either anadromous or katadromous. Anadromous fish, as exemplified by salmon or Acipencer or shad, are those that bread naturally in freshwater streams but spend the middle years of their lives in the sea. Katadromous forms, as exemplified by the eel, display the opposite kind of life cycle. These animals breed in the sea and spend the middle years of their lives in fresh water streams.

There are forms which restrict their migration between fresh water sections of the river and the estuary. Several species of palaeomonid prawns (_Macrobrachium rosenbergi; M. vollenhovenii_) are examples of shellfish which undergo such a life cycle. These forms breed in estuaries but spend the mid-years of their live in fresh waters. Then, there are forms which migrate back and forth between the estuary or a lagoon and the sea in different phases of their lives. A mullet _e.g. Mugil cephalus_ or a shrimp _e.g. Penaeus mododon, P. notialis_ are examples of finfish and shellfish which show such a pattern of migration. These forms breed in the sea but spend part of their juvenile and adult lives in the estuary where they form a sizeable fishery. Apart from salinity of the water, its temperature exercises a selective influence on fish that thrive there warmwater fish as contrasted with temperate or coldwater fish. Even in tropical countries, a river may have and usually does have a coldwater section in its upper reaches and a warmwater section in its middle and lower reaches. In temperate countries and in the upper reaches of tropical countries at high altitudes, coldwater fish _e.g._ trout, loach etc. live. Then warm waters have their distinctive fish fauna _e.g._ scores of species of carps and catfishes and several species of murrels etc. Notwithstanding the fact that the capacity of water to dissolved oxygen (DO) is negatively correlated with temperature, the oxygen content of water at a given temperature can vary a great deal depending on turbulance, photosynthesis and Biochemical Oolygen Demand. DO of water exercises a selective influence on quality of fish life. In water of low oxygen content, air-breathing fish thrive best _e.g._ Clarias, snakeheads etc. Fish that are used to living in well-oxygenated water _e.g._ trout, do not thrive in waters of low oxygen content.

Notwithstanding differences in the physioco-chemical characteristics of its habitats (viz. fresh water, brackish water and sea water) aquaculture systems are of several kinds. Most of the systems are highly variable in magnitude and intensity ranging to serve as one-family units or large scale commercial enterprises. The different kinds of aquaculture are:

i.   Static water ponds.

ii.   Running water culture.

iii.   Culture in re-circulating systems: in reconditioned water and in closed systems.

iv.   Culture in rice fields.

v.   Aquaculture in raceways, cages pens and enclosures

vi.   Finfish-culture cum livestock rearing.

vii.   Hanging, on-bottom and stick methods of oyster culture.

The snake head _Ophiocephalus obscurus_ is the common form in West Africa. Based on the number of species that are cultured in a system aquaculture may be classified into two Monoculture and Polyculture.

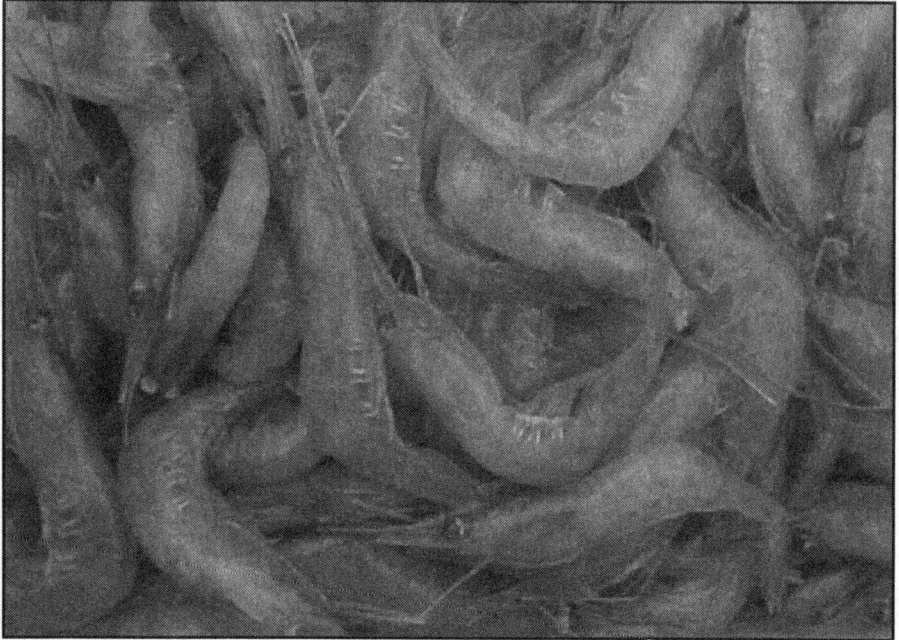

Figure 3.6: Prawn

Almost 400 species are reared in the aquatic environment with the aim of harvesting animal or plant protein. Basically aquaculture grouped into category marine aquaculture and freshwater aquaculture.

(a) *Marine aquaculture:* Also known as Mariculture, it is the branch of aquaculture that cultivates marine organisms either in the open ocean, an enclosed portion of the ocean or tanks or ponds filled with seawater. Finfish like flounder and whiting, shellfish like prawns and oysters and sea plants like kelp and seaweed are cultured in saltwater. Mariculture products are also used for cosmetics, jewelry such as cultured pearls and fish meal.

    i.   **Sea ranching:** Sea ranching is a culture method whereby juvenile animals, generally produced in hatcheries but could also be wild-caught, are introduced into the natural environment and allowed to grow without containment structures. The environment provides the animals with everything they need and no additional feed is required. Sea ranching of sea cucumbers and scallops, where hatchery produced juveniles are placed on the sea bed and allowed to grow to marketable size. Juvenile scallops and sea cucumbers are produced in hatcheries. Scallop and sea cucumber ranching is only viable if the culture area is closed to commercial trawl fishing while the animals grow and if the animals remain in the specified culture area until harvest. Scallops are normally grown in deep water and harvested using trawl boats. Sea cucumbers are normally harvested by hand either by diving or hand harvesting at low tide in shallow water.

ii. Surface lines: Surface line culture is generally used to grow shellfish - such as pearl oysters, scallops and mussels, tunicates, seaweeds and sponges in panel-style baskets, small cages *e.g.* lantern nets, pearl nets or on ropes that are suspended below floating surface lines. Each species has a well established method for growing. Line cultures systems comprise a series of parallel ropes buoyed at the surface with floats and are anchored to the substrate at each end. Rows of lines and floats are normally visible on the surface but are usually coloured so as to blend into the surroundings to minimize impacts on visual amenity. The sea bed remains free of obstacles and natural processes can take place beneath the farm. Environmental impact from line culture is reduced through correct location and adequate spacing of lines to minimize benthic (bottom) disturbance. Line aquaculture is also designed to minimize negative impacts to fauna. Lines are kept very taut and are well spaced to reduce risk of entanglement. Rack and line aquaculture is a collective term that involves growing primarily filter-feeding animals, such as edible oysters, pearl oysters and sponges, on structures placed in the water column, but without any addition of feed. Cultured species obtain their food by filtering naturally occurring phytoplankton and organic matter that is suspended in the water column. Structures used to support these animals in the water column include surface lines, subsurface lines and various designs of intertidal racks.

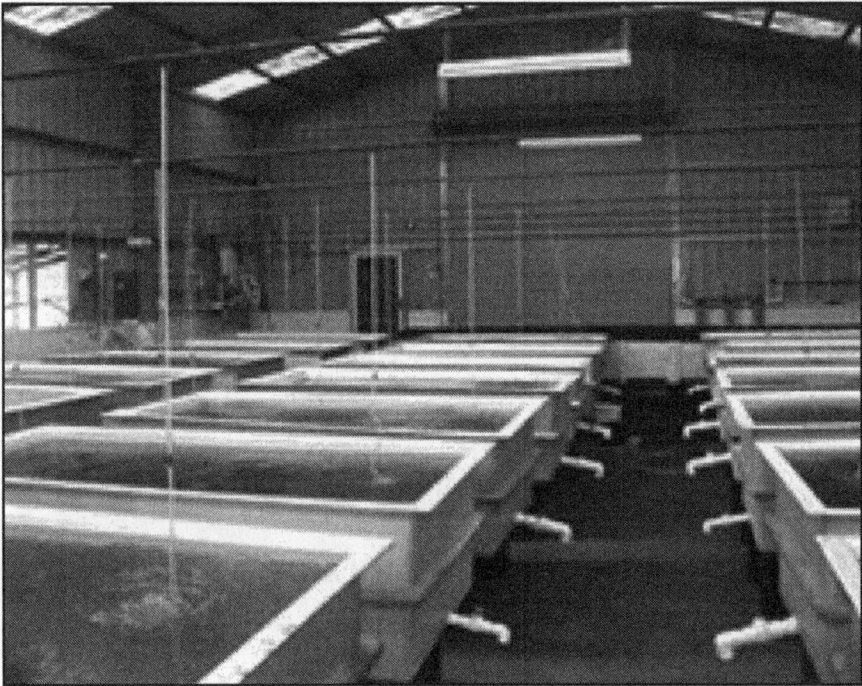

Figure 3.7: Tanks holding juvenile scallops or sea cucumbers Juvenile

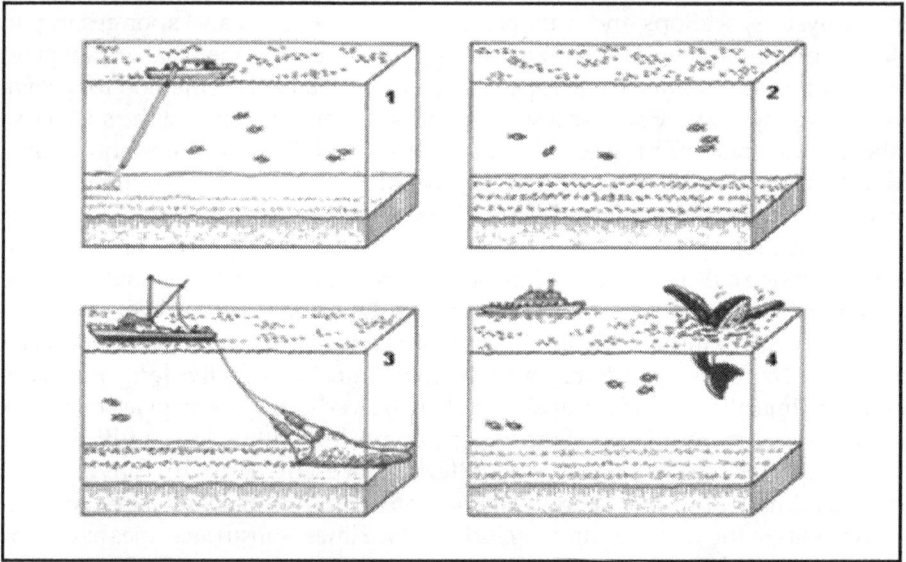

Figure 3.8: Sea Ranching: 1. Spat or juveniles are placed on the sea bed, usually in the form of a slurry delivered by a length of pipe or by hand. Most of time there is no activity. 2. Spat or juveniles feed naturally with no input from the farmer. 3. Some aquaculture product, such as scallops, is harvested by trawling. Others, such as sea cucumbers, are harvested by hand. 4. The timing of harvesting activities can be scheduled to reduce conflict with other commercial activities. Trawling can be undertaken at different times to other commercial activities so there is no overlap.

iii. Subsurface lines: Subsurface line culture, used for culturing pearl oysters or scallops, is similar to surface line culture except the horizontal mainlines and suspended culture panels are positioned well below the surface. Benefits of this type of configuration are reduced agitation of the cultured animals from wave action and allowing vessels to motor freely over the top of the farm. As the lines and supporting floats are submerged, the only structures visible on the surface are site corner markers and optional intermittent buoys marking the location of submerged lines and anchors. The culture panels are held off the bottom by a series of floats along the mainline. As with surface line culture, lines are maintained in a taut condition and well-spaced to allow for wildlife movements and to reduce risk of entanglement. Wide spacing of lines also allows for good flushing, good light penetration to the seabed and natural processes can take place beneath the lines.

iv. Racks: Rack culture in Australia is generally used to grow edible oysters such as the Sydney rock oyster, native flat oyster and Pacific oyster. Each species has a well-established method for growing. Oysters are suspended from small platform structures or post-and-line structures that are placed in the intertidal zone. Oyster racks are usually a combination of wood and plastic and are about the width of a walkway. The industry standard in Australia is an adjustable system where oysters are enclosed in plastic mesh bags that are hung from lines suspended between wooden or plastic posts. The benefits of an adjustable longline system lies with the ability to raise and lower the oyster bags on the line, thereby giving the oyster farmer a management technique to control shell growth, condition and cleaning.

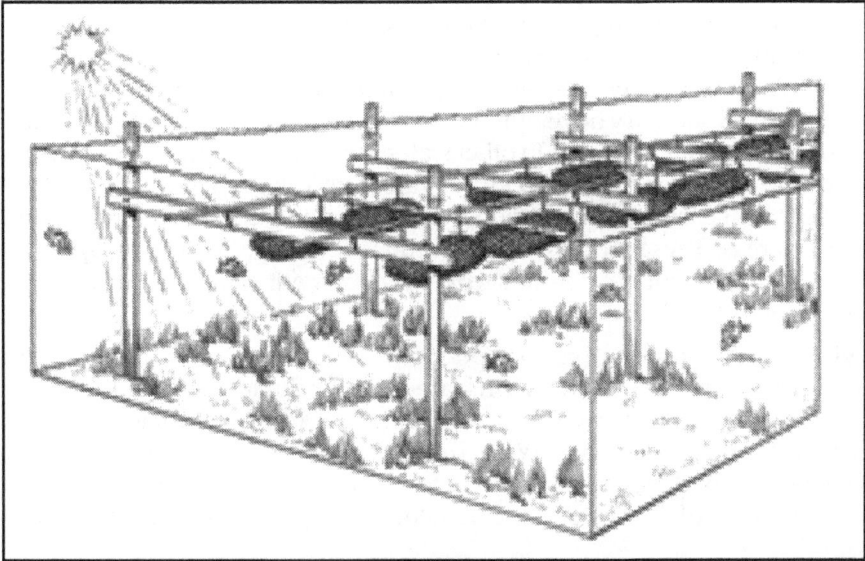

Figure 3.9: Adequate clearance and spacing of the oyster bags allows for good flushing, good light penetration and for natural processes to take place beneath the racks

Other systems are in use including growing oysters on sticks or trays. There is minimal environmental impact from rack culture, but correct location is important to minimize benthic (bottom) disturbance. Oyster bags are suspended high in the intertidal water column so natural processes can take place beneath. Because the structures are usually fairly narrow and well-spaced, light is allowed to penetrate and impacts to sea grass or other benthic plants and animals can be negligible.

v. Sea cages: Sea cages are a common production technology used for intensive marine aquaculture of fin fish. The type, size and design of cages are dependent upon a number of factors including the culture species, site conditions and environmental features.

Species grown in sea cage systems include:

- Atlantic salmon,
- Trout,
- Southern bluefin tuna,
- Cobia,
- Mulloway,
- Barramundi,
- Snapper.

There is also potential to culture other species in cage systems, such as coral trout, barramundi cod and lobster. Cage nets can be made of different materials but nylon mesh is most commonly used. However, alternatives include semi-rigid PVC coated polyester, brass and galvanized steel netting which have been shown to be more resistant to biofouling and prevent predation from sharks and seals. Sea cage fin fish culture has demonstrated significant economic benefits in other Australian states and internationally. Intensive cage aquaculture is a demonstrated driver of regional primary industry development worldwide and is one of the most successful and profitable farming systems. In other states fish farming industries have expanded rapidly, based on financial and technical innovation applied to sea cage culture that have contributed significant regional economic and social advantages to their respective areas. These industries have capitalised on value-adding opportunities and have made a major contribution to the development of their respective regions in a relatively short period.

vi. Pond: Purpose-built earthen ponds, constructed on coastal lands or adjacent to the estuarine parts of river systems, are used for the intensive culture of marine prawns and fin fish. Saline water is pumped onto the farm where it is then gravity fed to a series of production ponds. Water drains from the ponds and enters a treatment pond whereby solid wastes settle out before water is discharged back to the sea. In some cases, some of this water is recirculated back through the farm system.

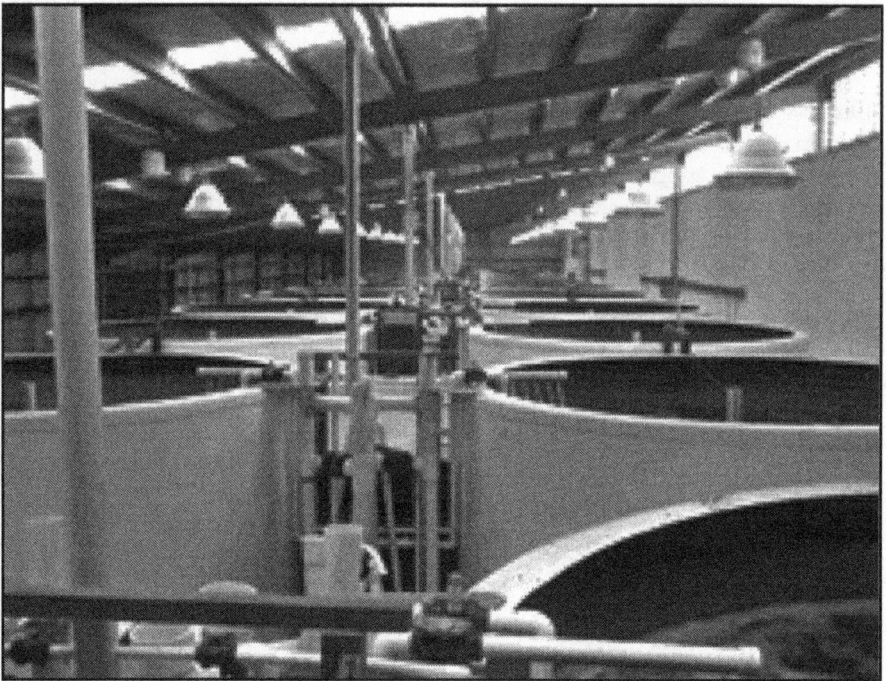

Figure 3.10: Indoor aquarium tank systems

The major species of prawn farmed in Australia is the black tiger prawn (*Penaeus monodon*), with the banana prawn (*P. merguiensis*) and kuruma prawn (*P. japonicus*) also under production. Barramundi are the primary species of fin fish farmed in saline ponds. Pond sizes are variable but most prawn ponds are about one hectare in size with barramundi ponds being about 0.4ha. Ponds are constructed with a gently sloping bottom to allow for draining and harvesting of the cultured product and to allow full draining for a dry-out period between crops. Pond depths vary from 1.5 to 2.0 meters.

Hatcheries: Marine hatcheries are involved in producing a diverse range of species for both the commercial aquaculture industry for on-growing as well as for the aquarium trade. Species produced in marine hatcheries include:

- Prawns,
- Pearl and edible oysters,
- Scallops,
- Barramundi cod,
- Cobia,
- Mangrove jack,
- Mullet,
- Aquarium fish,
- Seahorses,
- Corals,
- Sandfish.

Some growout aquaculture operations produce juveniles in their own hatchery facilities, while other growers rely on stock produced by independent hatcheries.

(b) Freshwater aquaculture

Freshwater aquaculture is the culture of aquatic species within and dependent on, the freshwater environment. The organisms are grown indoors in controlled conditions and temperature. Fish is a rich source of vitamins and fish oil is suggested by many physicians for the patients of aching bones. Due to increased production in aquaculture, the dietary requirements of people have also been taken care of. Fish contains a lot of essential minerals, proteins ad micro-nutrients that cannot be found in other kinds of meat all at once. Also fish has the lowest fat percentage as compared to other meats. Before aqua culturing, fish was very costly but now, as the production has increased, it has become very affordable and is within the budget of common person. In cold areas of the world, people prefer fish over other meats as it is easily available there. Freshwater aquaculture has also improved economies of many areas by providing new job opportunities. The fish produced there is mostly used by industries for processing which is then made available as canned food item. Due to stagnation in wild fish harvesting, many fishermen have moved to aquaculture farming and are earning more than before. Besides social benefits, aquaculture also has many environmental befits as well. The pressure on wild fish has decreased immensely which was a hot debate for many years that this must be done to save water life. Big species in water pray on small fish and by taking out fish from the sea, humans are endangering their existence. The older fishing methods were harmful for eco life of water. Some of the traditional techniques resulted in the death of untargeted species also and made the water unsafe for growth of species. Aquaculture is eco safe farming technique that does not harm the eco system. The controlled environment ensures that the environment remains pollution free.

Recirculation systems: Recirculating aquaculture systems are indoor, tank-based systems in which fish are grown at high density under controlled environmental conditions. Generally, farmers adopt a more intensive approach (higher densities and more rigorous management) than other aquaculture production systems. Recirculating aquaculture systems can be used where suitable land or water is limited or where environmental conditions are not ideal for the species being cultured. This type of aquaculture production system can be used in marine environments; however, it is more commonly used in freshwater environments. There is a large cost involved in setting up and running a recirculation system and you will need to consider a number of factors in designing the system that will fit the needs.

Characteristics of recirculating aquaculture systems

Water quality: The water in the system is recirculated through tanks and a series of water treatments to remove waste products. Unless the water is treated, fish will stress, resulting in retarded growth, increased pre-disposition to disease and finally death.

Tanks: Production tanks vary in size and shape. Smooth, round tanks with sloping bottoms are useful as solids can be concentrated and subsequently removed from a centre drain. This design facilitates thorough cleaning and ensures aeration is evenly distributed.

Filters: In simple recirculation systems, water may be treated by two processes: mechanical filtration to remove solids such as faecal matter, uneaten feeds, etc. and biological filtration to remove dissolved toxic wastes.

Other system components: Depending on the location and the species of planning on farming, one should consider including other components such as disinfection devices, foam fractionators or protein skimmers, dedicated aeration units and temperature control.

Support equipment and facilities: The access to water quality testing equipment, a purpose-built facility to accommodate bulk feeds and hygiene measures to limit the spread of disease are important consideration.

Suitable species for Recirculating systems

The design of recirculating aquaculture system will depend on the specific requirements of the species of culture. When designing a recirculating system, it is important to understand the impact of different factors on a species.

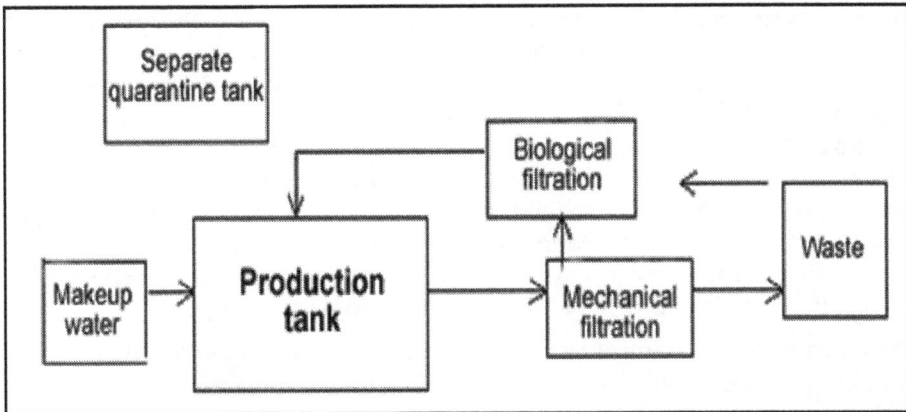

These factors include water quality requirements, stocking density and size of stock, feed types and disease. The costs of establishing and operating a viable recirculating aquaculture facility are usually much higher than most people anticipate.

BOX 3.4

DIFFERENT KIND OF AQUACULTURE

1. Pond Culture

Static freshwater ponds: Ordinary fresh water fish culture ponds are still-water ponds. They vary a great deal in water spread area and depth. Some are seasonal and some perennial. The ponds may be rainfed (sky ponds) and/or may have inlet and outlet systems. The water supply may be from a stream or a canal or from an underground source such as wells, tube-wells etc. The water retentivity of the ponds depends on soil composition of the pond bottom and subsoil water level. The natural biological productivity of such ponds depends on soil and water qualities. Homestead ponds are usually small and shallow. Commercial freshwater ponds have to have an assured water supply and inlet and drainage systems. In organized aquaculture, the carrying capacity of still-water ponds is enhanced by manuring and/or fertilizing and exercising water quality control. Fish are also fed from an extraneous source for obtaining fast growth. Science of freshwater pond fish-culture has made great strides in recent years and there is a fast advancing frontier of knowledge on every aspect of pond culture starting from farm designing and construction upto production of marketable fish of a wide variety of cultured fresh water species of finfish and shellfish. There is considerable competition with agriculture and other land-use agencies in this system of aquaculture and its success would, by and large, depend on comparative economics of land use. But much also depends on national policies on land use and the encouragement government gives to aquaculture as a means of producing fish protein.

Brackish water ponds: Not only are the species different from those cultured in freshwater ponds but the principle of operation of brackish water ponds is different from those of freshwater ponds. Here the pond or the farm is essentially located on a tidal creek or stream and there is a system of sluices to control the ingress and egress of water into and from the ponds. Examples are: Milkfish farms in Philippines, Taiwan, Indonesia etc. Brackish water fish farming is a fast growing science. Here also there is competition with other land use agencies, especially forestry, but the extent of competition with agriculture is relatively less because coastal land is generally not suitable for agriculture. The ARAC farm at Buguma is tidally fed and the salinity range is 5 – 21 ppt.

Mariculture: Mariculture is aquaculture in the saltwater of the sea. It may be in seas, bays, bayes, sounds etc. *e.g.* traditional mariculture in inshore and offshore waters by a large number of countries. Mariculture of finfish in cages is relatively recent. Though a new development, it has assumed considerable importance and has great potential *e.g.* mariculture of several species of salmonids; *Salmo salar*, *Oncorhynchus* sp; of yellow tail, *Seriola quinaueradiata*; of red seabream (*Pagrus major*) etc.

2. Running water culture

In Japan, at places where there is abundant supply of water, common carp is cultured in running water ponds. The most intensive common carp is cultured in running water ponds. A very high common carp production rate of 980 t/ha has been achieved at the Tanka Running water fish farm in Japan where there is plentiful supply of running water of high dissolved oxygen content and optimum range of temperature for feeding. Running water culture of common carp is done in a small way in Europe, Indonesia and Thailand.

3. Culture in Recirculatory systems

This system is comparable to running water culture system except that in the latter, water goes waste whereas here the same water is reused. In this system, water is filtered continuously and recirculated, often after aeration, to the fish pond. The filtering element is a biological filter comprising 3-4 cm diameter pebbles or honey-comb synthetic strips, designed to arrest faecal matter and to denitrify catabolic wastes through bacterial action. The Motokawa Fish farm in Japan is well known for carp production in recirculatory filtering ponds. This system has been tried experimentally for carp fry rearing at the Central Inland Fisheries Research Institute, Barrackpore (W.B.) India, with commendable results. There are several new developments in reusing water for fish culture, given in two volumes, by Tiews (1981). A recirculatory system is sometimes classified as a system of waste-water aquaculture and reducing biological oxygen demand (BOD) of the waste water. Several mechanisms of handling waste-water exist *viz.*

    i.   Pretreatment of waste water *e.g.* cascading through a series of ponds: air system etc.

ii.   Dilution of waste water,

iii. Pretreatment and dilution,

iv.   No treatment of waste water.

Advantages include increase in fish yields through increase in natural fish food, 5000 kg/ha at Aquaculture Research Station, Dor Israel from fluid cowshed manure; sewage fed system in Bengal and Tamil Nadu, India - 15,000 kg/ha/year and direct use of solid organic matter in natural waters by phytoplankton and zooplankton. Restraints in wastewater fish culture systems lie in:

i.   Do level in ponds,

ii.   Toxic material in wastewater,

iii. Tastes and odour in fish,

iv.   Parasites and diseases,

v.   Public health problems (Salmonella, Shigella) of other Enterbacteriacae,

vi.   Pond effluent standards,

vii. Public acceptance.

These lead to problems of fish pond management *i.e.* acquiring understanding of physioco-chemical dynamics of pond in relation to physiological requirements of cultured species. Polyculture system needs to be encouraged where productivity is based on natural foods *e.g.* ecological niche approach in the polyculture of Chinese and Indian carps in India.

Water reconditioning in aquaculture is necessary where there is inadequate water supply for the fish culture programme or where water quality requirements are such that reconditioning is indicated.

The different fish rearing systems using reconditioned water are:

i.   Simple flow-through (single pass) system *i.e.* ample water-supply of appropriate quality.

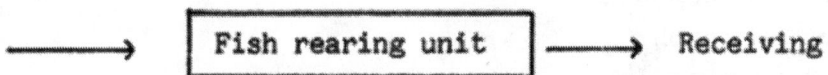

$$\longrightarrow \boxed{\textbf{Fish rearing unit}} \longrightarrow \textbf{Receiving}$$

i.   Single pass system with pre and post-treatment *i.e.* Water supply:

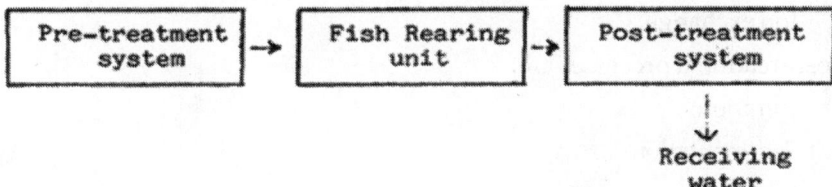

$$\boxed{\textbf{Pre-treatment system}} \rightarrow \boxed{\textbf{Fish Rearing unit}} \rightarrow \boxed{\textbf{Post-treatment system}}$$

$$\downarrow$$

$$\textbf{Receiving water}$$

iii. A system re-using water in fish rearing unit:

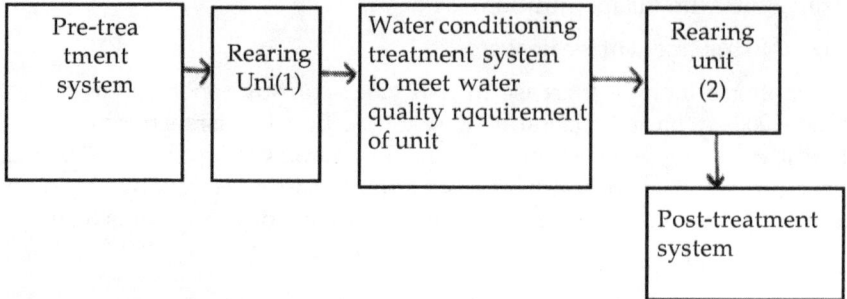

| Pre-trea tment system | → | Rearing Uni(1) | → | Water conditioning treatment system to meet water quality rqquirement of unit | → | Rearing unit (2) |

Rearing unit (2) → Post-treatment system

The pre-treatment processes used are:

i.   Sedimentation,

ii.   Screening,

iii. Shocking to kill aquatic life,

iv. Filtration,

v.   Sterilization,

vi. Aeration,

vii. Degassing (nitrogen, CO_2 removal),

viii. Heating or cooling if necessary,

ix. pH control.

The reconditioning processes are:

i.   Sedimentation,

ii.   Mechanical filtration,

iii. Biological filtration,

iv. Extended aeration,

v.   Activated sludge,

vi. pH control,

vii. Heating or cooling,

viii. Sterilization,

ix. De-gassing,

x.   Ion exchange.

Post-treatment processes are:

i.   Aeration,

ii.   Sedimentation,

iii. Filtration,

iv. Disinfection,

v. Activated sludge,

vi. Lagooning,

vii. Digestion or equivalent,

viii. Coagulation,

ix. Absorption taste or odour removal by activated carbon.

These systems are mostly applicable to sophisticated and intense aquaculture.

In Closed System: Fresh water model developed at Ahrenbury in Germany is a 50 m^3 in circuit for mirror carp, *Cyprinus carpio*, 6 m^3 in fish tanks and 44m^3 in purification unit. Temperature kept constant at 223°C and quantity of food (g of food/fish/day) has been kept equal. Rate of flow 25 m^3/hour; maximum carrying capacity, determined experimentally being 1.5t of fish and ratio of water volume to fish weight 30:1. Closed circuits have limited carrying capacity and when the capacity is exceeded, the system may break down. The highest production, an annual yield of 8.6t of carp is obtained using semi-monthly rather than monthly and 1.5 monthly stocking sequence, fish are harvested when 500 g in weight rather than 1000, 1500 or 2000 g and fed on fish having raw protein content of 36 per cent rather than 47 per cent. The cost of feeds is the main operating costs when using the system. The decrease in income is proportionately more rapid than decrease in production when the size of fish harvested increase and stocking sequence are prolonged.

4. Culture in Rice Fields

Culturing fish and growing rice together in the same paddy fields is an old practice in Asia and the Far East. Interest in producing rice and fish together had declined in recent years because of use of fish-toxic pesticides required to protect high yielding varieties (HYV) of rice introduced as part of green revolution in Asia. Now, newer HYV of rice strains are being developed with inbred resistance to insects and insect-transmitted diseases which decrease the need for pesticide protection or growing rice. Four trials conducted in Philippines on *Tilapia mosambica* and *Cyprinus carpio* stocking have resulted in standing crops of fish in paddy fields averaging 69-288 kg/ha at harvest time.

5. Aquaculture in Raceways: Cages, Pens and Enclosures

Marine aquaculture farms may be located at six possible sites *viz.* either on the shore with pumped sea-water supply, in the intertidal zone; in the sub-littoral zone or offshore with surface floating, mid-water floating or seabed cages. The first three are enclosures and the last three cages. The enclosures in Europe have by and large stemmed from those set up for yellow tail (*Seriola quinqueradiata*) farming in Japan of inter-tidal enclosure:

    a. Adoike near Takasu in Inland sea in Japan,

    b. Ardtoe in Great Britain. Since concrete seawalls or stone-pitched embankments are expensive, few intertidal enclosures are now built.

5.1 Rigid structures

A large number of rigid net enclosures have been built in Inland sea in Japan in recent years, but not all are successful: because of poor siting providing less circulation, others fouled by marine organisms which restrict circulation. More modern successful net enclosures have been positioned after hydrographic surveys to insure sufficient water exchange and research on building material. Most suitable galvanized chain-link and galvanized weldmesh, for example:

a.   Yellow tail 3.5 ha farm at Sakaide in Seto Inland Sea, Japan.

b.   Faery Isles, Lake sween, Scotland.

c.   Bamboo barricades for milkfish farming in Laguna de Bay, Philippines.

d.   Sub-littoral enclosures for salmon farming in Norway *e.g.* Flogoykjolpo (1.2 ha) and Volokjolpo (3.5 ha) near Movik, west of Bergen (Farming potential os salmon 1000 t.)

e.   Sub-littoral enclosure built in 1974 at Loch Moidart (40 m^3 capacity) (tidal range of 5m).

5.2 Flexible Structures

Buoyed fish net enclosure but resting on bottom *e.g.* 10 ha trial enclosure in Laguna de Bay, Philippines.

5.3 Floating Fish Cages

Most important development of the decade is aquafarming. Its merits lie on:

a.   can be used where seabed is unsuitable for shellfish.

b.   being off bottom, predators can be controlled more easily.

c.   can be towed out of danger if threatened by pollution.

5.4 Cages with Rigid Framework

a. 8m diameter 6m deep   Having galvanized steel collar, galvanized chain

b. 14m diameter 7m deep   link bag net for yellow-tail farming in Japan.

c. cages at Loch Ailort For Salmon farming in Scotland provided with

                             rigid 50 × 12m Salmon cage

(d) cages at Loch Moidart   collars and cat-walks for inspection of fish.

  (6 × 4 × 3. 1m)

5.4.1 Cages with Flexible Framework

a. 55m diameter and 25m deep chum salmon (*Oncorynchus keta*) in Lake Saroma at Hokkaido, Japan. Here netting material can be changed even when fish are in stock.

b. Midwater fish cage of the Hiketa Fishermen's Cooperative Association of Japan in Inland sea: 9m sq. × 8.25m deep with a buoyed feeding neck. These are grouped in 10– 12 cages. They can be raised in calm sea and lowered in rough sea.

c. Domsea Farm cage of Puget Sound, Washington U.S.A. 15.2 × 15.2 × 7.6m cage.

d. Floating fish cage of Kampuchea and Southern Vietnam.

5.4.2 Merits of Cage Culture

Advanced type of aquaculture having scores of advantages over pond culture.

a. 10-12 times higher yields than pond culture for comparable inputs and area.

b. Prevents loss of stock due to flooding.

c. No question of seepage and evaporation losses.

d. No need for water replacement.

e. No problem of pond excavation and dependence on soil characterics.

f. Avoids proximity of agricultural areas hence reduces hazards of pesticide contamination;

g. Can be conveniently located near urban markets avoiding the need for fish preservation and transportation.

h. Eliminates competition with agriculture and other land uses.

i. Affords easy control of fish reproduction in *Tilapia sp.*

j. Complete harvest of fish is effected.

k. Optimum utilization of artificial food.

l. Reduced fish handling.

m. Initial investment relatively small.

5.4.3 Limitations of Cage Culture

They are relatively few. They are:

a. Difficult to apply when water is rough,

b. High dependence on artificial feeding. High quality feed desirable especially in respect of protein, vitamins and minerals. Feed losses are possible through cage walls.

c. At times interferes with natural fish populations round cage.

d. Risk of theft is increased.

6. Monoculture

Monoculture in the culture of a single species of an organism in a culture system of any intensity, be it in any type of water, fresh, brackish or salt.

Fresh water

*   Common carp in East Germany.

*   Common carp in Japan.

*   *Tilapia nilotica* in several countries of Africa.

*   Rainbow trout (*Salmon gairdneri*) culture in several countries.

*   Channel catfish (*Ictalurus punctatus*) in U.S.A.

*   Catfish, *Clarias gariepinus* in Africa.

Brackish water

*   Milkfish, *Chanos chanos* in the Philippines.

*   Mullet culture in several countries.

Seawater

*   Yellowtail, *Seriola quinqueradiata* in Japan.

*   Kuruma shrimp, *Peneaus japonicas,*

*   Nori: *Porphyra* sp. in Japan

*   Scallop (*Patinopecten yessoesin*) in Japan

*   Red seabream (*Pagrus major*) in Japan

*   Pacific salmon (*Oncorhynchus* sp.) in Nort America

*   Eel (*Anguilla* sp.) in Japan.

Feeding with species specific feed is the main basis for monoculture in the case of finfish.

7. Polyculture

Polyculture, as the name implies, is the culture of several species in the same water body. The culture system generally depends on natural food of a water body sometime augmented artificially by fertilization and/or by supplementary feeding. If artificial food is given it is a common food acceptable to all or most species that are cultured.

Fresh water

- Polyculture of *Clarias gariepinus* and tilapias in Africa.
- Polyculture of several species of Chinese carps in China, Taiwan etc.
- Polyculture of several Indian major carp species in India.
- Polyculture in Indian major carps, Chinese carps and other fish in India called composite fish culture.

Brackish water

- Milkfish and shrimp culture in Philippines and Indonesia.
- Mullet and shrimp culture in Israel. In systems where production depends on natural fish pond zonation *i.e.* ecological niches assume great importance.

8. Hanging on bottom and stick methods of oyster culture

In the hanging method, oysters as they grow are suspended from rafts, long-lines or racks. Raft method is used in protected areas as in the Seto Inland sea of Japan. The long-line system has horizontal lines attached to wooden barrels or metal drums at or near the surface from which strings of seed oysters are suspended. The long-line system is used in offshore grounds. The system can withstand rough seas which might destroy rafts. The structures in the rack method consist of vertical poles or posts driven into bottom which support horizontal poles. Strings of seed oyster are tied to horizontal poles such that they do not touch the bottom. The trend of rack method is downward because of coastal pollution. In the sowing method, oysters are directly placed on the bottom. In the stick method, seed oysters are attached to wooden sticks riven into bottom in the intertidal zone. In both stick and on bottom method, crawling predators take a toll of oysters. Raft and long line methods are most productive as they minimize losses by predation and maximize production.

3.7 Pisciculture

Pisciculture is derived from two words Pisces which means fish or fishes and culture which means rearing, raising or breeding of living things. Therefore pisciculture is defined as a branched of animal husbandry that deals with rational deliberate culturing of fish or fishes to marketable size in a controlled water body. Whereas Aquaculture on the other hand is a branch of animal husbandry involving raising or breeding of living things either plants *e.g.* seaweed, plankton and algae or animals *e.g.* fin-fish, shell-fish, oyster shell, clams, cockles, shrimps, crayfish, periwinkles, turtles in a controlled water body to marketable size. Pisciculture can also be define as a branch of Aquaculture that deals with raising of fish to marketable size in a controlled water body or simply put fish farming. The species of fish which can be kept successfully in captivity throughout their lives from egg to adult is exceedingly limited in number. The various breeds of goldfish are familiar examples, but the carp is almost the only food-fish capable of similar domestication. Various other food-fishes, both marine and fresh-water, can be kept in ponds for longer or shorter periods, but refuse to breed, while in other cases the fry obtained from captive breeders will not develop. Consequently there are two main types of pisciculture to be distinguished the rearing in confinement of young fishes to an edible stage and the stocking of natural waters with eggs or fry from captured breeders. Fish farming can be classified into small scale fish farming and large scale fish farming or commercial fish farming based on the scale of production or permanent and mobile fish farm which is based on the durability or mobility of materials used in construction of the fish farm pond, concrete fish pond and earthen fish pond are examples of permanent fish farm.

Composite pisciculture is a scientific technology for getting maximum fish production from a pond or a tank through utilization of available food organisms supplemented by artificial feeding. Normally, the major species selected for composite fish culture are Katla, Rohu, Mrigal and exotic or common carps. A combination of Katla, Rohu, Mrigal can be considered in the ratio of 4:3:3. This has been done considering the fact that Katla is a Surface Feeder, Rohu Column Feeder and Mrigal Bottom Feeder. Protein is an essential ingredient of human food. It is also particularly essential for growing children both for their physical and mental growth. Protein deficiency leads to several diseases in human beings particularly children. Among sources of protein, animal meat is a vital source and fish is the cheapest and most easily digestible animal protein. Fish grows naturally in rivers and ponds but can also be produced under artificial conditions. Small entrepreneurs (farmers) can easily take up pisciculture in ponds and take it up as a source of livelihood or to supplement the family income. It also provides employment to skilled and unskilled youth. The pond/tank should have perennial fresh water source and water level in the pond is to be maintained up to depth of 2m. The water level should not be allowed to go down below 1m. It could be a new pond or existing pond which could be de-silted and deepened.

Integrated Fish Farming

The principle of integrated fish farming involves farming of fish along with livestock and/or agricultural crops. This type of farming offers great efficiency in resource utilization, as waste or byproduct from one system is effectively recycled. It also enables effective utilization of available farming space for maximizing production. The rising cost of protein-rich fish food and chemical fertilizers as well as the general concern for energy conservation has created awareness in the utilization of rice and other crop fields and livestock wastes for fish culture. Fish culture in combination with agriculture or livestock is a unique and lucrative venture and provides a higher farm income, makes available a cheap source of protein for the rural population, increases productivity on small land-holdings and increases the supply of feeds for the farm livestock. The scope of integrated farming is considerably wide. Ducks and geese are raised in pond and pond-dykes are used for horticultural and agricultural crop products and animal rearing. The system provides meat, milk, eggs, fruits, vegetables, mushroom, fodder and grains, in addition to fish. Hence this system provides better production, provides more employment and improves socio-economic status of farmers and betterment of rural economy. Integrated fish farming can be broadly classified into two viz. Agriculture-fish and Livestock-fish systems. Agri-based systems include rice-fish integration, horticulture-fish system, mushroom-fish system, seri-fish system. Livestock-fish system includes cattle-fish system, pig-fish system, poultry-fish system, duck-fish system, goat-fish system, rabbit-fish system.

Fisheries Department provides technical and financial assistance for integrated fish farming. The Integrated fish farming practices utilize the waste from different components of the system viz live stock, poultry, duckery, piggery and agriculture byproducts for fish production. 40-50 kg of organic wastes are converted into one kg of fish, while the pond silt is utilized as fertilizers for the fodder corps, which in turn is used to raise livestock. The system of integrated farming is very wide. The system provides meal, milk, eggs, fruit, vegetables, mushroom, fodder and grains in addition to fish. It utilizes the pond dykes which otherwise remain utilized for the production of additional food and income to the farmer. The possible integrated farming systems are given blow.

Fish cum Agriculture System	Fish cum Animal System
Fish cum Paddy Culture	Fish cum Dairy
Fish cum water chestnut	Fish cum Pig Farming
Fish cum Pappaya	Fish cum Rabbit Farming
Fish cum Mulberry	Fish cum Poultry
Fish cum Mushroom	Fish cum Duck Farming

Major factor of Pisciculture

(a) Location of pond

Soil should be water retentive, availability of assured water supply and the area, which is not prone to flood, may be identified.

(b) Pond management

- Before stocking, clear the pond of unwanted weeds and fish either by manual using fishnets or by using Mahua oil cake.

- Alkaline nature to be maintained by adequately adding lime in the ponds.

- Fertilize the ponds properly to improve the natural availability of phytoplantation.

(c) Stocking

- Ponds will be ready for stocking after 15 days of application of fertilizers.

- Fingerlings of 10 cm size should be used for stocking at the rate of 5000 numbers per hectare.

(d) Post stocking

- Apart from natural food, fish may be fed by rice bran or oil cake.

- The feed may be placed on bomboo tray or it may be sprayed at corner of the ponds.

- Organic manuring may be done at monthly intervals at the rate of 1000 kg/ha.

(e) Harvesting

- Generally done at the end of one year, when fish attain a weight of 750 grams to 1.25 kg.

- A production of 4-5 tons is possible in one-hectare pond.

Fresh Water Prawn Farming

There are more than 100 species of Freshwater prawn found in the world. There are more than 25 species are found in India. Out of these 10 species are important from commercial point of view. Out of them *Macrobrachium rosenbengii* is the main species which is used in culture practices. This is also known as giant prawn. This can be cultured in both fresh water as well as brackish water. It is fast growing animal and farmers can culture profitably. It contains 20-22 per cent animal protein and has less cholestrol. It has essential amino-acids and mineral which are very important for human beings. In culture practices, the freshwater prawn has two stages *i.e.* Nursery Pond and Growout Pond. Fresh water prawn is stocked in nursery pond for 45-60 days then it is shifted to grow-out ponds. The ponds are prepared by using manure and fertilizers. The stocking density in nursery pond is kept 2.00-2.50 lakh per hectare. Feed is provided 5 times at 8-10 gm per kg body weight at initial stage. Check trays are used to regulate the feeding. Prawn crop becomes ready for sale with 7-8 months. The expenditure about Rs. 1.50 lakh per hectare and income is Rs. 2.50 lakh. Thus net income is Rs. 1.00 lakh per hectare in 8 months.

BOX 3.5

ORNAMENTAL FISH BREEDING

Keeping colourful and fancy fishes known as ornamental fishes, aquarium fishes or live jewels is one of the oldest and most popular hobbies in the world. The growing interest in aquarium fishes has resulted in steady increase in aquarium fish trade globally. At present in India, hundreds of exotic and indigenous ornamental fish varieties are being bred under captive condition. Majority of the production goes to domestic market and to some extent for export. There are quite a large number of tropical aquarium fishes known to the aquarists. While many of the fishes are easy to breed, some of these are rare, difficult to breed and expensive. Most of the exotic species can be bred and reared easily since the technology is simple and well developed. It is advisable to start with common,

---

attractive, easily bred and less expensive species before attempting the more challenging ones.

Culture/rearing: The culture/rearing of these fishes can be taken up normally in cement tanks. Cement tanks are easy to maintain and durable. One species can be stocked in one tank. However, in case of compatible species two or three species can occupy the same tank. Ground water from dug wells/deep tube wells/ bore-wells are the best for rearing fish. The fishes reach marketable size in around 4 to 6 months. Eight to ten crops can be taken in a year.

Feeding: Young fish are fed mainly with Infusoria, Artemia, Daphnia , Mosquito larvae Tubifex and Blood worms. For rearing, formulated artificial or prepared feed can be used. Currently, no indigenous prepared feed for aquarium fish is available. The amount and type of food to be given depends on the size of the fry. Feeding is generally done twice in a day or according to the requirement. For rearing from fry stage dry/ prepared feed can be used.

Breeding: 95% of ornamental fish export is based on wild collection. Such capture based export is not sustainable and it is a matter of concern for the industry. In order to sustain the growth it is absolutely necessary to shift the focus from capture to culture based development. Moreover, most of the fish species grown for their ornamental importance can be bred in India successfully. Organized trade in ornamental fish depends on assured and adequate supply, which is possible only through mass breeding. The method of breeding is based on the family characteristics of the fish. The success of breeding depend on the compatibility of pairs, the identification of breeders which is a skill gained through experience. Generally the brooders are selected from the standing crop or purchased and reared separately by feeding them with good live food. However, it is always better to buy good brood stock and replace the breeders. Otherwise, the original characteristic of the species keeps on getting diluted because of continuous inbreeding. Brooders especially egg layers should be discarded after few spawnings.

Health care: Water exchange, is a must for maintaining water quality conducive for the fish health. Only healthy fish can withstand the effects of transportation and fetch a good price. Permitted chemicals / antibiotics, vitamins, etc can also be used for preventing/treating diseases.

3.8 Poultry farming

Poultry farming, raising of birds domestically or commercially, primarily for meat and eggs but also for feathers. Chickens, turkeys, ducks and geese are of primary importance, while guinea fowl and squabs are chiefly of local interest. Humans first domesticated chickens of Indian origin for the purpose of cockfighting in Asia, Africa and Europe. Very little formal attention was given to egg or meat production. Cockfighting was outlawed in England in 1849 and in most other countries thereafter. Exotic breeds and new standard breeds of chickens proliferated in the years to follow and poultry shows became very popular. From 1890 to 1920 chicken raisers stressed egg and meat production and commercial hatcheries became important after 1920. Poultry activity in India is graduated from backyard farming to Hi-tech, environmentally controlled poultry. The Bank is providing loans to all activities of poultry farming *i.e.* Layer farming, Broiler farming and Hatcheries. The entrepreneur should have thorough knowledge of poultry farming substantiated by training certificate/ experience certificate etc. The backward linkages like suitability of climates, availability of day old chicks, water and veterinary services will be the pre-requisite. The poultry farming in India is supported and financed by NABARD also.

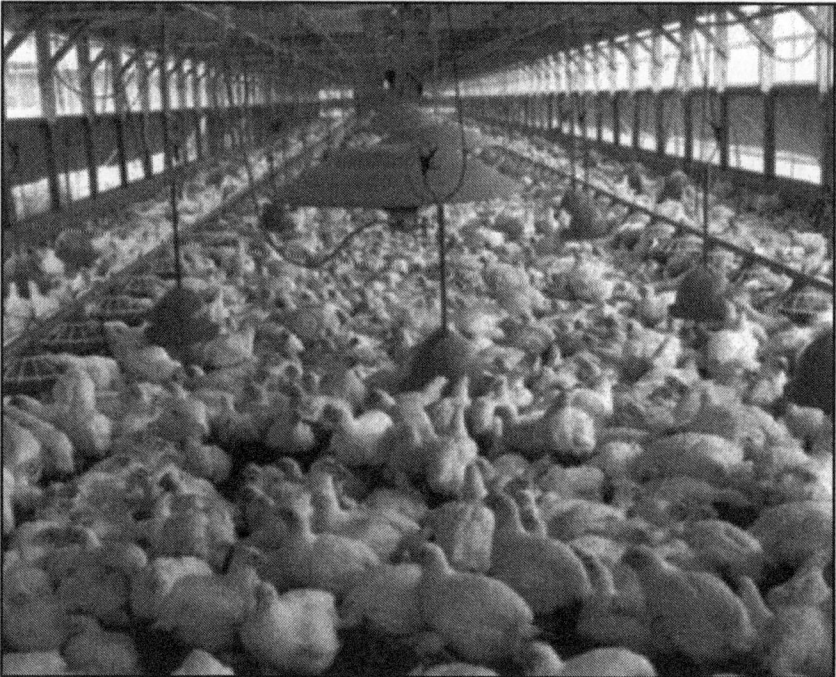

Figure 3.11: Poultry farm

3.8.1 Breeds

The breeds of chickens are generally classified as Asiatic, American, Mediterranean and English. The American breeds of importance today are Plymouth Rock, Wyandotte, Rhode Island Red and New Hampshire. The Barred Plymouth Rock, developed in 1865 by crossing the Dominique with the Black Cochin, has grayish-white plumage crossed with dark bars. It has good size and meat quality and is a good layer. The White Plymouth Rock, a variety of the Barred Plymouth Rock, has white plumage and is raised for its meat. Both varieties lay brown eggs. The Wyandotte, developed in 1870 from five or more strains and breeds, has eight varieties and is characterized by a plump body, excellent meat and good egg production. Only the white strain is of any significance today because it is used in broiler crosses where its white plumage, quality of flesh and rapid growth are highly desirable. Chicken breeding is an outstanding example of the application of basic genetic principles of inbreeding, line breeding and crossbreeding, as well as of intensive mass selection to effect faster and cheaper gains in broilers and maximum egg production for the egg-laying strains. Maximum use of heterosis or hybrid vigour, through incrosses and crossbreeding has been made. Crossbreeding for egg production has used the single-comb White Leghorn, the Rhode Island Red, New Hampshire, Barred Plymouth Rock, White Plymouth Rock, Black Australorp and White Minorca. Crossbreeding for broiler production has used the White Plymouth Rock or New Hampshire crossed with White or Silver Cornish or incrosses utilizing widely diverse inbred strains within a single breed. Rapid and efficient weight gains and high quality, plump, meaty carcasses have been achieved thereby.

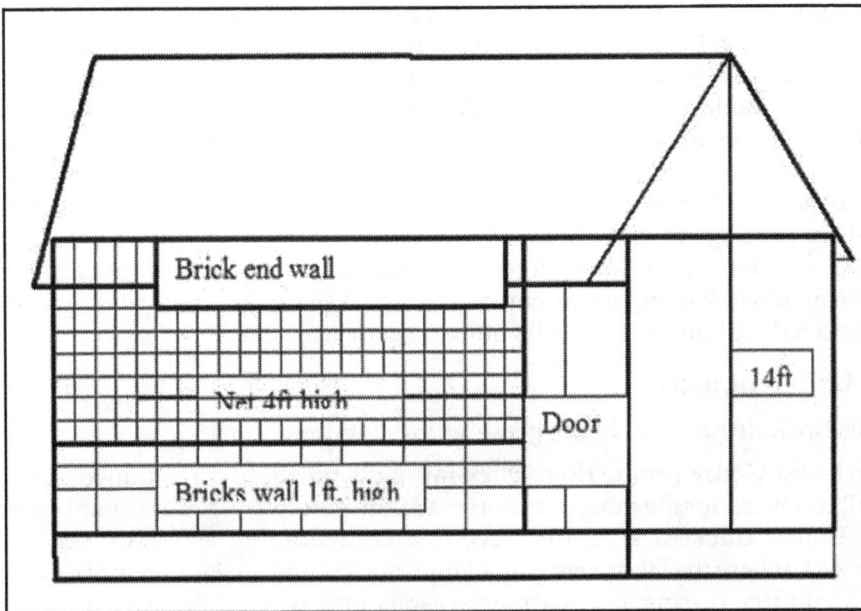

Figure 3.12: Poultry House

The male sperm lives in the hen's oviduct for two to three weeks. Eggs are fertilized within 24 hours after mating. Yolks originate in the ovary and grow to about 1.6 inches (4 cm) in diameter, after which they are released into the oviduct, where the thick white and two shell membranes are added. Then egg moves into the uterus where the thin white and the shell are added. This process requires a total of 24 hours per egg. The hatching of fertilized eggs requires 21 days, with the heavy breeds requiring a few more hours and the lighter breeds slightly fewer. Ideal hatching temperature approximates 100°F (38°C) with control of air flow, humidity, oxygen and carbon dioxide being essential. Standardized egg-laying tests and official random sample tests have been used for many years to measure actual productivity.

3.8.2 Feeding

Chicken feeding is a highly perfected science that ensures a maximum intake of energy for growth and fat production. High quality and well balanced protein sources produce a maximum amount of muscle organ, skin and feather growth. The essential minerals produce bones and eggs, 3 to 4% of the live bird being composed of minerals and 10 per cent of the egg. Calcium, phosphorus, sodium, chlorine, potassium, sulphur, manganese, iron, copper, cobalt, magnesium and zinc are all required. Vitamins A, C, D, E and K and all 12 of the B vitamins are also required. Water is essential and antibiotics are almost universally used to stimulate appetite, control harmful bacteria and prevent disease. Modern rations produce a pound of broiler on about 2 pounds (0.9 kg) of feed and a dozen eggs from 4.5 pounds (2 kg) of feed. A carefully controlled environment that avoids crowding, chilling, overheating or frightening is almost universal in chicken raising. Cannibalism, which expresses itself as toe picking, feather picking and tail picking, is controlled by debeaking at one day of age and by other management practices. The feeding, watering, egg gathering and cleaning operations are highly mechanized. The vast majority of chicks hatched each year are used for broiler production and the remainder for egg production. In egg production feed represents more than two-thirds of the cost. Pullet (immature hen) flocks predominate. Hens are usually housed in wire cages with two or three hens per cage and three or four tiers of cages superposed to save space. Cages for laying hens have been found to increase production, lower mortality, reduce cannibalism, lower feeding requirements, reduce diseases and parasites, improve culling and reduce both space and labour requirements.

3.8.3 Other poultry

These include turkeys, ducks, geese, guinea fowl and squabs.

Duck and Goose production: Duck raising is practiced on a limited scale in nearly all countries, for the most part as a small farm enterprise. Khaki Campbell and Indian Runner ducks are prolific layers, each averaging 300 eggs per year. In Indonesia, where the labour supply is large, duck herders take a flock of ducks to the high country during the warmer seasons and work their way down the mountainsides to the lowlands. Ducks are easily transported, can be raised in close confinement and convert some waste products and scattered grain *e.g.* by gleaning rice fields to nutritious and very desirable eggs and meat. In developed countries, commercial plants have been built exclusively for duck meat production. Goose raising is a minor farm enterprise in practically all countries, but in Germany, Austria, some eastern European countries (notably Poland), parts of France and locally elsewhere, there is important commercial goose production.

The two outstanding meat breeds are the Toulouse, predominantly gray in colour and the Embden, which is white. Geese do not appear to have attracted the attention of geneticists on the same scale as the meat chicken and the turkey and no change in the goose industry comparable to that in the others has occurred or seems to be in prospect. In some commercial plants, geese are fattened by a special process resulting in a considerable enlargement of their livers, which are sold as a delicacy.

Guinea fowl and Squabs: Guinea fowl are raised as a sideline on a few farms in many countries and eaten as gourmet items. In Italy there is a fairly extensive industry. There the birds are raised in yards with open-fronted shelters. The guinea fowl are marketed at 16–18 weeks of age. The market weight is usually about 1.0-1.5 kg (2.5-3.5 pounds), but food conversion is poor. Pigeons are raised not only as messengers and for sport but also for the meat of their squabs (nestlings), also a gourmet item. Squab production is rare in most countries with established poultry industries.

3.8.4 Poultry diseases

Poultry are quite susceptible to a number of diseases; some of the more common are fowl typhoid, pullorum, fowl cholera, chronic respiratory disease, infectious sinusitis, infectious coryza, avian infectious hepatitis, infectious synovitis, bluecomb, Newcastle disease, fowl pox, avian leukosis complex, coccidiosis, blackhead, infectious laryngotracheitis, infectious bronchitis and erysipelas. Strict sanitary precautions, the intelligent use of antibiotics and vaccines and the widespread use of cages for layers and confinement rearing for broilers have made it possible to effect satisfactory disease control. Parasitic diseases of poultry, including hexamitiasis of turkeys, are caused by roundworms, tapeworms, lice and mites. Again, modern methods of sanitation, prevention and treatment provide excellent control. Poultry diseases are a constant threat to the intensive poultry farm. Maintenance of quarantine facilities and procedures is vital in the prevention of disease on the farm. Quarantine, hygiene and vaccination should be the first choices in disease control and a failure in any of these primary areas will inevitably result in increased disease control costs. An important issue in the welfare and productivity of the poultry on the farm is the maintenance of the environment in which the birds live. Under intensive production systems, the poultry house design features to control the internal environment include insulation, fans, foggers, reflective paints, brooders, blinds and curtains. Given the dependence of many environmental control mechanisms on electricity and in the interests of animal welfare, intensive poultry farm operations should possess an alternate power supply in case of an emergency. This may be by way of power generating equipment or tractor operated pumps. At modern shed stocking densities the lives and welfare of poultry livestock do depend on a backup source of power supply.

3.8.5 Poultry waste

Effective waste management is a crucial element in the successful operation of any poultry enterprise. The waste issues are the management of dead birds, manure and spent litter. Poultry manure and litter are a valuable fertilizer. It is superior to conventional fertilizers under certain conditions as it has a high nutrient value; high organic matter, aiding physical soil structure and a slow release of nutrient, aiding in plant uptake and reducing the potential for nutrient leaching. Therefore, its management should reflect its value. Pests and vermin control strategies need to be designed and conducted efficiently and regularly. Starlings, sparrows, rats, mice, flies, mosquitoes, lice, mites and ticks all have implications in the transmission of poultry diseases and some have additional human health and product quality considerations. Free range farms have the additional problem of foxes, hawks, crows, cats and dogs to contend with. Control of pests is to be integrated with other site management operations.

3.9 Sericulture

The art of silk production is called sericulture that comprises cultivation of mulberry, silkworm rearing and post cocoon activities leading to production of silk yarn. Sericulture provides gainful employment, economic development and improvement in the quality of life to the people in rural area and therefore it plays an important role in anti poverty programme and prevents migration of rural people to urban area in search of employment. Hence several developing nations like India, China, Brazil, Thailand, Vietnam, Indonesia, Egypt, Iran, Sri Lanka, Philippines, Bangladesh, Nepal, Myanmar, Turkey, Papua New Guinea, Mexico, Uzbekistan and some of the African and Latin American countries have taken up sericulture to provide employment to the people in rural area. Sericulture is an agro-based, labour intensive, export oriented commercial activity. Producing silk is a lengthy, complex process. As men took responsibility for the mulberry trees, growing the only food silkworms eat, but women were responsible for the critical task of feeding the leaves to the silkworms. Silkworms do not spin cocoons on demand; timing and temperature have to be handled carefully and during the month between hatching and spinning the cocoons have to be fed every few hours, day or night. If properly coddled, the worms eventually spin cocoons for several days, each cocoon made up of a strand of silk several thousand feet long. Over two thousand silkworms are needed to produce one pound of silk. Silk is the fine strong soft lustrous fiber produced by silkworms. The word silk sounds luxury and class. Silk is the queen of textile and the naturally produced animal fiber. Till today, no other fabric can match it in luster and elegance. As long as human desire for silk garments continues, the demand for sericulture activity remains. Sericulture means cultivation of silkworms, which finally produces silk.

Sericulture is the cultivation of silk through rearing of silkworm. It involves the raising of food plants for silkworm, rearing of silkworm for production of cocoons, reeling and spinning of cocoon for production of yarn etc. for value added benefits such as processing and weaving. Sericulture also includes the practical aspects such as increasing productivity of land as well as labour, stabilization of cocoon production, improvement of silk yarn, fabric and generating profitable income for rural poor and backward people. Silk is an animal protein fibre secreted (produced) by the silkworm larva for spinning of the cocoon. This cocoon provides a protective shell (shelter) for the soft and delicate caterpillar to pass the pupal stage inside it and metamorphose into an imago (moth). Silk yarn is obtained from the silk cocoons.

3.9.1 Sericulture in Karnataka

The Mysore Silk is synonymous with splendor and grandeur. Mysore silk has been registered as Geographical Indicator under Intellectual Property Rights. Karnataka is the homeland of Mysore Silk. Karnataka sericulture has a history of more than 230 years. In 1785, the Tiger of Mysore Tippu Sultan established sericulture in Mysore kingdom. He wanted Mysore to be the foremost among silk producing nations. The dream of this great ruler became true during later period. During these years Karnataka sericulture has seen many ups and downs in its long journey. It has transformed into a model in mulberry sericulture in the country. During early 19th century while the world sericulture was collapsing, Mysore Sericulture industry sustained. Though, most of the exotic silkworm varieties perished remained stable through this period and even today it is the back bone of mulberry sericulture in India. In 1800, the Mysore Royal Government established sericulture in Mogenahalli near Channapatna, which became the center of sericulture activities soon. In 1860, first silk filature was established in Bangalore by an Italian industrialist. During this period many exotic Italian or Chinese or Japanese races were used to produce cross breed layings by this filature. In 1896, great industrialist Sir J.N.Tata established a Silk Farm with a filature attached to it in Japanese pattern, in Bangalore, with the help of Sri K. Sheshadri Ayyar, the Diwan of Mysore. He got the technical expertise from Japanese couple Mr and Mrs Odzu, who gave scientific outlook for the Sericulture industry. Mr. Odzu trained Sri V.M. Appadhorai Mudaliar and Sri Laxman Rao for a period of one year in this farm.

The Architect of Mysore Sir M.Vishveshwaraiah gave much importance to Sericulture in rural development. He hired the services of Signor Washington Mari from Italy to organize and develop silk industry in Mysore in 1913. Signor Mari made available 12 varieties of pure European and Chinese silkworm to conduct experiments. Under the guidance of Signor Mari, Appadhorai Mudaliar conducted native environment breeding experiments in Channapatna.

They successfully developed many cross breed combinations between females of Mysore Local (Pure Mysore) and males of European and Chinese races, which were far superior to their parents. In 1914, Signor Mari shifted his headquarters to Bangalore and Mudaliar continued to carry out the breeding experiments in Channapatna Farm. In 1914, independent Department of Sericulture was established and Signor Washington Mari became the first Director of Sericulture. In 1919, Government hired the services of Japanese expert, Mr. Yonemura for conducting research and imparting training in sericulture. Government started Silk filature in 1922 and Silk weaving factory in 1931-1932 at Mysore. During later part of 1970s under ISDP and during 1980s under World Bank aided two sericulture projects Department of Sericulture took up extensive expansion programmes. Infrastructures like drainages, Technical Service Centers cocoon markets, were established.

This boosted the raw silk production to 9236 MT during 1997-98. Directly and indirectly sericulture is providing jobs for about 10.67 lakh people. One hectare of Mulberry provides year long continuous job for 13 persons. Karnataka has well established Multivoltine and Bivoltine Seed areas. They cater to the demand of parental seed cocoons required for the production of cross breed and bivoltine hybrid layings. Almost 88% of Karnataka sericulture is spread in southern part of Karnataka, which is fast modernizing. Factors like urbanization, industrialization, depleting water table, scarcity of agriculture labour have affected sericulture in this part.

Table 3.1 Sericulture in Karnataka (District wise)

S.No. District	Taluka	Silk Farms	Total Area (acre)	Mulberry Area (acre)
1. Bangalore Urban	Anekal	1.Kumbarahalli	20.00	2.20
2. Bangalore Rural	Devanahalli	2.Mallenahalli	3.12	-
	Doddaballapura	3.Doddaballapura	26.16	-
	Hoskote	4.Hindiganal	6.13	-
		5.Sulibele	20.00	-
3. Bagalakote	Bagalakote	6.Bagalakote	7.20	-
4. Belgaum	Athani	7.Ainapura	13.30	2.00
	Belgaum	8.Hirebagewadi	29.18	3.20
	Gokak	9.Gokak	12.00	1.20
	Hukkeri	10.Hedakal	64.13	-
	Khanapura	11.Khanapura	32.16	2.30
	Parasagada	12.Soundatti	31.10	-
	Ramadurga	13.Ramadurga	10.02	2.30
	Raybag	14.Kankanavadi	13.30	2.00
5. Bellary	Bellary	15.Sridharagadda	20.20	-
		16.Kolagallu	48.28	1.00
	H.B.Halli	17.Hampasagara	22.30	-
		18.Sovenahalli	19.26	-
	Kudligi	19.Machihalli	32.28	-
		20.Kandagal	39.29	-
6. Bidar	-	-	-	-
7. Bijapur	Bijapur	21.Sindagi	21.23	1.10
8. Chamaraja NagaraNagara	Chamaraja nagara nagar	22.Kuderu	5.00	-
		23.ChamarajaNagar	7.35	-
		24.Umattur	1.26	0.20
		25. Mangala	9.38	0.27
	Kollegal	26.Kollegal	16.06	2.20
	Yelandur	27.B.R.Hills	42.06	1.00
9. Chikkaballpur	Chintamani	28.Madikere	18.00	0.30
		29.Yenigadele	6.16	-
	Siddlagatta	30.Chowdasandra	25.00	-
	Gowribidanur	31.Karekallahalli	30.00	1.04
10. ChikkaMagalur	Kadur	32.Linglapura	35.31	-
	Tarikere	33.Sollapura	18.19	2.10

Contd...

Table 3.1 Contd...

S.No.	District	Taluka	Silk Farms	Total Area (acre)	Mulberry Area (acre)
11.	Chitradurga	Challakere	34.Na.MahadevaPura	17.14	-
		Chitradurga	35.Maragatta	20.00	0.20
		Hiriyur	36.Nandihalli	13.28	-
		Holelakere	37.Kotehala	10.10	-
		Molakalmur	38.Rayapura	148.00	-
12.	DakshinaKannada	Beltangadi	39.Garukatte	20.17	1.15
		Puttur	40.Koila	50.00	1.15
13.	Davanagere	Channagiri	41.B.R.T Colony	30.00	-
14.	Dharwar	-	-	-	-
15.	Gadag	Mundragi	42.Mundragi	25.10	-
		Rona	43.Rona	5.00	-
16.	Gulbarga	Gulbarga	44.Hedagimudra	12.07	-
			45.Kavadimatti	4.05	-
17.	Hassan	Arakalagud	46.Rudrapatna	25.00	2.00
		Arasikere	47.Jajur	25.24	1.00
		ChannarayaPatna	48.Jambur	60.00	-
		Hassan	49.Ambuga	46.31	1.00
		Holenarasi pura	50.Tatanahalli	44.33	-
18.	Haveri	Haveri	51.Haveri	43.10	-
		Ranebennur	52.Ranebennur	64.04	1.00
19.	Kodagu	Somaverpet	53.Kudege	25.00	2.00
20.	Kolar	Bangarpet	54.Kuppanahalli	10.00	2.00
		Mulbagal	55.DevarayanaSamudra	29.00	-
		Srinivasapur	56.Panasamakanahalli	10.00	-
21.	Koppal	Yelburga	57.Chikkoppa	33.03	-
		Kustagi	58.Narabenchi	21.11	2.00
22.	Mandya	K.R.Pet	59.Chikkonahalli	34.28	2.00
		Maddur	60.Maddur	12.16	2.10
		Mandy	61.H.Malligere	100.00	5.10
23.	Mysore	Hunasur	62.Dharmapura	20.00	-
		Nanjanagud	63.Nanjanagud	14.26	2.00
			64.Thandavapur	43.17	2.15
		Periyapatna	65.Kaggundi	49.24	2.04
		T.Narasipura	66.Mugur	5.15	1.04
			67.Horlahalli	33.01	1.00

Contd...

Table 3.1 Contd...

S.No.	District	Taluka	Silk Farms	Total Area (acre)	Mulberry Area (acre)
24.	Ramanagar	Ramanagar	68.K.P.Doddi	24.34	0.30
			69.Sugganahalli	4.35	-
		Channapatna	70.Iggalur	30.00	-
			71.Kanva	27.35	-
25.	Raichur	Lingsugur	72.Kannapurahatti	33.12	2.00
			73.Kesarahatti	65.00	1.00
26.	Shimoga	-	-	-	-
27.	Tumkur	Chikkanayaknahalli	74.Byraganahalli	12.00	1.00
		Gubbi	75.Herur	20.00	0.16
		Madhugiri	76.Kempapura	56.12	-
			77.Jogihalli	19.30	-
		Sira	78.Sira	20.00	1.32
		Tiptur	80.Huchhagodnahalli	26.15	2.25
28.	Udupi	-	-	-	-
29.	Uttara Kannada	Haliyala	81.Haliyala	20.04	-
30.	Yadagir	-	-	-	-
Mysore Seed area					
		Magadi	82.Magadi	11.16	1.20
			83.Solur	16.18	1.00
		Kunigal	84.Bilidevalaya	38.39	2.00
			85.Kunigal	11.24	1.20
			86.Hosegakaval	50.00	2.10
			87.Kempnahalli	14.00	2.00
			88.Santhemavthur	25.00	1.31
		Tumkur	89.Hebbur	20.00	2.00
		Turuvekere	90.Segehalli	36.15	2.05

Source: Dept. of Sericulture GOI

3.9.2 Silkworm Germplasm in India

The domesticated silkworm species, *Bombyx mori* L. evolved almost 4600 years ago from the wild species, *Bombyx mandarina* Moore, which is a native of China and Palaearctic region. The eggs of silkworm, *B. mori* were first introduced from China into Japan and Korea in the first century and subsequently into Middle Eastern and European countries and later into the neighboring countries around China in the sixth century. The historical background of silkworm entry into India is still a mystery; and the historical evidence indicates that a flourishing silk trade was practising between India and Rome/Greece during Kaniska period (56 BC). This is the authentic historical record of silk production and trade in India, which indicates the early history of Indian sericulture. The rich tradition of silk and silk use are evident from ancient sacred literature like the Rigveda, the Ramayana and the Mahabharatha, which are more than 2000 years old, but the information about indigenous silkworm races and their stock maintenance are not well documented. Silkworm rearing was prevalent in Kashmir and North Eastern states during sixteenth century, the Moghul period where the univoltine and multivoltine silkworms were respectively reared and the Tippu Sultan introduced silkworm rearing in south India in 1785. During eighteenth century, the British rule in India, quite a few univoltine and bivoltine races were imported from Italy, France, Russia and China and the races were bred and maintained by the farmers and there was no systematic maintenance of the silkworm germplasm and hence only few races survived under Indian climatic condition. At present, only few old indigenous races are surviving viz. Barapolu, Chotapolu, Nistari, Sarupat and Moria, whereas the indigenous univoltine Kashmiri races are almost extinct. Systematic silkworm stock maintenance and breeding started in the early nineteenth century. Prior to 1922, only pure races were reared and hybrid silkworms were introduced later, Pure Mysore × *C. nichi* was probably the first hybrid in Karnataka and exploitation of hybrids in West Bengal and Kashmir came much later during 1956 and 1959 respectively. Silkworm genetic stock maintenance started during 1940 in an organised way at Sericultural Research Station, Berhampore in West Bengal and subsequently temperate silkworm germplasm stocks were established at Univoltine Silkworm Seed Station, Pampore in Kashmir and multivoltine and bivoltine silkworm stocks were established at Central Sericultural Research Institute, Mysore in Karnataka and Coonoor in Tamil Nadu.

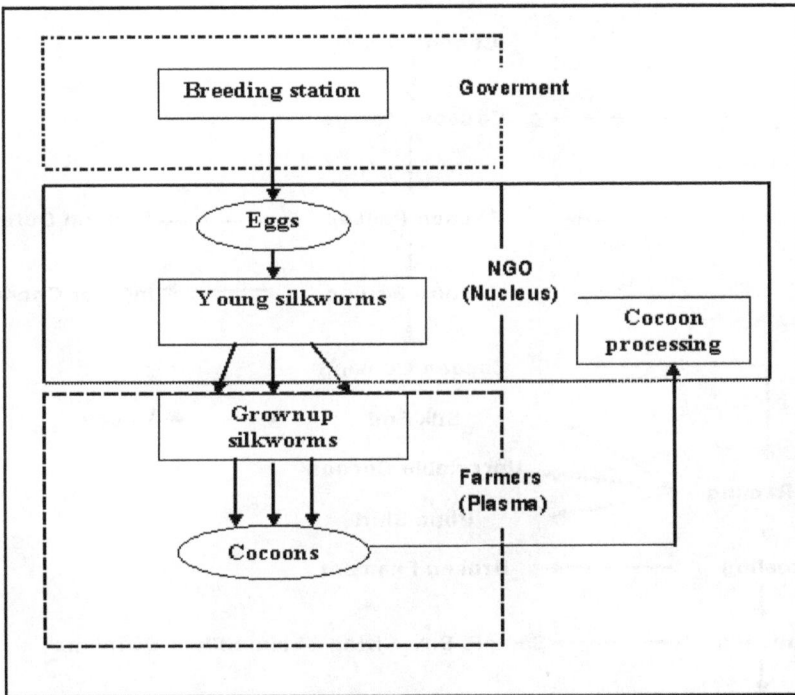

Figure 3.13: Silk production and supporters

3.9.3 Production of Silk

India and China are the two main producers, together manufacturing more than 60% of the world production each year. Silkworm larvae are fed by mulberry leaves and, after the fourth moult, climb a twig placed near them and spin their silken cocoons. This process is achieved by the worm through a dense fluid secreted from its structural glands, resulting in the fibre of the cocoon. The silk is a continuous filament fiber consisting of fibroin protein, secreted from two salivary glands in the head of each larva and a gum called sericin, which cements the two filaments together. The sericin is removed by placing the cocoons in hot water, which frees the silk filaments and readies them for reeling. This is known as the degumming process. The immersion in hot water also kills the silkworm pupae. Single filaments are combined to form thread. This thread is drawn under tension through several guides and wound onto reels. The threads may be plied together to form yarn. After drying the raw silk is packed according to quality.

Stages of Production

The stages of production are as follows:

i.   The silk moth lays thousands of eggs.

ii. The silk moth eggs hatch and the larvae feed on the mulberry leaves.

iii. First, it weaves a net to hold itself

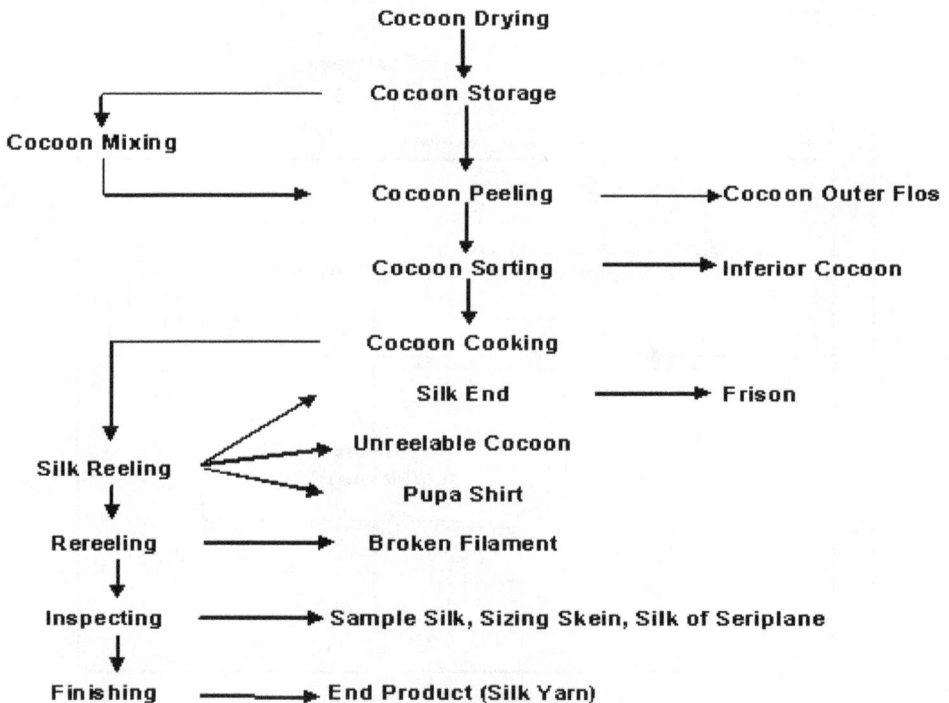

Figure 3.14:Sericulture process

iv. Next, it swings its head from side to side in the way of the number 8.

v. The silk solidifies when it comes in contact with the air.

vi. The silkworm spins approximately 1 mile of filament and completely encloses itself in a cocoon in about two or three days but due to quality restrictions, the amount of usable silk in each cocoon is small. As a result, 5500 silkworms are required to produce 1 kg of silk.

vii. The silk is obtained from the undamaged cocoons by brushing the cocoon to find the outside end of the filament.

viii. Then silk filaments are wound on a reel. One cocoon contains approximately 1,000 yards of silk filament. The silk at this stage is known as raw silk. One thread consists of up to 48 individual silk filaments.

3.9.4 Mulberry Cultivation

Mulberry is a hardy plant capable of thriving under a variety of agroclimatic conditions. At the same time, it is also sensitive responding extremely well to optimum agricultural inputs but showing practically no growth when plant nutrients and moisture begin to operate as limiting factors. This is evident from the fact that under the poor rainfall conditions of 25-30 (625-750 mm) prevailing in South India, the current leaf yield is of the order of only 3,000-3,500 kgs per hectare whereas under assured irrigation and appropriate fertilizer application, it can be stepped upto 30,000 kgs or so or nearly ten times. Further, mulberry under South Indian conditions, unlike in temperate regions like Japan, Korea and USSR, gives continuous growth almost throughout the year, because of optimum temperature conditions and good sunshine available.

Soil and climatic conditions: Mulberry can grow practically on any type of land except on very steep lands. Good growths are obtained when it is raised on either flat land or gently sloping or undulating lands. On more slopy or steep lands, necessary attention to proper soil conservation methods as contour drains, contour planting or even bench terracing should be given. Mulberry grows in a wide range of soils, but best growth is obtained in loamy to clayey loam soils. The mulberry plant can tolerate slightly acidic conditions in the soil. In the case of too acidic soils with pH below 5, necessary corrective measures through application of Dolomite or Lime should be adopted. In case of alkaline soils, application of Gypsum should be resorted to for correction of the soil alkalinity. Since, mulberry is a deep rooted plant; the soil should be sufficiently deep upto about two feet in depth. In respect of elevation, mulberry thrives well upto about 4,000 feet, above growth will be retarded because of the cooler temperature. Mulberry falls under the category of perennial crops and once it is properly raised during the first year, it can come to full yielding capacity during the second year and lasts for over 15 years in the field without any significant deterioration in the yield of leaf. It is very important that the initial planting and establishment of the crop is carried out according to scientific methods for obtaining best yield results in the subsequent years.

Land preparation: Land should be prepared by deeply ploughing with heavy mould board plough upto depth of 30-35 cm in order to loosen the soil before planting, taking advantage of the pre-monsoon showers during April-May. Thereafter, the land may be ploughed once or twice with a light plough or country plough to bring the soil to a fine tilth. Afterwards, a basal dose of organic manure like compost or cattle manure should be applied at the rate of atleast 10 tonnes per hectare for rainfed mulberry and 20 tonnes per hectare for irrigated mulberry. Finally, the manure should be properly incorporated into the soil by ploughing and the land leveled and made ready for planting during the monsoon rains of June-July. It must be stressed here that application of basal dose of organic manure like compost or cattle manure is essential for successful initial establishment of the plantation. Under very exceptional circumstances, where these are not at all available, an alternative may be resorted to by growing nursery raised plants and transplanting them into the main field. Generally, pit system of planting with wider spacing should be adopted for rainfed mulberry while row system with closer spacing can be adopted for irrigated mulberry. Therefore, for planting mulberry under rainfed conditions pits should be dug at a spacing of 3 x 3 (0.9 m x 0.9 m). The pits should be of the size 35 cm x 35 cm and at least 35 cm deep. These pits are filled with soil, preferably mixed with some cattle manure and in the pits the cuttings or rooted saplings are planted. In the case of irrigated gardens, the prepared land is thrown into ridges and furrows by using a ridge former or working with manual labour. It may be noted that there is only one irrigation channel for every two rows of mulberry plants. This helps in both saving and more effective use of the irrigation water.

Planting material and planting: In tropical conditions as in South India, mulberry can root easily and can be easily propagated through cuttings with minimum of time and expenditure. The cuttings should be prepared from 4-8 months old hard wood branches which are brown in colour and at least 10-12 mm in diameter. The cuttings should be at least 18-20 cm long with a minimum of three buds. The ends of the cuttings should be clean cut with a sharp knife, without splits or bark peeling off. It is in the selection of planting material that mistakes are often made which result in poor establishment of the plants with lots of failures and resultant gaps. Cuttings either thin in diameter or green in colour should be avoided as the chances of their success are poor. Therefore, for successful rooting of the cuttings, every care should be taken to see that the cuttings of the desired maturity, thickness and length alone are selected for planting. Because, only such cuttings provide necessary nutrients for the buds to sprout and grow till such time adequate root formation takes place. It is also to be remembered that the soil should be very fertile containing adequate quantities of organic matter. Therefore, it is absolutely necessary that whenever straight planting of cuttings is resorted to, the soil should receive a basal dose of manure like compost or organic manure at the rate indicated already. The manure should be thoroughly mixed with the soil before planting is undertaken. At the time of planting, it is important to see that the cuttings are placed deep and the soil around well compacted, leaving just one inch alone of the cutting exposed. This ensures the cuttings being planted sufficiently deep in the soil resulting in the formation of roots below the ground level. Further, this will prevent the cuttings from drying up. While planting, the cuttings should be planted either upright or with only a very slight tilt. In places where compost or cattle manure is not available, it is highly risky to resort to direct planting of cuttings. Under such conditions, it will be found necessary to raise rooted plants, in nurseries and transplant 2-3 months old rooted plants with about 3 inches growth and a stem thickness of about 10 mm in the main field. While transplanting nursery raised plants, it is important to see that the original cutting from which the plants have grown are buried deep in the soil at least one to two inch below ground level and the soil around pressed hard as in the case of planting cuttings. This ensures better anchoring of the plants. In all the new plantings with either cuttings or nursery raised plants, it should be so timed that there is 1-2 months of rainfall following the planting operation, particularly in the case of rainfed mulberry.

Spacing: In the case of rainfed mulberry gardens, the aim should be to raise mulberry plant with a sturdier frame so that it is able to withstand prevailing drought conditions, better. Therefore, the spacing should be atleast 3 x 3 (0.9 m x 0.9 m) as is being currently practiced. When cuttings are planted in the pits prepared for the purpose, they should be planted in threes at a spacing of 15 cm from each other, forming an equilateral triangle. When nursery raised rooted plants are transplanted, they may be planted as single plants. In the case of irrigated qualitative mulberry, the overall advantage in raising mulberry for both quantitative and qualitative harvest is in favour of planting mulberry with a spacing of 2 (0.6 m)d between the rows and 9-10 (23-25 cm) within the row. This slightly wider spacing as compared to the existing Kolar system of row cultivation helps to produce better quality leaves from the point of view of silkworm rearing. In the case of irrigated gardens, where the practice of leaf picking instead of whole shoot harvest is followed, it would be found necessary to adopt a wider spacing namely 2 x 2 (0.6 m x 0.6 m). Upto 3 x 3 (0.9 m x 0.9 m) is also practiced sometimes, but in this case, the plants tend to become almost small trees and present problems of harvest.

Manuring: The application of a basal dose of organic manure like compost or cattle manure is necessary for successful establishment of the garden. Thereafter, the young growing plants should be assisted to put forth vigourous and maximum growth through periodical fertilizer applications. In the case of the rainfed garden, which is planted in June-July during the South-West monsoon season, the mulberry will receive sufficient rains from both the monsoons and this fact should be taken full advantage of, to achieve maximum growth and build up a huge sturdy frame so that the plant may stand the following drought months, from January to April, very well. This is achieved by applying two doses of nitrogenous fertilizers such as Ammonium sulphate or Urea at the rate of 25 kg of N/ha for the first application after 2 to 3 months of growth and again, another 40 kg of N/ha as the second dose after an interval of another three months. This should enable the plants to reach a growth of about 2 m in about 6 to 8 months time. In the case of irrigated mulberry, where the plants will grow vigorously due to assured irrigation, the first dose of nitrogenous fertilizer should be given after 2 months of planting at the rate of about 40 kg N/ha. In another 2 to 2 months the plants would be ready for first harvest of leaves. Thereafter, the normal fertilizer application programme could be resorted to.

Weeding and inter-cultivation: During the initial stage of plant establishment in the field, weed growth should be kept to the minimum, so that the growing young plants are not smothered by the weeds. Atleast two weedings should be carried out during the first six months after planting of cuttings, once after two months of planting and again after an interval of 2 to 3 months. The weeding operation should be thorough and the soil should be dug deep to remove the weeds with roots. This deep digging is carried out as part of the weeding operation and results in necessary loosening of the soil and a stimulation to the plants to grow vigorously. Thus special care should be taken to reduce the weed growth as much as possible in the first year of planting. Thereafter, the shade effect of the fully grown mulberry will tend to keep the weeds down. Similarly, periodical inter-cultivation should be resorted to particularly in the case of dry mulberry gardens during the first year so that soil loosening results in better aeration and stimulation of plant growth. This also helps in catching the rain water and its deep penetration for better retention of soil moisture. During the first year, all attention should be concentrated on establishing the mulberry field properly as indicated above. One should not be in a haste to take early leaf harvests before the plants attain full growth. In the case of mulberry under rainfed conditions, it will take 10 to 12 months before first pruning is resorted to and systematic cultivation is taken up. On the other hand, in about six months time, the plants will reach full growth under the irrigated conditions and thereafter, systematic cultivation can be taken up.

The present low yields of leafy under rainfed mulberry are mainly due to poor rainfall and lack of or inadequate application of manures or fertilizers. Even under the limitations of scanty rainfall prevalent in South India, scope exists to improve leaf yields through optimum mannuring of the fields. Therefore, manure should be applied in the form of both bulk organic manure like compost or cattle manure and chemical fertilizers. Organic manure should be applied at the rate of ten tones per hectare, immediately after pruning and inter-cultivation and thoroughly incorporated in the soil. This should be carried out systematically once in the year so that the organic content in the soil is improved and as a result, the fertilizer application is more effectively utilized. Alternatively, where organic manure is not available, a green manure crop like sunhemp can be raised annually during the rainy seasons and incorporated into the soil to serve the same purpose. In addition to bulk organic manure, chemical fertilizers should also be applied at the rate of 100 kg N, 50 kg P and 50 kg K per hectare per annum, which may be applied in two equal split doses. The first dose should be applied sometime in late August *i.e.* 6-8 weeks after the application of the organic manure and the second dose sometime in late November during the North-East monsoon rains. The first dose may be in the form of complex manure like 15:5:15 or 17:17:17. About 300 kg or 6 bags of 17:17:17 will be required to meet the requirements of the first dose of 50 kg N, 50 kg P and 50 kg K. The second dose maybe given as 50 kg N only which is available in 250 kg or 5 bags of Ammonium sulphate or about 100 kg or 2 bags of Urea. While applying the fertilizers, it should be spread close to the plant in either side along the row. After application, the fertilizer should be incorporated well into the soil by digging with spade or forking in with a digging fork for good results. This is very important operation; as otherwise, the fertilizer would be wasted and would not be effectively utilized by the plant.

Harvesting of leaves: Leaf harvest commences after about 10 weeks from the time of pruning in June and upto 6 harvests can be taken during the year at an interval of roughly 7-8 weeks in between harvests. The quantum of harvests will depend on the precipitation received in the different seasons, being more during rainy seasons (more than $2/3^{rd}$ of the total harvest) from August to December during the first three harvests and comparatively poorer during the drought months from

January to May, except the Mungaru season when pre-monsoon showers are received resulting in a slightly improved harvest. Picking of leaves should be carried out in time *i.e.* when the leaves are at the correct stage of maturity for harvest. Otherwise, part of the leaves will become over mature course and suffer in quality from the point of view of nutritive value for the silkworms. Also part of the leaves may turn yellow, shed and be lost. Therefore, timely harvest, as the leaves reach the required stage of maturity, will lead to fuller harvest of the available leaves without wastage and realization of maximum yield. It is also important to stress here that while harvesting, the terminal buds of branches should not be picked but allowed to grow till the plant reaches its full frame of growth upto about 6 inches or so. Thereafter, the tips of the branches may be picked so as to encourage the formation of secondary branches. Unfortunately, the current practice is to strip the entire branch from top to bottom at every harvest which results in serious setback to the growing plant. This is also one of the main factors responsible for reduced harvests in the case of rain fed mulberry at present.

3.9.5 Mulberry Pest and Diseases

Powdery mildew

Causal organism: *Phyllactinia corylea*

Symptoms

- White powdery patches appear on the lower surface of leaf which is gradually increased and cover whole leaf surface.

- Affected leaves turn yellowish and defoliate prematurely.

Peak season: October-November

Control measure: Foliar spray of 0.2% Sulfex 80 WP 2 g/l. Lower surface of the leaves should be thoroughly drenched.

Safe period: 15 days

Leaf rust

Causal organism: *Peridiospora mori*

Symptoms

- Several small pin head shaped brown postules appear on the lower surface of mature leaves

- Reddish brown spot appear on the upper surface of the infected leaves.

- Severely infected leaves turn yellowish and margin of the leaves become dry.

Peak season: February-March

Control measure: Foliar spray of 0.2% Blitox 50 WP or 0.2% Bavistin 50 WP.

Safe period: 15 days.

Leaf spot

Causal organism: *Cercospora moricola*

Symptoms: Circular light brown spots appear on both sides of the leaves.

- The adjacent spots unite together to form a larger spot
- The necrotic tissues of such spots drop out and form the characteristics shot holes.
- Highly infected leaves defoliate prematurely

Peak season: Rainy and winter season.

Control measure:

- Avoid dense planting.
- Collect and burn unused infected leaves after pruning.
- Spray 0.1% Bavistin when disease symptom appears 2-3 times at ten days interval. Safe period: 7 days.

Sooty mould

Causal organism: A group of ascomycetes and deuteromycetes fungi.

Symptoms: Thick black coating developed on the upper surface of the leaves.

Peak Season: August-December.

Bacterial blight

- Foliar spray of 0.02% Monocrotophos on 15th and 30th day of pruning to control.
- Spray 0.2% Indofil M-45 75 WP to check the growth of saprophytic fungi.

Safe Period: 15 days

Foliar diseases of mulberry reduce the yield and quality of leaf thereby affecting silkworm rearing especially during rainy and winter seasons. The cumulative loss due to major foliar diseases is upto 15-18%, besides deteriorating the leaf quality. The following technologies were developed for the control of major foliar diseases to avoid the leaf yield loss.

Leaf spot: The disease caused by a fungus, *Cercospora moricola* is more prevalent during rainy and winter seasons. The symptoms are brownish necrotic, irregular spots on the leaf surface which enlarge, coalesce and leave the characteristic shot hole. Foliar spray of 0.2% Bavistin (Carbendazim 50% WP) solution (2 g Bavistin in 1 litre water) has been found effective.

Root knot Disease

It is caused by a bacteria, *Pseudomonas syringae* pv. mori/*Xanthomonas campestri* sp. v. mori and is common during rainy season when there is high humidity and temperature. It shows numerous blackish brown irregular water soaked patches on the leaves resulting in curling and rotting of leaves. Step-up pruning (30 cm above the ground) during rainy season in high rainfall areas and spraying 0.2% Streptomycin or Dithane M45 (Mancozeb 75% WP) with safe period of 2-3 days are recommended. 150-180 litres of fungicide solution is required for one-acre garden. The quantity is obtained by dissolving 300-320 g/ml of chemicals in 150-180 litres of water. First spray is to be given 30-35 days after pruning/leaf harvesting. 2nd spray has to be given 10-15 days after first spray, if the disease is not controlled. Safe period is 5 days. Root knot is one of the major diseases limiting crop production throughout the world. It can occur any time of the year mainly in sandy soils low in organic matter. The severity of the disease increases with increased age of the garden. The estimated yield loss due to the disease is 15-30 per cent. Infected plants become weak and predisposed to other diseases while severely infected plants ultimately die.

Causative organism: The organism causing root knot disease is a nematode *Meloidogyne incognita*, an endoparasite inhabiting mulberry roots.

Symptoms

i.   Stunted growth.

ii. Poor and delayed sprouting.

iii. Reduced leaf size and yield.

iv. Chlorosis and marginal necrosis of leaves, yellowing and wilting of leaves in spite of adequate soil moisture availability.

v.   Death of plants in severe cases.

Symptoms on the underground parts :

i.   Formation of gall/knots on roots.

ii. Reduced and stubby root system.

iii. Retarded root growth.

iv. Necrotic lesions on the root surfaces and death of active rootlets.

Chemical control: Chemical methods of nematode management become necessary in sick soils and heavily infested gardens as they give quick results. Furadon 3 G (40 kg/ha) can be applied either in furrows or broadcast to the soil after light harrowing followed by irrigation. The leaves from treated plots can be fed to silkworms after 45 days.

Botanical control: A water soluble compound, isolated from a plant is dissolved in water and the solution is applied by foliar spray on mulberry plants twice at an interval of 7 days. The treatment reduces root-knot and tukra disease of mulberry. No residual toxicity exists in mulberry leaves of treated plants after a couple of weeks. Then leaves could be fed to silkworm larvae safely.

3.9.6 Silkworm Diseases and Pest Control

Diseases are the behavioral and physiological changes induced by pathogens in an organism. All diseases have specific symptoms and characteristics. Similarly, silkworms are also affected by various types of diseases caused by protozoa, fungi, bacteria and viruses. Since they cause substantial financial loss to the industry, their prevention and control assumes utmost importance.

Pebrine: Pebrine is caused by a protozoan called *Nosema bombycis*. In the initial stages the larvae appears to be healthy, but when observed under a microscope we can see oval, shinning spores of Nosema. Pebine disease is infected to the silkworms in two methods; peroral and transovarial infection. In advanced stages of infection, silkworms stops feeding resulting in unequal size larvae, they become sluggish and die. The dead larvae turn black in colour due to secondary bacterial infection. If infection occurs in late V instar, the larvae spin the cocoons and the moth may also emerge. Infected female moths lay pebrine contaminated eggs in lumps one above the other. The number of eggs per laying is also drastically reduced. Pebrine is commonly observed during rainy and winter season. The spores spread through the faecal matter and digestive secretions of the infected larvae, contaminate the mulberry leaves, rearing equipments and rearing environment. Pebrine disease can be controlled by disinfecting the rearing room, equipments and rearing surroundings. During rearing, unequal size worms and faecal matter should be microscopically examined for the presence of pebrine spores and if observed, larvae, cocoons and layings should be collected and burnt or buried. In the grainages, scientific methods of mother moth examination should be employed. If pebrine disease is detected, effective disinfection should be undertaken before starting the next rearing or grainage operations. Microscopic smears are to be prepared by crushing the abdominal region of the mother moth in 2ml, 0.6% Potassium carbonate solution. Similarly, smears can be prepared from dead and unequal larvae, layings, facial matter and also from the rearing room dust. The smears should be subjected to microscopic examination and if pebrine spores are detected, the crop should be destroyed followed by disinfection.

Flacherie: Flacherie is a syndrome associated with infectious flacherie, Densonucleosis (DNV), Cytoplasmic polyhedrosis (CPV) and Bacterial diseases and several types of bacteria. The disase is caused by Infectious flacherie virus, densonucleosis virus and kenchu virus. Flacherie may be caused by virus individually as well as in association other virus or bacteria. There are different types of flacherie, white flacherie, red flacherie, chained faecal matter. The body of the infected larvae become flaccid, pale in colour and become soft. Sometimes, the facial matter is execrated in a chain form. The infected larvae stop feeding, become weak and retarded growth, fail to settle for moult and starts vomiting releasing contaminated body fluid. Dead larvae putrefying on the rearing bed and start emitting bad smell. If the infection is during the late larval stage, larvae spin the cocoon, but they die inside the cocoons, some larvae fail to spin the cocoons and die and hang on the mountage. Flacherie is observed throughout the year, but incidence is very high during rainy season. To control flacherie, the rearing room, equipments and surroundings should be disinfected. During rearing, the rearing bed should be disinfected with recommended bed disinfectants. If the incidence is high, the rearing bed should be dusted with active lime powder before feeding. Diseased, weak larvae are to be separated from the rearing bed and disposed into a bowl containing lime water. Feeding the larvae with good quality leaves, good ventilation in the rearing room and adequate bed spacing helps to prevent the incidence of flacherie. Maintenance of recommended temperature and humidity also helps to contain flacherie.

Muscardine and Aspergillosis: This is a fungal disease caused by *Beauveria bassiana*, *Aspergillus flavus*, *A. oryze* and *A. tameri*. Fungal disease in silkworms is caused mainly through cross infection. Initially the infected larvae appears normal and do not show any external symptoms. As the disease spreads, the feeding rate reduces and larvae go below the bed. The body become flaccid and soft, after death, the fungal conidia grow on the body surface and larvae become hard like white chalk. If the infection is during the fifth instar, the larvae spin the cocoons, but die inside the shell. Aspergillosis infected larvae also show the same symptoms of white muscardine but on death of the larvae, they turn green in colour. Generally fungal disease is seen during rainy season but incidence is very high during winter. High temperature and humidity required during chawki stage is also highly congenial for fungal spores to multiply. Therefore, chawki stage is also highly congenial for fungal spores to multiply. Therefore, care should be taken in observing the worms frequently. To control the spread and incidence of muscardine, disinfection of rearing room and appliances should be done scientifically. Muscardine infected larvae should be immediately separated from the bed and disposed into bowl containing lime water. Maintenance of hygiene during rearing, dusting of active lime powder on the rearing bed during moulting periods, good ventilation in the rearing room and providing adequate spacing in the bed helps to prevent the occurrence of muscardine. Dusting of 1-2% Dithane M45 in Kaolin or Captan in claked lime on silkworm body immediately after every moult and on the 4th day of fifth instar at 3-5 g/sq.ft. Old news paper or paraffin paper is covered for 30 min. feeding should be given afterwards.

3.10 Apiculture

3.10.1 Prefixture

Apiculture is derived from the honeybee's Latin name *Apis mellifera*, meaning honey gatherer. Since bees do not collect honey but nectar from which honey is made, the scientific name should actually be *Apis mellifica* meaning honey maker. Although apiculture refers to the honeybee, the vital role all bees play in the pollination of crops and flowering plants has caused apiculture to also include the management and study of non-Apis bees such as bumblebees and leafcutter bees. Some 90 million years ago, flowering plants first appeared on earth. The wasp-like ancestors of bees took advantage of the food made available by flowers and began to modify their diet and physical characteristics. Since then, flowering plants and bees co-evolved. This eventually led to a complete interdependence, meaning that flowering plants and bees cannot live and reproduce without each other. The genus Apis is comprised of a comparatively small number of species including the western honeybee *Apis mellifera*, the eastern honeybee *Apis cerana*, the giant bee *Apis dorsata* and the small honeybee *Apis florea*. Honeybees are indigenous to the Eurasian and African continents and were introduced to the Americas and Australia by European settlers. The western honeybee is comprised of some 24 races or sub-species. The African honeybee, sometimes referred to as Killer bee, is a race of the western honeybee and can cross-breed. Bees collect pollen and nectar. Pollen is the protein source needed for bee brood development while nectar is the carbohydrate source providing energy. Nectar is a sugar solution produced by flowers containing about 80 per cent water and 20 per cent sugars. Foraging bees store the nectar in the honey sac where the enzyme invertase will change complex sugars into simple sugars called mono-saccharides. Upon return to the hive, the foraging bee will disgorge the partially converted nectar solution and offer it to other bees. Housekeeping bees will complete the enzymatic conversion, further removing water until the honey solution contains between 14-20per cent water. Honey is too dry for any microbes to live in. Honey is non-perishable and can be kept indefinitely in a cool, dry place. The flavor, aroma and color of honey are determined by the floral source. For example, buckwheat honey is almost black while fireweed honey is almost colorless. Unlike other bees, honeybees can communicate details about the location, quality and quantity of food sources. This allows honeybees to access and utilize food sources efficiently at great distances. Honeybees maintain temperatures in the brood nest of between 30 and 34°C, even in the middle of winter. The honeybee colony is comprised of one queen, thousands of worker bees and a few hundred male bees called drones. Colony size varies according to season and condition of the colony. Several diseases including viruses, various microbes and mites can affect the honeybee.

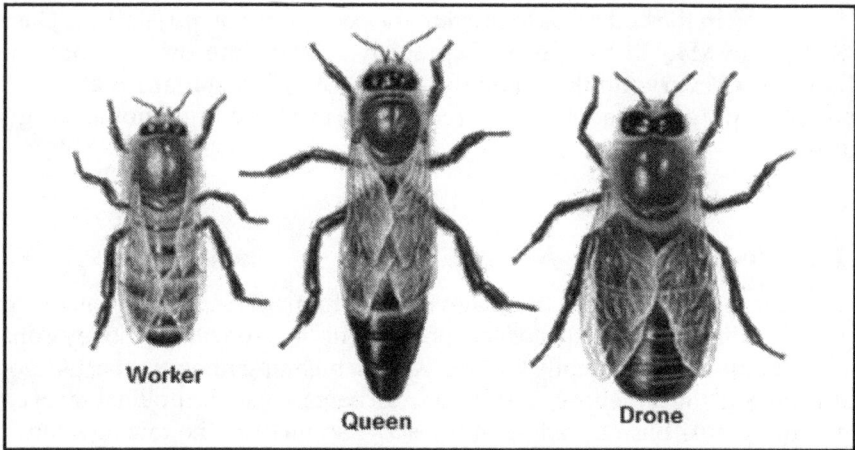

Figure 3.15a: Honey bees

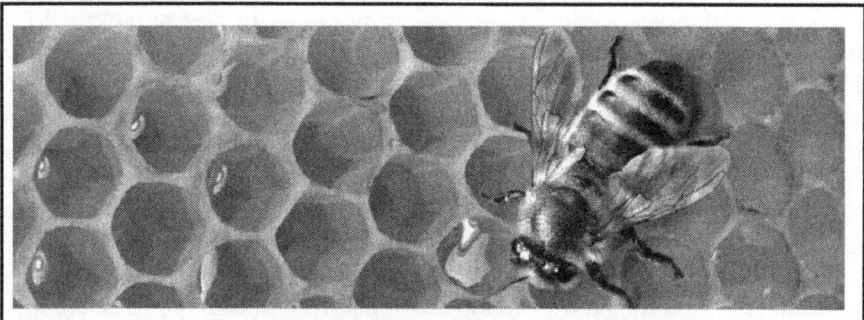

Figure 3.15b: Honey bee in Honey comb

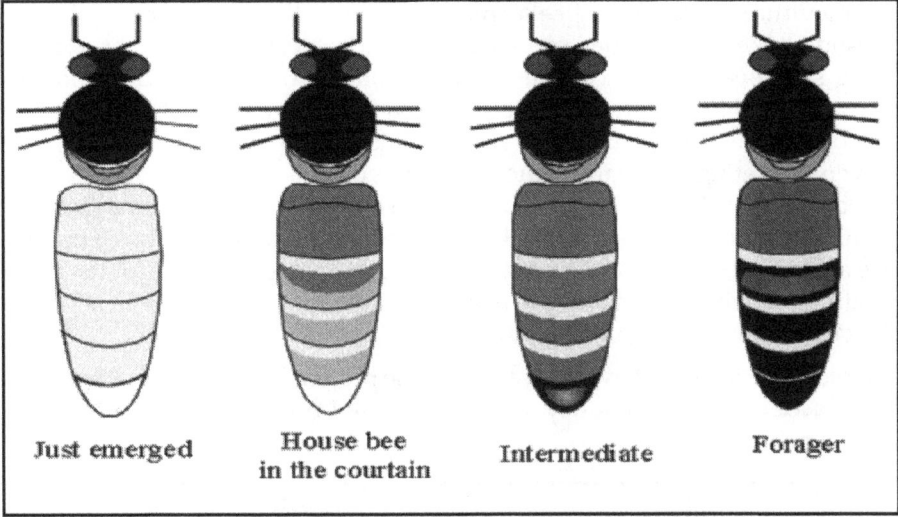

Figure 3.15c: Workers of *Apis dorsata*

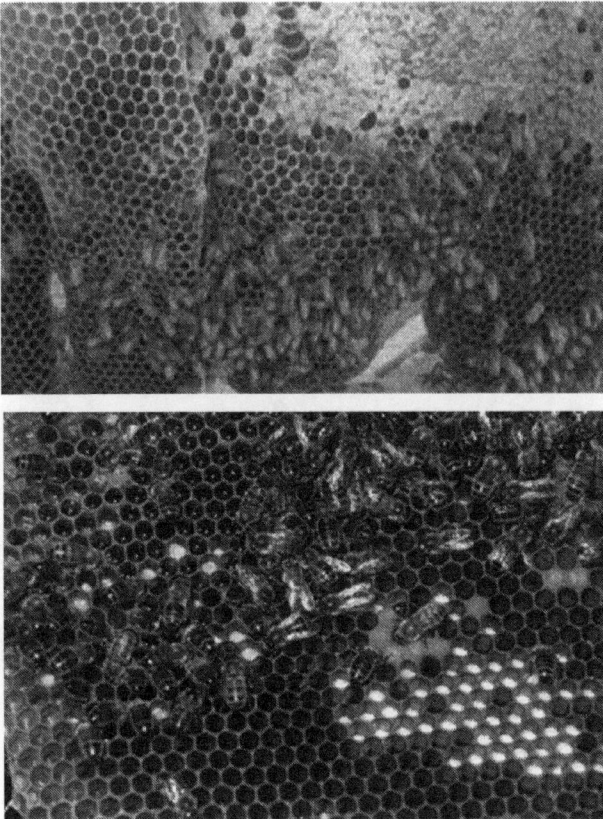

Figure 3.15d: Honey comb

Apiculture is the art of beekeeping, but more than just keeping hives and harvesting honey, it includes setting up properly located and constructed hives, making sure bees have access to plentiful sources of nectar and preparing the harvested liquid honey after it has been taken from the hive. It also includes being aware of local laws governing the keeping of bees and processing of their products and even marketing the final products. Colonies of bees are highly socialized groups of insects that create their own ecosystems in and around their hives. Before even beginning to set up a beekeeping hobby or business, gaining a thorough knowledge of bee anatomy, behavior and ecology can build an invaluable basis for the business. An individual who undertakes the responsibility of keeping a hive is taking on an entire civilization of creatures.

Apiculture does not have to be a large scale project. Keeping a few hives can give families access to endless honey as well as related products like beeswax candles and fresh honeycombs.

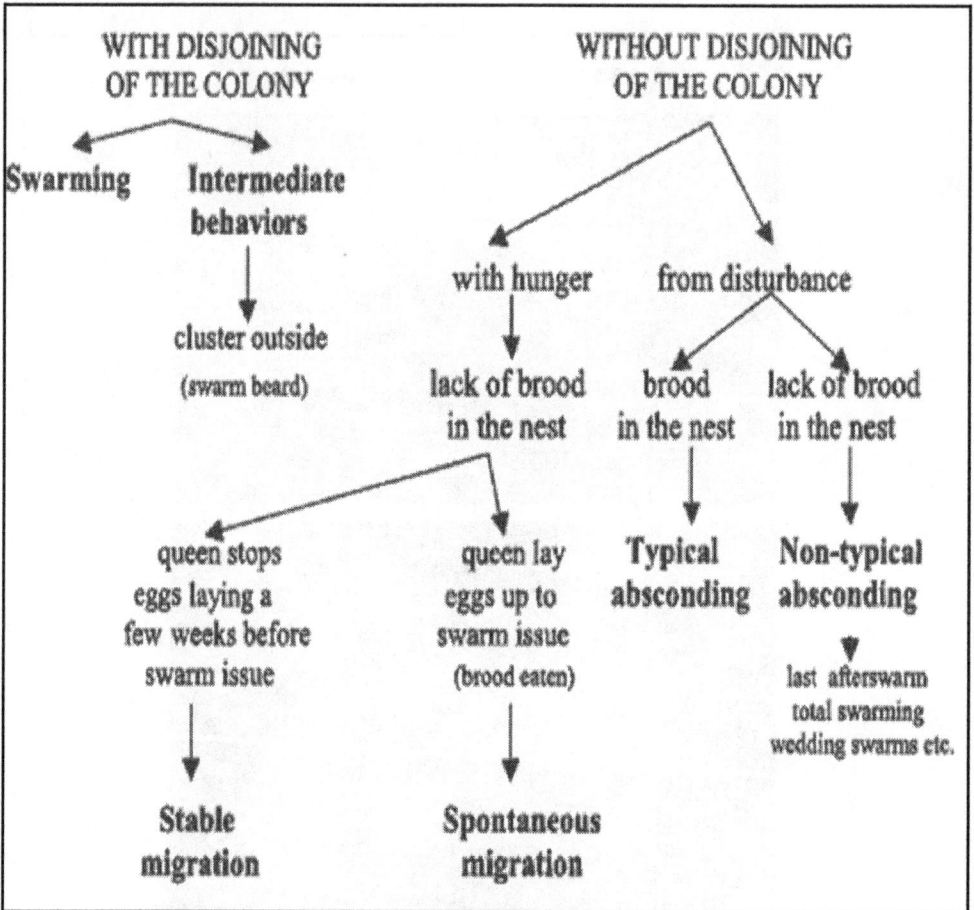

Figure 3.16: Nest abandonment by Swarms

It can also go hand-in-hand with other activities, such as gardening, as a few properly managed hives can provide invaluable pollination services to flowers, fruit trees and vegetables.Some of the hands-on processes of apiculture include constructing the hives and upkeep on these outdoor structures that can become weathered by the elements. Handling the bees can be one of the most difficult tasks. A smoker and proper clothing can help the beekeeper keep from getting stung while removing honeycombs or carrying out the delicate procedures of replacing the hive's queen bee. While it may seem strange to relate management techniques to bees, it is a vital skill. Beekeepers must know what the bees require before they can build a successful hive, including providing consistent sources of fresh water, nectar and pollen. An individual who is both aware and respectful of the natural cycle of bees will find handling them much easier and he or she will also be alert to pests and threats to the hive before they become a real problem. Keeping an eye on rainfall charts, temperatures, climate changes and information on area vegetation can help the alert beekeeper avoid or prepare for potential problems. An important part of keeping bees is knowing regional and national regulations regarding beekeeping. Honey is a food product and as such, its preparation is subject to regulations. There are also rules about where hives can be placed in residential areas and insurance concerns to be investigated as an ongoing part of the business.

3.10.2 Production Process

a. Equipment requirements for Bee keeping

- **Hive:** It is a simple long box covered with a number of slats on top. The rough measurements of the box should be around 100 cm of length, 45 cm of width and 25 cm in height. The box should be 2 cm thick and the hive must be glued and screwed together with entrance holes of 1 cm wide. The slats (top bars) must be as long as the hive is wide in order to fit across and the thickness of about 1.5 cm is sufficient to support a heavy honey comb. The width of 3.3 cm needs to be given to give the bees the natural spacing they need to easily build one comb to each separate top bar.

- **Smoker:** It is the second important piece of equipment. This can be made from a small tin. We use the smoker to protect ourselves from bee stings and to control the bees.

- **Cloth:** To protect our eyes and nose from stings at the time of work near the apiary.

- **Knife:** It is used to loosen the top bars and to cut off the honey bars.

- **Feather:** To sweep the bees from the comb.

- **Queen Excluder:** It is a selective barrier inside the beehive that allows worker bees but not the larger queens and drones to traverse the barrier.

- **Match box:** A matchbox is a box made of cardboard or thin wood designed to hold matches. It usually has a coarse striking surface on one edge for lighting the matches contained inside.

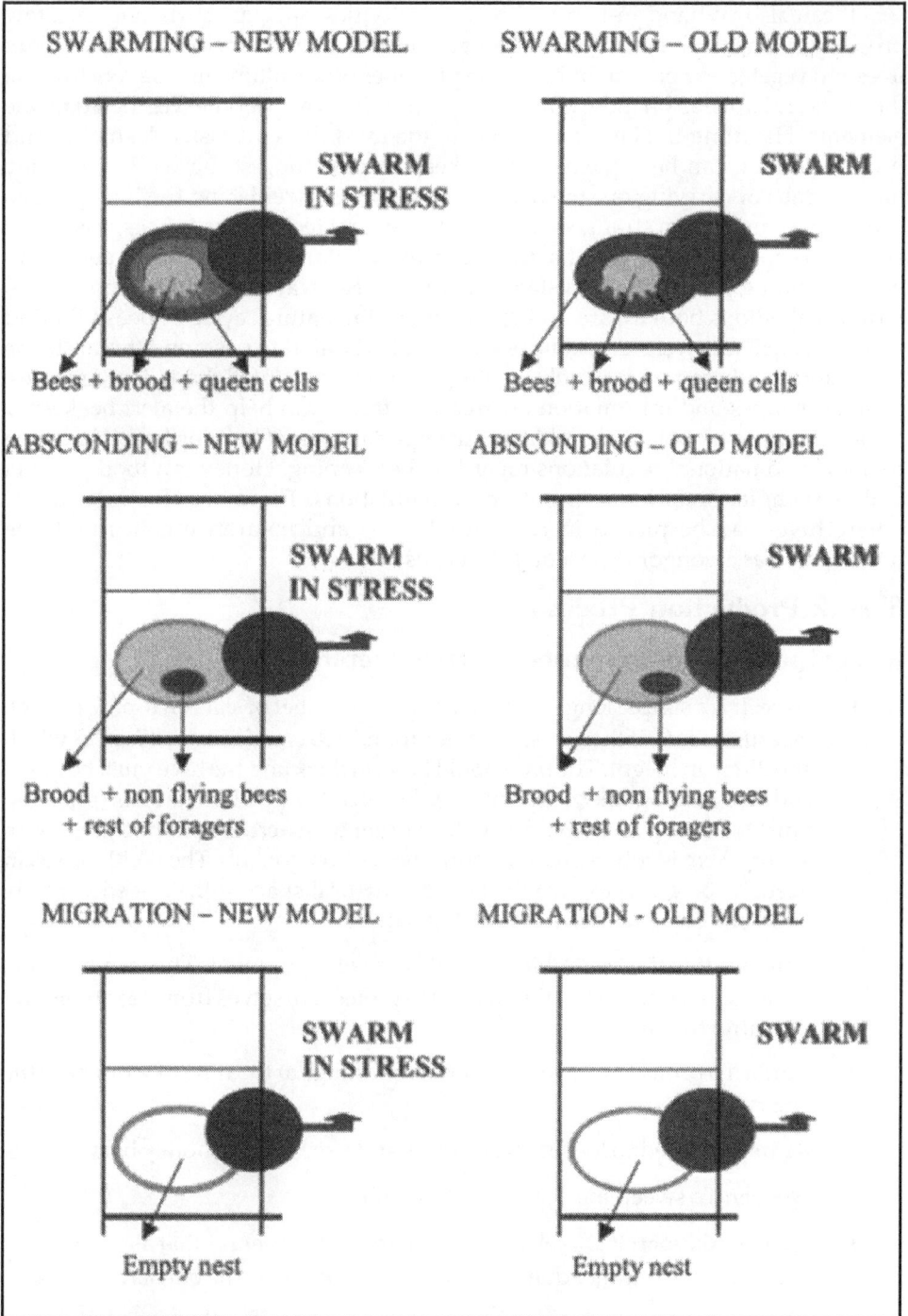

SWARMING – NEW MODEL

SWARM
IN STRESS

Bees + brood + queen cells

SWARMING – OLD MODEL

SWARM

Bees + brood + queen cells

ABSCONDING – NEW MODEL

SWARM
IN STRESS

Brood + non flying bees
+ rest of foragers

ABSCONDING – OLD MODEL

SWARM

Brood + non flying bees
+ rest of foragers

MIGRATION – NEW MODEL

SWARM
IN STRESS

Empty nest

MIGRATION - OLD MODEL

SWARM

Empty nest

Figure 3.17: Models of Nest for honey bee

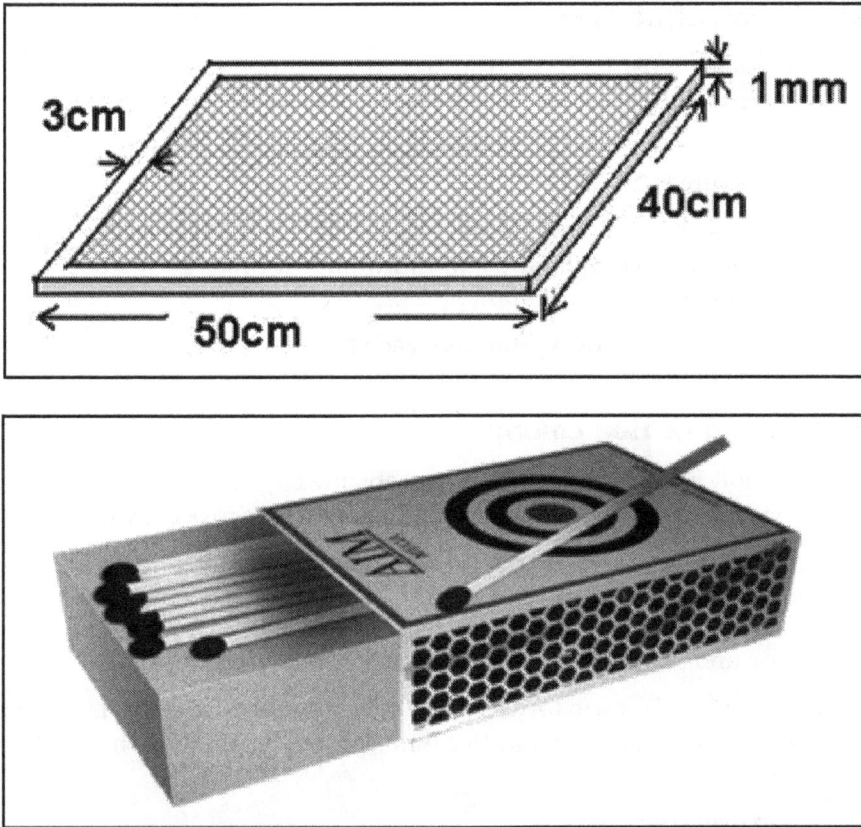

Figure 3.18: Queen Excluder and Match Box

b. Species of Honey bees

There are four species of honeybees in India. They are:

- **Rock bee** (*Apis dorsata*): They are good honey gathers with an average yield of 50-80kg per colony.

- **Little bee** (*Apis florea*): They are poor honey yielders and yield about 200-900g of honey per colony.

- **Indian bee** (*Apis cerana indica*): They yield an average honey yield of 6-8 kg per colony per year.

- **European bee** [Italian bee] (*Apis mellifera*): The average production per colony is 25-40 kg.

- Sting less laip present in Kerala known as stingless bees. They are not truly stingless, but sting is poorly developed. They are efficient pollinators. They yield 300-400 g of honey per year.

c. Establishment of hives

- The apiary must be located in well-drained open area, preferably near orchards, with profuse source of nectar, pollen and water.

- Protection from sunlight is important in order to maintain an optimum temperature in the hive.

- Ant wells are fixed around the hive stand. The colonies must be directed towards east, with slight changes in the directions of the bee box as a protection from rain and sun.

- Keep the colonies away from the reach of cattle, other animal, busy roads and streetlights.

d. Establishing of Bee colony

- To establish a bee colony, bees can be obtained by transferring a wild nesting colony to a hive or attract a passing swarm of bees to occupy it.

- Before putting a swarm or even a colony in a prepared hive, it would be beneficial to make the hive smell familiar by rubbing old brown comb pieces or some bee wax. If possible, the Queen bee can be captured from a natural swarm and placed under a hive to attract the other bees.

- Feed the hived swarm for a few weeks by diluting a half cup of white sugar in half a cup of hot water as this will also help in building the comb along with the bars rapidly.

- Avoid over crowding

e. Management of colonies

- Inspect the beehives at least once in a week during the honey-flow seasons preferably during the morning hours.

- Clean the hive in the following sequence, the roof, super/supers, brood chambers and floorboard.

- Observe the colonies regularly for the presence of healthy queen, brood development, storage of honey and pollen, presence of queen cells, bee strength and growth of drones.

Look for the infestation by any of the following bee enemies

- Wax moth (*Galleria mellonella*): Remove all the larvae and silken webbings from the combs, corners and crevices of bee box.

- Wax beetles (*Platybolium* sp.): Collect and destroy the adult beetles.

- Mites: Clean the frame and floorboard with cotton swabs moistened with freshly made potassium permanganate solution. Repeat until no mites are seen on the floorboard.

Management during lean season

- Remove the supers and arrange the available healthy broods compactly in the brood chamber.

- Provide division board, if necessary.

- Destroy queen cells and drone cells, if noted.

- Provide sugar syrup (1:1) at the rate of 200 g sugar per colony per week for Indian bees.

- Feed all the colonies in the apiary at the same time to avoid robbing.

Management during honey flow season

- Keep the colony in sufficient strength before honey-flow season.

- Provide maximum space between the first super and the brood chamber and not above the first super.

- Place queen excluder sheets in between brood and super chamber to confine the queen to brood chamber.

- Examine the colony once in a week and frames full of honey should be removed to the sides of the super. The frames, which are $3/4^{th}$ filled with honey or pollen and one-fourth with sealed brood should be taken out of brood chamber and in its place empty combs or frames with foundation is added.

- The combs, which are completely sealed or $2/3^{rd}$ capped may be taken out for extraction of honey and returned to supers after honey extraction.

f. Harvesting of honey

- Harvest the honey by smoking the bees off the parts which needs to be harvested and cut the combs carefully.

- Harvests are normally possible during and shortly after the two main flowering seasons, namely October/November and February-June.

- A ripe comb is light in colour and filled with honey. More than half of the honey cells on both the sides are sealed with wax.

3.10.3 Beekeeping in India

Honey and beekeeping have a long history in India. Honey was the first sweet food tasted by the ancient Indian inhabiting rock shelters and forests. They hunted bee hives for this gift of God. India has some of the oldest records of beekeeping in the form of paintings by prehistoric man in the rock shelters. With the development of civilization, honey acquired an unique status in the lives of the ancient Indians. They regarded honey as a magical substance that controlled the fertility of women, cattle, as also their lands and crops. The recent past has witnessed a revival of the industry in the rich forest regions along the sub-Himalayan mountain ranges and the Western

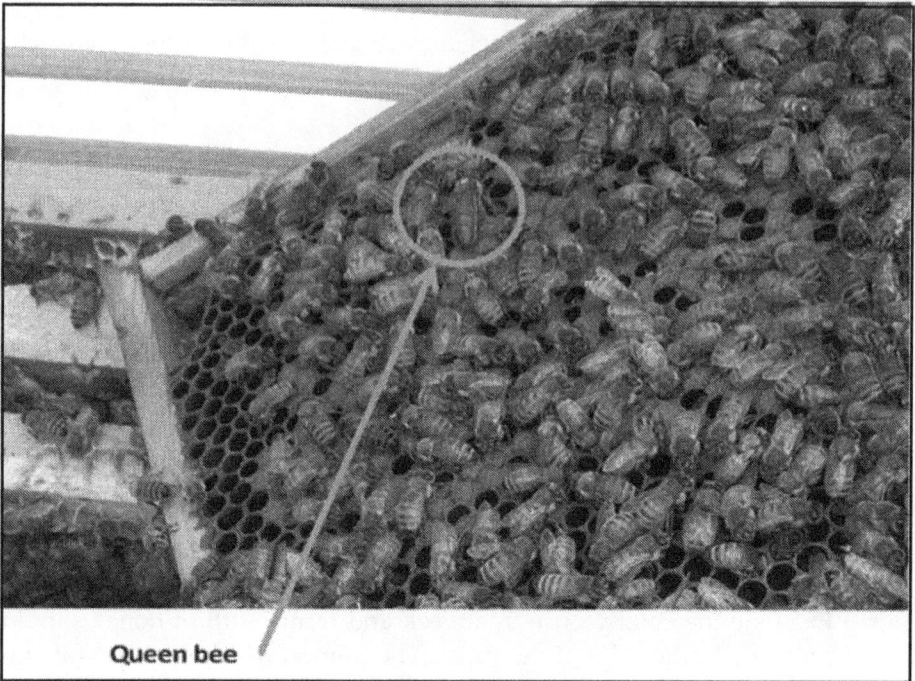

Figure 3.19a: Queen Bee

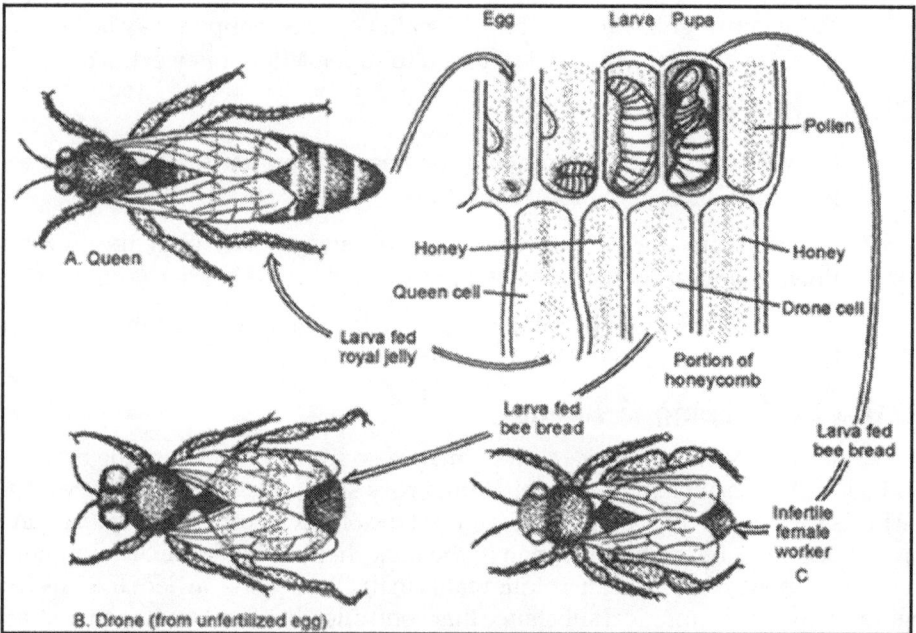

Figure 3.19b: Life Cycle of Honeybee

In India beekeeping has been mainly forest based. Several natural plant species provide nectar and pollen to honey bees. Thus, the raw material for production of honey is available free from nature. Bee hives neither demand additional land space nor do they compete with agriculture or animal husbandry for any input. The beekeeper needs only to spare a few hours in a week to look after his bee colonies. Beekeeping is therefore ideally suited to him as a part-time occupation. Beekeeping constitutes a resource of sustainable income generation to the rural and tribal farmers. It provides them valuable nutrition in the form of honey, protein rich pollen and brood. Bee products also constitute important ingredients of folk and traditional medicine. The establishment of Khadi and Village Industries Commission to revitalize the traditional village industries hastened the development of beekeeping. During the 1980s, an estimated one million bee hives had been functioning under various schemes of the Khadi and Village Industries Commission. Production of apiary honey in the country reached 10,000 tons, valued at about Rs. 300 million. Side by side with the development of apiculture using the indigenous bee, *Apis cerana*, apiculture using the European bee, *Apis mellifera*, gained popularity in Jammu and Kashmir, Punjab, Himachal Pradesh, Haryana, Uttar Pradesh, Bihar and West Bengal. Wild honey bee colonies of the giant honey bee and the oriental hive bee have also been exploited for collection of honey. Tribal populations and forest dwellers in several parts of India have honey collection from wild honey bee nests as their traditional profession. The methods of collection of honey and beeswax from these nests have changed only slightly over the millennia. The major regions for production of this honey are the forests and farms along the sub-Himalayan tracts and adjacent foothills, tropical forest and cultivated vegetation in Rajasthan, Uttar Pradesh, Madhya Pradesh, Maharashtra and Eastern Ghats in Orissa and Andhra Pradesh.

The raw materials for the beekeeping industry are mainly pollen and nectar that come from flowering plants. Both the natural and cultivated vegetation in India constitute an immense potential for development of beekeeping. About 500 flowering plant species, both wild and cultivated, are useful as major or minor sources of nectar and pollen. There are at least four species of true honey bees and three species of the stingless bees. Several sub-species and races of these are known to exist. In recent years the exotic honey bee has been introduced. Together these represent a wide variety of bee fauna that can be utilized for the development of honey industry in the country. There are several types of indigenous and traditional hives including logs, clay pots, wall niches, baskets and boxes of different sizes and shapes. In modern beekeeping, the combs are built on wooden frames that are moveable. This facilitates inspection and management of bee colonies. Three types of moveable frame hive are in common use; the Newton type along with its standardized version ISI Type A, the Jeolikote Villager and its counterpart ISI Type B and the Langstroth type. Besides the hives, the beekeepers need equipment and implements like the hive stand, nucleus box and smoker. The industry also needs equipment and machinery for handling and processing of honey, beeswax, for manufacture of comb foundation sheets and for other operations. India has a potential to keep about 120 million bee colonies that can provide self-employment to over 6 million rural and tribal families. In terms of production, these bee colonies can produce over 1.2 million tons of honey and about 15,000 tons of beeswax. Organized collection of forest honey and beeswax using improved methods can result in an additional production of at least 120,000 tons of honey and 10,000 tons of beewax. This can generate income to about 5 million tribal families.

Modern beekeeping also includes production of beeswax, bee collected pollen, bee venom, royal jelly, propolis, as also of package bees, queen bees and nucleus colonies. All these are possible only with a proper management of bees, utilizing the local plant resources and adapting to the local climatic conditions. Modern beekeeping makes heavy use of beekeeping equipment and honey processing plant. This results in high efficiency and also ensures the quality of the processed honey. Seasonal management of bee colonies varies in different parts of the country although the basic management methods are the same.

Flow management, dearth management, provision of feeding and control and cure of bee disorders, bee diseases, pests and enemies, are some of the routine measures to keep bee colonies healthy and strong. There are special management techniques like queen rearing, migration for honey production or for colony multiplication, which the beekeeper takes up after he gains sufficient knowledge and experience in handling bee colonies. About 10,000 tons of forest honey is produced annually. Apiary honey produced under the KVI sector is estimated to be a little less than 10,000 tons in 1990-1991. Over 95% of this was from the *A. cerana* colonies, the rest being from the European bee colonies. Forest honey, mostly from rock bee hives, is usually collected by tribals in forests and is procured by forest or tribal corporations as a minor forest produce. Quite a large quantity is also collected by groups or individuals on their own. Forest honey is usually thin, contains large quantity of pollen, bee juices and parts, wax and soil particles.

The honey collector gets between Rs. 10 and Rs. 25 per kilogram of the forest honey. Forest honeys are mostly multifloral. Apiary honey is produced in bee hives and is harvested by extraction in honey extractors. Other types of beekeeping equipment like queen excluder, smoker, hive tool, pollen trap, honey processing plant are also used. Beekeepers sell the honey to the co-operative society, if one exists in the area. In many parts of India, the beekeeper gets a much higher price if he sells it directly to the consumer. Apiary honeys are usually multifloral when marketed by state level marketing organizations, because honeys from different sources are mixed while pooling, storage and processing. Several unifloral honeys are available in markets restricted to small areas within the state where it is produced. Rubber plant contributed to over 60 % of the total apiary honey production during 1990-1991. Besides this, jamun, hirda, beheda, arjun, neem, litchi, palmyrah palm, eucalyptus, lagerstroemias, tamarind, cashew tree, scheffleras, tun, karanj, false acacia, wild shrubs like shain, crops of different varieties of mustards, sesame, niger, sunflower, berseem clover, khesari, coriander orchard trees including different types of citrus, apple, puddum, cherry and other temperate fruit trees, coconut tree and coffee plantations are some important sources that provide unifloral honey.

Much of the forest honey is sold to the pharmaceutical, confectionery and food industries, where it is processed and used in different formulations. Apiary honey is usually processed at the producer's level. This consists mainly of heating the honey and filtering. A few beekeepers or honey producers co-operative societies have better processing facilities that involve killing of honey fermenting yeasts. About 50 % of the apiary honey under the KVI sector is graded and marketed under AGMARK specifications. In 1985 the consumption of honey was estimated to be about 8.4 g per capita, while in other countries this was 200 g. presently this would be about 2.5 g. Honey has so far been consumed mainly as a medicine and for religious purposes. A small quantity has been used in kitchen as an ingredient of pickles, jams and preserves. With the increasing production in recent years, there is an increasing trend to use honey in food.

This is obviously the case with the affluent segments of the population. Forest honey is used in pharmaceutical, food, confectionery, bakery and cosmetic industries. One often finds a good demand for local honeys like honeys from Mahabaleshwar. People in Maharashtra have a strong liking for jamun, hirda or gela honeys which have acquired special individual medicinal significance. Similarly, kartiki honey in Kumaon, Uttar Pradesh is locally much favored. Some honeys have an essentially non-local market. Rubber tree honey can only be sold in non-local markets. Coorg honey with its characteristic flavour was well known during 1950s and 1960s. Shain or sulah honey from Kashmir has been very popular. Presently litchi honey from Bihar and other northern states is in great demand. The price structure is regulated by the market forces of supply and demand. Beekeepers in well-known hill stations and other places of tourist attraction take advantage of the popularity of honey and can market their produce at remunerative prices. Indian honey has a good export market. With the use of modern collection, storage, beekeeping equipment, honey processing plants and bottling technologies the potential export market can be tapped.

Honey

Honey is a supersaturated sugar solution with approximately 17.1% water. Fructose is the predominant sugar at 38.5%, followed by glucose at 31%. Disaccharides, trisaccharides and oligosaccharides are present in much smaller quantities. Besides carbohydrates, honey contains small amounts of protein, (including enzymes), vitamins and minerals. Honey yields 64 calories per tablespoon, making it a more concentrated source of energy than other common sweeteners. While the amino acid content is minor, the broad spectrum of approximately 18 essential and nonessential amino acids present in honey is unique and varies by floral source. Proline is the primary amino acid with lysine being the second most prevalent. Other amino acids found in honey include phenylalanine, tyrosine, glutamic and aspartic acids. The glutamic acid is a product of the glucose oxidase reaction.[13] Proline and other amino acids are contributed by pollens, nectar or bee themselves.

The past two decades have brought a resurgence of interest in learning more about antimicrobial and wound healing properties of honey. Studies conducted in various parts of the world indicate the following:

Table 3.2 Nutrients (%) in Honey

Nutrient	Percentage
Water	17.20 %
Fructose	38.29 %
Glucose	31.28 %
Sucrose	1.31%
Maltose	7.21 %
Carbohydrates	1.54 %
Acid	0.57 %
Protein	0.26 %
Minerals	0.17 %
Enzymes, Vitamins etc.	2.21 %

- Honey is a natural source of energy for the body. Sugars are the fundamental unit of energy for our bodies. Honey is high in monosaccharide glucose and fructose. These sugars are quickly absorbed, providing the body with boost of energy. Doctors say that these sugars works best to enhance athletic performance and prevent fatigue.

- Dr. Susan Percival of University of Florida's Department of Food Science and Human Nutrition found the honey is rich in vitamins, amino acids, calcium, iron, magnesium and zinc-, all of which are essentials to good health. Honey contains several compounds that function as antioxidants. Antioxidants perform the role of eliminating free radicals, which are reactive compounds in our bodies. Free radicals are created through the normal process of metabolism and are believed to contribute too many serious diseases when left unchecked. Antioxidants play a large role in the prevention of cancer and heart disease.

- Research by Peter C. Molan, has shown that honey stops the growth of dental plaque bacteria and reduces the amount of acid produced, which stops the bacteria from producing dextran (a component of dental plaque).

- Honey has anti-inflammatory effects. It is used to relieve sore throat pain.

- Honey is a carbohydrate and will increase the level of tryptophan, an amino acid that is used in the production of serotonin, which is a neurotransmitter in the brain that will induce a sense of calm and drowsiness. That is why some people drink a cup of water with a spoonful of honey before sleep.

- A regular administration of honey helps to prolong and to give a better life quality to the seniors. The famous Chinese doctor, Tao Hongjing believes that People that want to have a long and healthy life should use honey daily. In recent research, it was demonstrated that in a survey of 100 people aged over 100 years old, over 80% of them regularly consumed honey. Honey benefits human longevity due to its high energy action and the presence of chemical elements, vitamins and enzymes that are important for the good operation of the human body.

3.11 Lac-culture

Lac culture is the cultivation of lac insects for the production of lac. The important lac producing countries are India and Thailand. The important centers in India are Bihar accounting 40 % of the country's total production, Madhya Pradesh, West Bengalorissa, Assam and Uttar Pradesh. Lac is a natural resinous substance of profound economic importance in India. It is the only resin from animal origin lending itself to diverse applications *e.g.* as a protective and decorative coating in the form of thin films, adhesives and plastics. It makes a small but significant contribution to the foreign exchange earning of the country, but the most important role that the lac plays in the economy of the country is that roughly 3-4 million tribal people, who constitute the socioeconomically weakest link of Indian population earn a subsidiary income from its cultivation. India is the major producer of lac, accounting for more than 50% of the total world production. It virtually held a monopoly in the lac trade during the period of the world war-I, producing nearly 90% of the world's total output. Today an average of about 20-22 thousand tons of stick lac (raw lac) is produced in the country per year. Most of the lac produced in India is from homestead land and wasteland. Usually host trees standing on rayyati lands are used for lac cultivation and in some areas trees on Government land are taken on lease or rental basis.

3.11.1 Lac

Lac is a resinous exudation from the body of female scale insect. Since Vedic period, it has been in use in India. Its earliest reference is found in *Atherva Veda*. There, the insect is termed as Laksha and its habit and behavior are described. The great Indian epic *Mahabharata* also mentions a Laksha Griha, an inflammable house of lac, cunningly constructed by Kauravas through their architect Purocha for the purpose of burning their great enemy Pandavas alive.

The English word lac synonyms Lakh in Hindi which itself is derivative of Sanskrit word Laksh meaning a lakh or hundred thousand. It would appear that Vedic people knew that the lac is obtained from numerous insects and must also know the biological and commercial aspects of lac industry. It is also worth to mention that a laksh griha would need a lot of lac which could only come from a flourishing lac industry in that period. Since ancient times, Greeks and Romans were familiar with the use of lac. The cultivation of lac insects has a long history in Asia, with some suggestion that it is as old as 4000 years in China where its cultivation accompanied the development of the silk industry. Lac is Nature's gift to mankind and the only known commercial resin of animal origin. It is the hardened resin secreted by tiny lac insects belonging to a bug family. To produce 1 kg of lac resin, around 300,000 insects lose their life. The lac insects yields resin, lac dye and lac wax. Application of these products has been changing with time. Lac resin, dye etc. still find extensive use in *Ayurveda* and *Siddha* systems of medicine. With increasing universal environment awareness, the importance of lac has assumed special relevance in the present age, being an eco-friendly, biodegradable and self-sustaining natural material. Since lac insects are cultured on host trees which are growing primarily in wasteland areas, promotion of lac and its culture can help in eco-system development as well as reasonably high economic returns. It is a source of livelihood of tribal and poor inhabiting forest and sub-forest area.

Lac is a natural, biodegradable, non-toxic, odourless, tasteless, hard resin and non-injurious to health. Lac is a resinous protective secretion of tiny lac insect, *Kerria lacca* (Kerr.) which belongs to the family Tachardidae in the super family Coccoidea of the order Hemiptera. The lac insect is a pest on a number of plants both wild as well as cultivated. The tiny red–coloured larvae of lac insect settle on the young succulent shoots of the host plants in myriads and secrete a thick resinous fluid which covers their bodies. The secretions from the insects form a hard continuous encrustation over the twigs. The encrusted twigs are harvested and the encrusted twigs scraped off, dried and processed to yield the lac of commerce which is regarded as Non Wood Forest Product (NWFP) of great economic importance to India. If lac crops are harvested by cutting down the lac bearing twigs a little before the larval emergence, that lac is known as ARI LAC (immature lac) or after the emergence is over, that is called phunki lac (empty lac).

Forms of Lac

- **Stick lac**: The lac encrustations is separated by knife or broken off with finger from the twig of host plants and is known is stick lac or crude lac or raw lac.

- **Seed lac**: The stick lac, after grinding and washing, is called seed lac or chowri.

- **Shellac**: The manufactured product prepared from stick lac after washing and melting, which takes the form of yellow coloured flakes, is called shellac.

- **Button lac** : After melting process, lac is dropped on a zinc sheet and allowed to spread out into round discs of about 3 inches diameter and ¼ inches thickness is called button lac

- **Garnet lac**: It is prepared form inferior seed lac or kiri by the solvent extraction process. It is dark in colour and comparatively free from wax.

- **Bleached lac**: It is a refined product obtained by chemical treatment. It is prepared by dissolving shellac or seed lac in Sodium carbonate solution, bleaching the solution with Sodium hypochlorite and precipitating the resin with sulphuric acid. Bleached lac deteriorates quickly and should be used within 2-3 months of manufacture.

Composition of Lac

The major constituents of stick lac or crude lac are resin, sugar, protein, soluble salt, coloring matter, wax, volatile oils, sand, woody matters and insect bodies. The resin is always associated with an odoriferous principle, a wax and a mixture of three dyes. Removal of both wax and dye results in a marvelous colourless and transparent resin having all the characteristic properties of the resin. Chemical analysis has revealed that the resin is made of at least six major chemical components of different molecular complexities. The building blocks of lac are mainly hydroxyaliphatic and sequiterpenic acids which are present in the proportion of 50:50. The basic blocks are aleuritic and jalaric acids. The former is 9, 10, 16-trihydroxy palmitic acid and the later adihydroxymonocarboxylic sesquiterpenic acid having an aldehyde functions.

Composition of stick Lac

Lac resin- 68%

Lac wax- 6%

Lac dye- 1%

Others- 25%

Lac resin: It is an ester complex of long chain hydroxy fatty acids and sesquiterpenic acid.

Lac dye: It is an anthraquinone derivative.

Lac wax: It is the mixture of higher alcohol, esters, acids and hydrocarbons.

Properties of Lac

The important properties of lac are as follows:

(i) Soluble in alcohol and weak alkalis,

(ii) Capacity of forming uniform durable film,

(iii) Possess high scratch hardness,

(iv) Resistance to water,

(v) Good adhesive nature,

(vi) Ability to form good sealers, undercoat primers,

(vii) Capacity to allow quick rubbing with sandpaper without slicking or gumming.

No other single resin, both natural and synthetic, possesses so many desirable properties and so lac is also termed as multipurpose resin.

Uses of Lac: Because of its unique combination of properties, lac finds a wide variety of application in paint, electrical, automobile, cosmetic, adhesive, leather, wood finishing and other industries. Earlier about half of the total output was consumed in gramophone industry. Lac has long been in use both for decorative and lacquers of various kinds and insulating varnishes. It is usually used as a first coating on wood to fill the pores and also applied to seal knots likely to exude resin and disfigure or spoil finished paint work. Lac is used in manufacture of glazed paper, printing and water proofing inks, lac bangles, dry mounting tissue paper, dental plates and optical frames. It is also used as a coat for metal ware to prevent tarnishing and for finishing various products such as playing cards, oil cloth and linoleum and for preserving archeological and zoological specimen. In electrical industry, lac is used as coating of insulator, coating of spark plugs, cement of sockets of electrical lamp, ant tracking insulating etc. In Pharmaceutical industry, lac is used in coating of tablets, micro-encapsulation of vitamins and coating of medicines. Lac dye is used in dying of wool and silk, soft drink formulation, pill coating, confectionary and chocolate coating. Lac wax has wide variety of uses in manufacturing shoe polishes, tailor's chalk, lipstick, crayons (for writing in glass). Now days it is also used in fruit coating.

Lac Production in India: India and Thailand are the two major producers of lac. The main lac producing states in India are Chhattisgarh, Jharkhand, Madhya Pradesh, West Bengal, Uttar Pradesh orissa, Maharashtra and Gujarat. The cultivation of lac is at present mainly confined to the conventional lac hosts trees of Palas, Ber and Kusum. At present total annual average production of stick lac in India is approximately 20-22 thousand tons which forms the raw material for lac industries. Chhattisgarh ranks 1st among the states followed by Jharkhand, Madhya Pradesh Maharashtra and West Bengal in lac production. These five states contribute around 95 % of the national lac production. .Nearly 75-80% of the finished product is exported and only a small portion nearly 20 to 25 % is consumed within the country. Area wise host plant for lac culture is listed below.

i. Palas *(Butea monosperma):* It is commonest lac host throughout the greater part of India, extending from North West Himalaya up to 900 m in hills of South India upto 1200 m.

ii. Kusum *(Schleichera oleosa):* Throughout Central and South India, Jharkhand, Madhya Pradesh orissa and parts of Karnataka and Tamilnadu.

iii. Ber *(Zizyphus mauritiana):* Important lac host in Murshidabad and Malda districts of West Bengal and Hoshiarpur district of Punjab State, Jharkhand and Chhattisgarh

iv. Khair *(Acacia catechu):* Only Jharkhand State (Chotanagpur area)

v. Ghont *(Zizyphus zylopyra):* Mainly cultivated in some parts of Northern Madhya Pradesh and Southern Uttar Pradesh.

vi. Jallari *(Shorea talura)*: It is the host plant in parts of Mysore and Chennai

vii. Galwang *(Albizia lucida):* It is an important lac host in Assam and has also given good results in Chotanagpur area in Jharkhand.

viii. Ficus sp. *(F. religiosa, F. bengalensis, F. infectoria):* These are universal in occurrence and from which occasionally lac is collected here and there throughout India.

ix. Arhar *(Cajanus cajan)* Grewia sp. *(G. glabra* and *G. serruleta) Leea sp. (L. aspera, L. crispa* and *L. robusta), Ficus cunia* are the favoured host plants in Assam.

3.11.2 Lac Hosts

The lac insects thrive on the sap of certain plants called lac hosts. So far, over four hundred species of plants have been recorded as hosts of which those are of importance from the commercial stand point are Palas *(Butea monosperma)*, Kusum *(Schleichera oleosa)*, Ber *(Zizyphus mauritiana)*. Other important lac host plants are Khair *(Acacia catechu)*, Ghont *(Zizyphus zylopyra)*, Barh *(Ficus bengalensis)*, Peepal *(Ficus religiosa)*, Arhar *(Cajanus cajan)*, Galwang *(Albizia lucida)* etc. There are other species of trees which are used in particular regions like *Crewia sp., Leea sp.* and *Cajanus cajan* in Brahmaputra valley, *Ficus sp.* in parts of Assam, U.P. and Punjab and *Shorea talura* in Karnataka and Salem area of Tamil Nadu.

Important Lac Host Plants: A bushy host plant species, *Flemingia semialata* Roxb. (Leguminaceae : Papilionacae), has been identified and field tested as a potential fast growing host for intensive lac cultivation during winter season lac crop of *Kusmi* Strain *(Aghani)* for increasing lac production to match with the growing global demand of lac.

Essential Characteristics of lac host: The factor that determines whether the lac insect will flourish on a particular host species or not is the character of the sap of host plant. It is believed that the sap reactions of a good lac host should be near about neutral or slightly acidic *e.g.* pH values between 5.8 and 6.0 and that the sap density of good lac host plants in lower than that on non-lac hosts. The sap reactions of non-lac hosts show distinct acidity or alkalinity.

3.11.3 Strains, Taxonomy and Life cycle of Lac insect

Strains of Lac and Lac Crops: Two strains of the lac insects are recognized in India, Rangeeni and Kusumi. Each strain completes its life cycle twice a year but the seasons of maturity differ considerably. In Mysore, the Rangeeni strain completes their life cycle in 13 months on Jallari *(Shorea talura)*. There are four lac crops in a year that are named after the Hindi months. Lac is not always left on the trees until it matures fully, particularly in case of *Baisakhi* crop. When it is not mature, it (*Baisakhi – ari*) is cut, leaving a certain amount on the tree to act as brood for the next crop. In *Rangeeni*, three crops can be obtained from the host tree such as Jalari *(Shorea talura)* mostly found in Karnataka (Mysore region) and Rain tree *(Samanea saman)*, mostly located in coastal region of West Bengal. These crops are commonly known as Trivoltine crop in which the lac insects pass through three life cycles in thirteen months. Seeds of Kusum tree are sown directly whereas those of other hosts like Palas and Ber are sown in nurseries and seedlings are transplanted. Though lac is cultivated under natural or jungle conditions, the lac insects prefer and yield better returns under orchards or plantation conditions.

Lac Insect Taxonomy: The first scientific account of the lac insect was given by J. Kerr in 1782 which was published in Philosophical Transaction of Royal Society of London (vol. 71, pp.374-382). The first scientific name given to it was *Tachardia lacca* following the name of French Missionary Father Tachardia. It was later changed to *Laccifer lacca* Kerr. The other name given to it has been *Kerria Lac* Kerr.

Phylum - Arthropoda

Class - Insecta

Order - Hemiptera

Suborder - Homoptera

Super family - Coccoidea

Family - Lacciferidae

Genus- *Laccifer*

Species - *lacca*

Lac insect belongs to super family Coccoidea which includes all scale insects. Scale insect is a common name for about 2000 insect species found all over the world. Scale insects range from almost microscopic size to more than 2.5 cm. These insects attach themselves in great numbers to plants. The mouth part of these insects is piercing and sucking type. They can be very destructive to tree-stunting or killing twigs and branches by draining the sap. There are six genera of lac insects, out of which only five secrete lac and only one *i.e. Laccifer* secretes recoverable or commercial lac. The commonest and most widely occurring species of lac insect in India is *Laccifer lacca* (Kerr) which produces the bulk of commercial lac. Lac insect of South East Asia is referred to as *Kerria chinensis*.

Life history of lac insect: The lac insect (*Kerria lacca*) starts its life as minute soft bodied nymphs, ovate in outline, slightly pointed posteriorly, nearly 0.6 mm. long excluding antennae and anal setae and about 0.25 mm across the thorax. It is crimson coloured, though yellow and white forms are also found in nature. The nymphs emerge in large number at certain times of the year from the lac cells of the female insect depending on the strains and crop seasons and crawl over the twigs and branches of the plants in search of suitable places for settlement. They settle very gregariously.

A healthy female produces 130 to 400 nymphs. The nymphal emergence from a female continues for a fortnight but from a twig comprising of many lac females, it continues for slightly more than 3 weeks and is controlled by the climatic conditions prevailing at that time. The lac nymphs usually emerge in greater number during 8.0 to 12.0 hrs. They thrust their hair like proboscis upto phloem region to derive their nutrition. Once settled, the female never moves during its life time, while the male moves out only during the last phase of its life. The female insect then spends its entire life alone in the lac cell. The larval settlement is very dense at first often completely covering the lower surface of the twigs and sometimes extending to the upper surfaces as well. Density of settlement ranges from 150 to 180 sq. cm. A day or so after settlement, the nymph start secreting resin from the glands, distributed under the cuticle all over the body except near the mouth parts, the breathing pores and the vent. The nymphs thus get encased in cells of their own secretion, which increases in size with the increase in the size of the insect.

The male and the female among the young larvae are not easily differentiated by the naked eye. In most cases, the females are preponderant, their population being about three times greater than that of the males. In some progenies the males may be in excess. After secretion of lac, the cell of the male is elongated and shaped like a cigar, while that of the female is more or less oval is shape. The lac formed by the male is relatively small and therefore, the occasional preponderance of the males makes a poor crop.

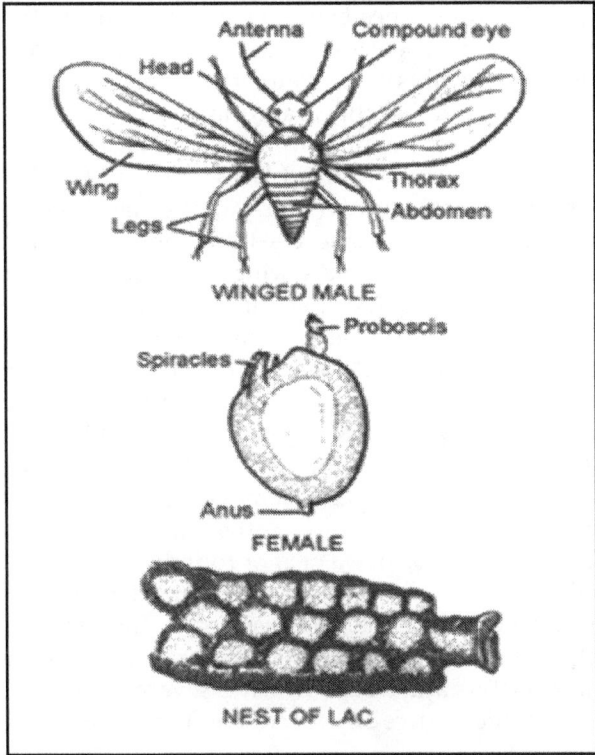

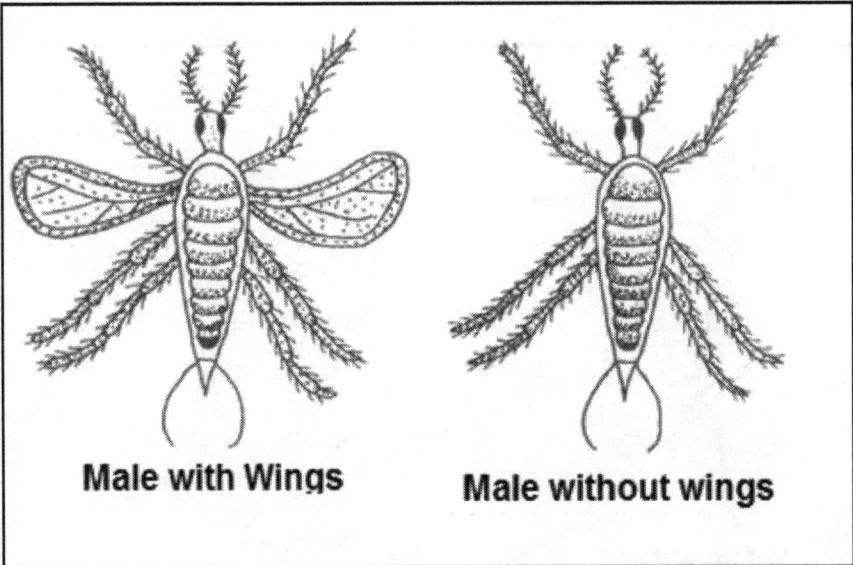

Figure 3.20 Lac Insect

The insect moults three times before reaching maturity, the duration of each instar depending on the host species and the environmental factors. After the first moult, both the female as well as male nymphs lose their legs, antennae and eyes. The male lac cells assume slipper like appearance and a loose operculum at the rear end is clearly seen after the second moult. During the last stage the male insects no longer feed as the mouth parts become atrophied. Subsequently after the second moult, the nymph passes through the prepupal and pupal stage when appendages which ultimately develop into legs, antennae, eyes and wings (except in apterous males), aedeagus etc. are seen. The adult males, winged or wingless emerge with the hind end of the body first by pushing the operculum. Normally the winged males occur during the summer crops and the relative number of the two forms in a colony varies considerably in different seasons. A male has life of 62-92 hrs. After emergence and copulate with the female which continues to remain enclosed in the lac cell. A male insect is capable of fertilizing 45 females. The female nymphs unlike the male do not develop the organs cast off earlier after the first moult except the rudimentary antennae and the organs peculiar to the females become conspicuous. During the subsequent instars the female nymphs become swollen in form and loose all traces of segmentation. They assume form of a pear or roundish bag and completely occupy the space inside the lac cells. After the final and the third moult, the female is sexually mature and is fertilized by the male. Lac secretion by the females continues and the size of the insects as well as that of the enveloping lac cells increase at faster space. The female lac insects thus attain size, which is several times that of a male lac cell and are therefore, the chief source of lac secretion. The females continue to secrete lac until eggs are laid.

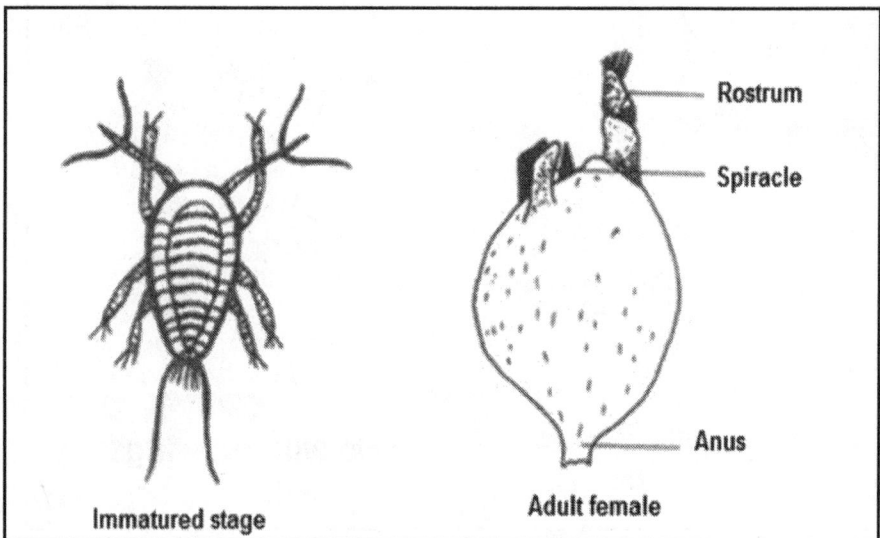

Figure 3.21: Showing loss of vegetative parts in adult female lac-insect

As the time of egg laying approaches, the female insects contract at one side, gradually vacating space inside the enveloping lac-cells. The powdery wax and wax filaments are secreted and shed in the vacated space, possibly to provide dry dressing and cushion for the future young nymphs. The anal tubercle is gradually withdrawn inside the cells for laying eggs, which hatch into nymphs immediately after laying. Egg laying ceases if the temperature falls below 17°C in summer and 15°C in winter. The lac nymphs inside the lac cells become inactive below the temperature of 20°C but their capacity to produce lac subsequently under favorable condition is not impaired. The bio-features of females in the progeny are not adversely affected by subjecting the brood lac (lac encrustation on a twig containing gravid females) to temperature below 20°C for short period.

3.11.4 Cultivation of Lac

Local Cultivation Practices of Lac

The cultivation practices followed by the lac cultivators are essentially the same throughout India except for slight deviation here and there to suit local conditions. It consists of taking repeated partial lac crop on the same tree after allowing a few shoots, carrying lac for self-inoculation every time or when the crop is harvested. Keeping the trees under continuous lac inoculation and heavy pruning of brunches repeatedly to collect lac crop, leads to general loss of vitality of the trees. Also the self inoculation of the trees lead to over-infection on the twigs and this quite often results in whole sale mortality of the crop in season of extreme summer. Besides, this helps multiplication of enemy insects of lac resulting in failure of crops, which ultimately forces the cultivator to abandon cultivation on most of the lac host trees. In such seasons brood lac is not readily available for purchase and if at all, a very high price has to be paid which the cultivator cannot afford to pay. The cultivator usually purchases his brood to the extent he can afford at that time and puts it on a few trees and start cultivation cycle afresh. In favorable seasons, he reaps his crops and inoculates more of his trees and continues the self inoculation repeatedly till the crop fails again. Thus production is unsteady and usually a bumper crop is obtained in cycles of 3 to 4 years. Being a subsidiary crop, lac cultivation is carried on a casual manner and the cultivator is generally satisfied with whatever he gets.

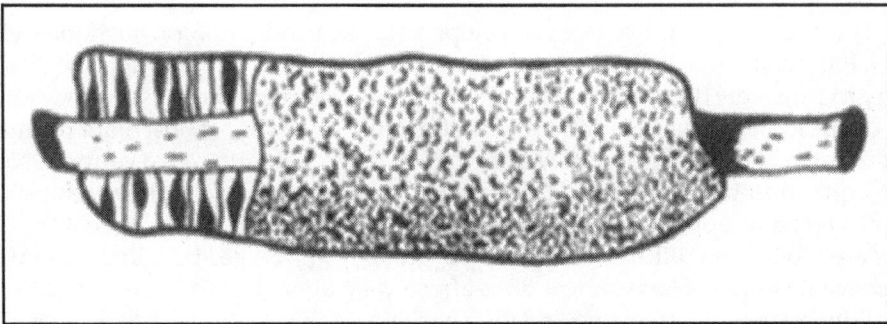

Figure 3.22: Lac incrustation

Scientific Method of Lac Cultivation

To start lac cultivation, two things are mainly to be taken into consideration:

(a) The suitable host plant on which the lac insect thrives.

(b) Availability of healthy brood lac in time.

Brood lac (in common parlance seed of other agricultural crops) is mature lac where from the young insects are ready to come out within the time specified. For getting the best result out of lac cultivation, the work should be planned on systematic basis. Such planning will aim at a sustained annual yield and also ensure that area under cultivation acquires self sufficiency of brood lac. Under systematic working, the host plants are cultivated and rested in turn in coupe system. The host trees should be properly pruned to put forth young succulent shoots before inoculation. Only enemy insect free brood lac should be used for inoculation. Lac crops being highly sensitive to climate vagaries, care has to be taken to provide optimum conditions for successful results.

Selection of Suitable Host plants

Selection of suitable host plants for lac cultivation is of paramount importance because quality and yield of lac depend on this. Selected lac hosts should have the following salient features:

(i)   Fairly quick growing.

(ii) Lower sap density.

(iii) Well adapted to pollarding.

Selection of Suitable site for Lac Cultivation

As lac can grow only in open areas, the sites for lac host plantation should be in such a place where free circulation of air around the host species is assured. Cultivation should not be attempted at places where fire susceptibility is there. When starting cultivation in new areas having lac host species, it is always desirable to prune them before infection to ensure good lac production.

Coupe System: A Sustained Yield Basis of Lac Cultivation

The coupe system has been developed for lac production on sustained yield basis. If the same tree is continuously inoculated, its vitality suffers and the yield of crop progressively diminishes. It is important that host plants are given periodic rest. The coupe system of cultivation provides for a maximum use of host plant resources consistent with their vigor and well being. In Rangeeni farms, two coupe systems with equal number of palas (*Butea monosperma*) trees in two coupes having six (6) months rest is adopted for raising *Baisakhi-cum-Katki* crops in alternate seasons. The trees are inoculated with about 500g of *rangeeni* brood lac per tree, in the month of October-November. Harvesting is done after a year, after allowing self-inoculation in June-July by partial harvesting and then harvesting the combined *Baisaki-cum-Katki* crop in next Oct. Nov. In the *Kusumi* farms, Kusum (*Schleichera oleosa*) is the major lac host plant species of *Kusumi* stain of lac insect. Five coupe systems with equal number of trees in each coupe having 18 months rest in between pruning and inoculation is adopted. The trees are pruned 18 months prior to inoculation. Thereafter, in the subsequent crops, harvesting will serve the purpose of pruning. The harvesting of crop is done after 6 months of inoculation.

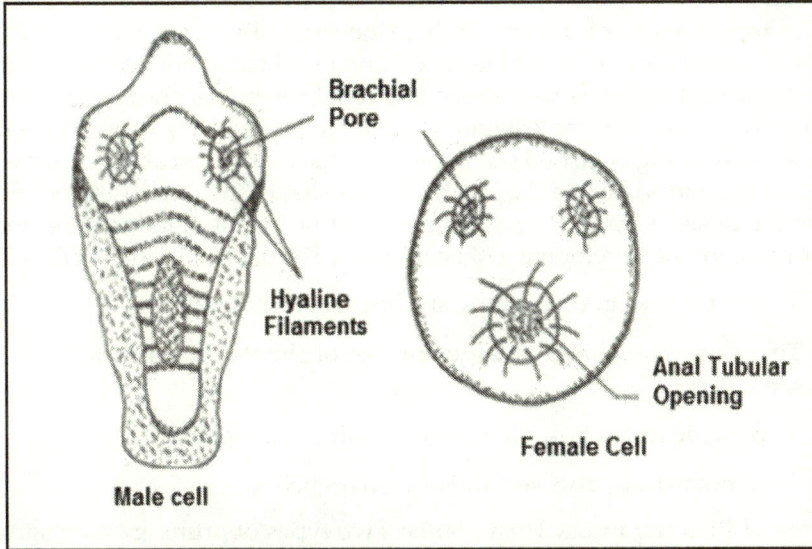

Figure 3.23: Different forms of Lac cell

Preparation of Feeding Ground for Lac Insects

To get a good quality lac through cultivation, it is necessary to ensure proper type of feeding ground to the lac insects. The insects have to be provided with succulent shoots, as it cannot drive its slender proboscis through thick bark. For getting a good number of requisite succulent shoots the most essential operation is pruning.

Pruning Operation

The lac hosts should have plenty of new growth with tender branches for feeding of the lac insect. Hence the trees can be pruned to get sufficient tender growth. As a separate process it is done before initial inoculation only but in subsequent years pruning is identical and one and the same as the cropping. Branches more than 2.5 cm in thickness are not cut, branches 1.25 cm or less in thickness are completely cut away at the places where they arise from the main shoots, while branches between 1.25 and 2.5 cm in thickness are cut leaving a stalk about 45 cm length. All the host trees should not be cultivated continuously with lac as this will have adverse effect on the vigour of the trees.

Pruning at proper time is one of the important operations where the branches/ twigs are cut in order to get the maximum numbers of succulent shoots to facilitate feeding of the lac insects.

Improvised scientific method of pruning which is done in the brood lac farms is as follows:

Pruning is done lightly, because light pruning avoids stunted growth and allows gradual increase in the frame of the tree. Branches more than 2.5 cm in diameter (more than thickness of one's thumb) are not cut. Branches 1.25 cm or less in diameter are cut flush with a branch or trunk from where they arise. Branches between 1.25 cm to 2.5 cm in diameter are cut, so as to leave behind a stalk of about 30-45 cm in length. Dead and diseased branches are removed, split or broken branches are cut below the split. If trees are old and have lost their capacity to produce vigorous shoots of new flush, heavier pruning is carried out to produce the new wood at the expense of the old. Such operation will bring the tree to a better shape, so that subsequent pruning will give the desired flush. Proper pruning should result a good shape and give plenty of room for the development of new shoots. The main objectives of Pruning are:

- To ensure new, good, healthy and succulent shoots.

- To ensure availability of large number of shoots (larger area for lac insect settlement).

- To provide rest to host plant for maintaining it vigour.

- To remove dead, diseased and broken branches.

Types of Pruning in Lac Host plants: Two types of pruning/ coppicing have been recommended for lac culture.

(i) **Apical/light pruning:** Branches less than 2.5 cm diameter should be cut from base and branches more that 2.5 cm diameter should be sharply cut leaving a stump of 30-45 cm from the base. Diseased and dead portion of branches should be removed completely. Light pruning is recommended for slow growing conventional tree host species like palas, kusum and ber.

(ii) **Basal/heavy pruning:** Branches having less than 7 cm thickness should be removed from the base, whereas thicker branches should be cut at a place where it has a diameter of 7 cm. In quick growing bushy host, pruning should be done at a height of 10-15 cm from the ground level *e.g. Flemingia macrophylla, F. semialata.*

Pruning time: It has been found that the best results are obtained by pruning in February for raising the Katki crop and in April for raising the *Baisakhi* crop in the case of major *Rangeeni* host, ber and palas. Pruning in these months will give shoots four and six months old respectively for the lac larvae to feed on. In case of kusum, pruning is best done in the month of June-July and January-February. These months coincide with those in which the crops mature and so harvesting of the mature crop serves the purpose of pruning also. Pruning time will, however need to be adjusted to suit local conditions. Under Chhotanagpur (Jharkhand) condition the following pruning times for different lac hosts have been found suitable for lac culture.

- **Kusum (*Schleichera oleosa*):** Prunning should be done either in January/ February or in June /July.

- **Khair (*Acacia catechu*):** Pruning is to be done in March. However, harvesting of lac crop during February may be used to serve as pruning also.

- **Ber (*Zizyphus mauritiana*):** Pruning should be done in February for inoculation in July and in

- April / May for inoculation in October-November. For *Kusmi* lac crop, ber should be pruned 5 months before inoculation. However, recent observations have shown that harvesting of *Aghani* crop during February may also serve as pruning for inoculation in June-July.

- **Palas (*Butea monosperma*):** Pruning should be done in February for lac inoculation in July and April for inoculation in October-November.

- *Ficus sp.*: Pruning is to be done in April for inoculation in July and in May for inoculation in October.

Pruning instruments: Most of the lac cultivators do pruning with axes. Proper pruning cannot be done with the axe. If branches are cut with axe, they will either break or split. In both the cases damage to tree will be caused at cutting place in form of scraping of bark or splitting, giving opportunity for insect pest attack. The ideal pruning instruments are secateurs and long handled tree prunners. Of these instruments, the most valuable are the long handled tree prunners. There are two types of secateurs. These are Roll cut secateur and the French secateur. The former is better and easier to use but is easily damaged by careless handling Pruning is also done with pruning knife and Dauli. The use of pruning shear and pruning saw fitted in long handle makes the operation easier as the pruning is done directly by standing on ground and climbing is avoided.

Collection of brood Lac: Lac sticks, having mature female insects ready to give rise to the next generation are called brood lac. As the female lac insect is capable of giving rise to a large number of larvae and to get the maximum benefit, it is essential that the brood should be cut at the proper time, so as to secure the emergence of the maximum possible number of larvae from it. For quality of brood lac, lac crops should be harvested only when mature. The cutting of brood lac should be taken up at the correct time keeping in view the swarming period *i.e.* the expected date of larval emergence. The ideal time of cutting would be that which will result in the swarming, starting immediately or within a couple of days of tying the brood on the host plant.

Selection of brood Lac: After the brood lac has been cut from the plants, it is necessary to subject it to proper examination, so that only healthy lac with the minimum signs of predator and parasite damage is selected for use as brood lac. This is necessary to minimize the chances of propagation of the insect enemies of lac insects.

Inoculation of brood Lac: This operation includes putting of bundles of brood lac (lac sticks containing gravid females) in the host twigs for allowing young lac larvae (crawlers) to come out of their mother cells and settle on the host plant. Brood lac should be cut from the parent tree when the lac cell is red in the anterior half and orange in the anal region. The brood lac should be thick and it should have continuous encrustation. The selected brood lac branches are cut into sticks of 15 to 30 cm. They are tied by means of a banana or jute fiber either singly or in bundles of two or three sticks each and either longitudinally or interlaced between two host branches. Longitudinal inoculation allows maximum contact between the brood and the host. Inoculation has to be done on a non rain day. The alternate host trees like *Acacia castechu Ougeinia oojeinensis* and *Moghania macrophylla* are used to rear the brood for maintaining the vigor, similarly if two common hosts are available in a locality for a strain like Palas and Ber for Rangeeni, brood from one host can be used for inoculation the other. Following aspects should be taken into consideration during inoculation operation:

(i)   Pest -free healthy brood lac should be used.

(ii) Unwanted portions of the brood lac sticks should be removed.

(iii) Bundles of brood lac (about 100 g. by weight) are to be prepared and put these bundles inside 60 mesh nylon netting bags (approx. size 30 x 10 cm). These will entrap all the predators and parasites but allow the lac larvae to come out.

(iv) The brood lac bundles are tied onto the branches parallel to shoots.

(v)   One meter long brood lac is sufficient to inoculate 10-15 m. long shoots of equal length.

(vi) During the period of inoculation, there are chances of brood bundles falling off and one should go round the inoculated trees in each branch and put such bundles back on the tree.

(vii) Attempts should be made to see that the brood lac bundles are not kept on the tree for more than the minimum period required for complete inoculation. Ordinarily, this period will be two to three weeks. If the brood lac is kept even after the lac larvae have completely emerged, there is the danger of a larger number of enemy insects emerging from the empty (phunki) brood lac sticks and infestating the field heavily.

Table 3.3: Inoculation Period in different Lac crops

Strain	Crop	Time of inoculation	With brood lac from	Time of harvesting
Rangeeni	Baisakhi	Oct- Nov.	Katki crop	June-July
	Katki	June-July	Baisakhi	Oct.-Nov.
Kusumi	Jathwi	Jan- Feb	Aghani	June-July
	Aghani	June- July	Jathwi	Jan-Feb

Phunki Removal: The operation pertains to the removal of brood lac bundles used for inoculation purposes and the used up brood lac after complete emergence of lac larvae from female cells is called phunki removal. Ordinarily the emergence of lac larvae from the brood lac ceases after three weeks. The phunki lac so removed is scrapped off thereafter in the brood lac for more than three weeks from the start of larval emergence to avoid emergence of enemy insects. Phunki bundles are pulled down from the trees with the help of pole mounted Phunki hook or by climbing on trees.

Harvesting: The crop is harvested earlier than the swarming is due but in the case of crop required for brood it is harvested later just before swarming is due to occur. The general symptoms of swarming are dried out appearance of encrustation two weeks before swarming and appearance of cracks on the encrustation at a later date. However, the appearance of an orange yellow area in the vicinity of the anal tubercle is the accurate indication for swarming. The crop for manufacture of shellac is spread out after harvest in a pucca floor without allowing them to stick together. Yield of *ari lac* harvesting is about 25% less than mature crop harvesting. Harvested branches are collected and scrapped to get stick lac. Pruning instruments are used in harvesting. Secateur or long handle tree prunners are better equipments for harvesting lac crop. If there is a surplus brood lac on the host, partial harvesting is done.

3.11.5 Enemies of Lac insects

Damage to lac crops may be due to both insects and causes other than insects, like monkeys, squirrels, rats, birds and lazards, adverse climatic conditions and bad pruning. The insect damage alone accounts for about 60 to 70% loss. There are many natural enemies of lac insects which include vertebrates, invertebrates (insect predators and parasites) and microbial flora.

Vertebrate enemies of lac insects

The important vertebrate enemies are squirrels and rats and the damage caused by those enemies can be as serious as 50% of brood sticks in worst condition. Squirrels are active during the day time and the damage by them is more common under forest condition. Rats are active at night time and the damage usually occurs near about the villages. Towards the crop maturity, these pests either gnaw the mature lac encrustation on the tree and the brood lac tied to trees for inoculation or consume the full grown lac female insects with plenty of eggs inside them. The damage to brood lac tied to trees interferes with the inoculation, as the brood bundles and lac encrustations drop to the ground while the larval emergence is taking place. Besides squirrels and rats, monkeys also cause some damage to lac encrustations and to the newly developing shoots from pruned trees by breaking them.

Control: It is difficult to control the squirrels and rats under the open field conditions where lac is cultivated. However scaring away of these animals or poisoning them may be adopted to keep the rodents under attack.

Insect enemies of Lac insect

It has been estimated that on an average, up to 30-40% of the lac cells are destroyed by insect enemies of lac crop. At times, the enemy attack can be so serious as to result in crop failures. There are two kinds of enemy of lac insect are parasite and predators.

(i) Parasites: All parasites causing damage to lac insect belong to the Order Hymenoptera of class Insecta. A list of parasites associated with lac insect *Kerria lacca*) is presented in table below.

Table 3.4 Parasites of Lac insect

S.No.	Name of the parasite	Family
1	*Anicetus dodonia*	Encyrtidae
2	*Atropates hautefeuilli*	Encyrtidae
3	*Aphrastobracon flavipennis*	Encyrtidae
4	*Bracon greeni*	Encyrtidae
5	*Campyloneurus indicus*	Encyrtidae
6	*Coccophaqus tchirchii*	Aphelinidae
7	*Erencyrtus dewitzi*	Encyrtidae
8	*Eupelmus tachardiae*	Eupelmidae
9	*Eurymyiocnema aphelinoides*	Aphelinidae
10	*Lyka lacca*	Encyrtidae
11	*Marietta javensis*	Aphelinidae
12	*Parageniaspis indicus*	Encyrtidae
13	*Parechthrodryinus clavicornis*	Encyrtidae
14	*Protyndarichus submettalicus*	Encyrtidae
15	*Tachardiaephagus tachardiae*	Encyrtidae
16	*Teachardiobius nigricans*	Encyrtidae
17	*Aprostocetus/Tetrastichus purpureus*	Eulophidae

Among the parasites listed above *Tachardiaephagus tachardiae* and *Tetrastichus purpureus* are the most abundant lac associated parasites. They lay their eggs in the lac cells and the grubs (larvae) hatching out feed on the lac insect within its cell.

(ii) Predators: The predators on the other hand, are more serious and may cause damage up to 30-35% to the cells in a crop. The list of predators of lac insects is given in table below.

Table 3.5 Predators of Lac insect

S.No.	Insect Predator	Order	Family
1	*Eublemma amabilis*	Lepidoptera	Noctuidae
2	*E. coccidiphaga*	Lepidoptera	Noctuidae
3	*E. cretacea*	Lepidoptera	Noctuidae
4	*E. scitula*	Lepidoptera	Noctuidae
5	*Pseudohypatopa pulverea*	Lepidoptera	Blastobasidae
6	*Catablemma sumbavensis*	Lepidoptera	Blastobasidae
7	*Cryptoblabes ephestialis*	Lepidoptera	Blastobasidae
8	*Phroderces falcatella*	Lepidoptera	Cosmopterygidae
9	*Lacciferophaga yunnanea*	Lepidoptera	Momphidae
10	*Chrysopa madestes*	Neuroptera	Chrysopidae
11	*C. lacciperda*	Neuroptera	Chrysopidae

Contd....

S.No.	Insect Predator	Order	Family
12	Berginus maindroni	Coleoptera	Mycetophagidae
13	Silvanus iyeri	Coleoptera	Cucujidae
14	Tribolium ferrugineum	Coleoptera	Tenebrionidae
15	Phyllodromia humbertiana	Dictyoptera	Blattellidae
16	Ischonoptera fulvastrata	Dictyoptera	Blattellidae

Eublemma amabilis and *Pseudohypatopa pulverea* are the most destructive key pests of lac insects and are in regular occurrence but their incidence may vary from season to season, place to place and crop to crop.

(i). **Eublemma amabilis:** It is the most destructive predator of lac insect and causes most damage during *katki* and *aghani* lac crops *i.e.* during the rainy season in comparison to the other two crops.

Life history: A single female moth lays grayish, flat and rounded eggs singly on the test of lac insect. The newly hatched larvae, 0.51 to 0.54 mm long, get at the lac insect either through the opening of the test or by tunneling a hole through encrustation. A single larva can destroy 40-60 lac insect cells in its whole larval period. It has six generations in a year and the duration of the generations is about 37, 45, 42, 125, 80 and 40 days respectively. Attacked lac cells can easily be identified because of its pinkish colouration due to presence of pink coloured discs of excreta inside the hollow lac cells.

(ii) *Pseudohypatopa pulverea*: It is also destructive predator of lac insects and found in all lac growing areas of the country. It feeds on the live and dead lac insects and is found in large numbers in stored lac and so it is responsible for the qualitative and quantitative deterioration of stored lac.

Life history: It lays oval (0.5 mm X 0.3 mm), colourless eggs, singly on the test of lac insects. Larvae pass normally through 5 instars but the hibernating larvae have nine instars. The newly hatched larva is about 1.35 mm long whereas a mature larva is 10-12 mm in length and 2 mm in breadth. Larval stages feed on the lac larvae and spin a loose web. A single larval predator is capable of destroying 45-60 mature lac cells.

Prevention and Control of Insect enemies

Preventive measures

(i) Parasite and predator free brood lac should be used for inoculation.

(ii) Self inoculation of lac crops should be avoided as far as possible.

(iii) Inoculated brood bundles should be kept on the host tree for a minimum period only.

(iv) Phunki (empty brood lac sticks) should be removed from the inoculated trees in 2 – 3 weeks time.

(v) All lac cut from the tree and all phunki brood lac (after use as brood lac) not required for brood purpose should be scraped or fumigated at once.

(vi) Cultivation of Kusmi strain of lac should be avoided in predominantly rangeeni area and vice versa.

Mechanical control: Use of 60 mesh synthetic netting (brood bag) to enclose brood lac for inoculation purposes can reduce infestation of enemy insects of lac. The emerging lac larvae easily crawl out from the minute pores of the net and settle on the twigs of the lac host plants, whereas the emerging adult predator enemies cannot move out of the brood bags and get entrapped within the net. This can check the egg lying by the predator moths on the new crop.

Chemical control: Application of 0.05% endosulfan at 30-35 days stage of crop has been identified as the most effective dose of insecticide without any adverse effect on the economic attributes of the lac insect.

Microbial control: Use of bio-pesticide, Thuricide (*Bacillus thuringiensis*) at 30-35 days stage of crop is the effective microbial control measure for important enemy insects of lac in field condition.

Biological control: Two ant predators' viz. *Camponotus compresus* and *solenopsis geminate rufa* are the most important and promising for biological control of predator enemies of lac in field condition. Egg parasitoids viz. *Trichogramma pretiosum*, *T. chilonis*, *T. poliae*, *Trichogrammatoidea bactrae* and *Telenomus remus* have been found to be effective in management of lac predators.

Microbial flora associated with Lac insects: Two types of microflora viz. bacteria and fungi are associated with the lac insects. Bacteria act through lac hosts and could be symbiotic or pathogenic whereas effect of fungi is direct either as symbiotic or as an adversary. Microbial studies conducted have revealed that four species of micro-organisms viz. *Micrococcus varians*, *M. conglomerates*, *Clostridium sp.* and *Bacillus subtilis* are found is permanent association with various stages of lac insects. Presence of various symbiotic microflora is considered beneficial for good yield of lac particularly during rainy season crop. Association of fungi with lac insect is not always beneficial. Besides insect enemies, lac crop yield suffers significant loss due to other biotic agents particularly fungi. Fungal infection in lac culture causes severe losses of lac yield by:

(i) Killing the lac insects by inhibiting respiration,

(ii) Hindering mating process,

(iii) Blocking larval emergence,

(iv) Affecting lac host efficiency.

Lac culture during rainy season is prone to fungal attack particularly when grown on Ber (*Ziziphus mauritiana*), Kusum (*Schleichera oleosa*) due to their steady and spreading crown. Three species of fungi belonging to family Eurotiaceae and Aspergillaceae viz. *Aspergillus awamori*, *Aspergillus terricola* and *Penicillium citrinum* are reported to cause maximum loss in lac crop. *Aspergillus awamori* and *Penicillium citrinum* are black and greenish in colour respectively were observed to make a continuous cover on lac insect culture and thereby blocking their breathing pores and ultimately leading to mortality of lac insects. A pathogenic fungus, *Pythium sp.* in female tests, causes a heavy mortality on the larvae which fail to enclose satisfactorily and lie dead in clusters within the female resinous cell.

Prevention and control: Application of fungicides, Bavistin (carbendazim 0.05%) and Dithane M-45 (mancozeb, 0.18%) by both dipping of brood lac before inoculation and spraying on standing crop gives significantly better yield of lac. Significant reduction (75% to 84%) in mortality of 2nd inster lac nymphs/larvae can be done by the application of different concentration of carbendazim and aureofungin on kusmi stain of lac insect.

Summary

1. Breeding is inherent in the keeping of animals, because it is the animal keeper who determines which animals will produce offspring. Breeding is the selection and mating of animals for the purpose of changing the characteristics of the next generation to better correspond to a breeding goal formulated by humans.

2. Animal breeding, as an applied field of population genetics, has a well-developed mathematical foundation that was laid early in its development.

3. A breeder is an individual animal keeper who selects animals and mates them for the purpose of producing offspring.

4. Genetic engineering is the name of a group of techniques used for direct genetic modification of organisms or population of organisms using recombination of DNA. The most accepted purpose of genetic engineering is focused on the direct manipulation of DNA sequences.

5. In mammals, techniques for reproductive manipulation of gametes and embryos such as obtaining of a complete new organism from adult differentiated cells (cloning) and procedures for artificial reproduction such as *in vitro* fertilization, embryo transfer and artificial insemination, are frequently an important part of these processes.

6. Most experiments on QTL detection in animals allow only the estimation of wide chromosomal regions (practical maximum resolution is of about 1 cM, but usual resolution is about 30 cM) that harbour a QTL in a statistical sense, estimated from the effects of some marker haplotypes on quantitative traits.

7. Theoretically, it is possible to predict accurately the breeding values of animals using many markers. From this knowledge, it is possible to develop a model for *in vitro* genetic improvement of animals. This is known as velogenetics.

8. Important applications of genetic markers in animal improvement include the optimization of mating strategies for non-additive genetic effects (estimation and managing of inbreeding and heterosis), parentage determination, genetic characterization of diverse animal breeds and populations using studies of between and within population (breeds) diversity and marker-assisted introgression of particular alleles.

9.   Cloning an animal is the production of a genetically identical individual, by transferring the nucleus of differentiated adult cells into an oocyte from which the nucleus has been removed.

10. Use of cloning in animal genetic improvement may increase the rates of selection progress in certain cases, particularly in situations where artificial insemination is not possible, such as in pastoral systems with ruminants.

11. Microinjection of DNA and now nuclear transfer, are two methods used to produce transgenic livestock successfully.

12. The technology of transgenesis is potentially useful to modify characters of economic importance in a rapid and precise way. Contrary to the classical selection programs, it is necessary a knowledge of the genes that control these characters and their regulation.

13. The techniques for obtaining transgenic animals in species of agricultural interest are still inefficient. Some approaches that may overcome this problem are based on cloning strategies.

14. Selective breeding utilizes the natural variations in traits that exist among members of any population. Breeding progress requires understanding the two sources of variation; genetics and environment.

15. Heritability is the proportion of the additive genetic variation to the total variation. Heritability is important because without genetic variation there can be no genetic change in the population.

16. Types of selection are individual or mass selection, within and between family selection, sibling selection and progeny testing, with many variations.

17. Methods of ranking animals for breeding purposes have changed as statistical and genetic knowledge has increased.

18. Progeny testing is used extensively in the beef and dairy cattle industry to aid in evaluating and selecting stock to be bred. Progeny testing is most useful when a high level of accuracy is needed for selecting a sire to be used extensively in artificial insemination.

19. Mating animals that are related causes inbreeding. Inbreeding is often described as narrowing the genetic base because the mating of related animals results in offspring that have more genes in common.

20. Deoxyribonucleic acid (DNA) is the genetic material that contains the instructions in each cell of organisms. DNA determines the genome and thus the genetic code, which is a blueprint for development of all body organs and structures. The structure of DNA can be visualized as a spiral staircase.

21. The connection between an organism's genetic makeup and its immune system, as well as applications of that knowledge, forms the young science of immunogenetics.

22. Genetic control of the immune system is based on the DNA of the individuals. Histocompatibility genes that serve several functions are on one area of a

chromosome, called the major histocompatibility complex (MHC), which exists in all higher vertebrates.

23. Cloning, an asexual method of reproduction produces an individual with the same genetic material (DNA) as another individual. Probably the best-known examples of clones are identical twins, which result when cells in the early development stage separate and develop into different individuals.

24. Aquaculture is most commonly known for the production of food organisms such as fish, prawns and shellfish.

25. Aquaculture on the other hand is a branch of animal husbandry involving raising or breeding of aquatic living things either plants *e.g.* seaweed, plankton and algae or animals *e.g.* fin-fish, shell-fish, oyster shell, clams, cockles, shrimps, crayfish, periwinkles, turtles in a controlled water body to marketable size.

26. Fish farming is the primary form of aquaculture. Fish farming is cultivation of fish for commercial purposes in man-made tanks and other enclosures.

27. Mariculture is the branch of aquaculture that cultivates marine organisms either in the open ocean, an enclosed portion of the ocean or tanks or ponds filled with seawater.

28. Algaculture is the type of aquaculture that cultivates algae. Most algae harvested are either microalgae (phytoplankton, microphytes or planktonic algae) or macroalgae, commonly known as seaweed.

29. Integrated multitrophic aquaculture (IMTA) is a more advanced system of aquaculture. In a multitrophic system, different species with various nutritional needs are combined into one system.

30. Sea ranching is a culture method whereby juvenile animals, generally produced in hatcheries but could also be wild-caught, are introduced into the natural environment and allowed to grow without containment structures.

31. Surface line culture is generally used to grow shellfish - such as pearl oysters, scallops and mussels, tunicates, seaweeds and sponges in panel-style baskets, small cages *e.g.* lantern nets, pearl nets or on ropes that are suspended below floating surface lines. Each species has a well established method for growing.

32. Subsurface line culture, used for culturing pearl oysters or scallops, is similar to surface line culture except the horizontal mainlines and suspended culture panels are positioned well below the surface.

33. Rack culture in Australia is generally used to grow edible oysters such as the Sydney rock oyster, native flat oyster and Pacific oyster. Each species has a well-established method for growing.

34. Purpose-built earthen ponds, constructed on coastal lands or adjacent to the estuarine parts of river systems, are used for the intensive culture of marine prawns and fin fish.

35. Freshwater aquaculture is the culture of aquatic species within and dependent on, the freshwater environment.

36. Pisciculture is derived from two words Pisces which means fish or fishes and culture which means rearing, raising or breeding of living things. Therefore pisciculture is defined as a branched of animal husbandry that deals with rational deliberate culturing of fish or fishes to marketable size in a controlled water body.

37. Composite pisciculture is a scientific technology for getting maximum fish production from a pond or a tank through utilization of available food organisms supplemented by artificial feeding.

38. Poultry farming, raising of birds domestically or commercially, primarily for meat and eggs but also for feathers. Chickens, turkeys, ducks and geese are of primary importance, while guinea fowl and squabs are chiefly of local interest.

39. The breeds of chickens are generally classified as Asiatic, American, Mediterranean and English. The American breeds of importance today are Plymouth Rock, Wyandotte, Rhode Island Red and New Hampshire.

40. Chicken feeding is a highly perfected science that ensures a maximum intake of energy for growth and fat production. High quality and well-balanced protein sources produce a maximum amount of muscle organ, skin and feather growth.

41. Poultry are quite susceptible to a number of diseases; some of the more common are fowl typhoid, pullorum, fowl cholera, chronic respiratory disease, infectious sinusitis, infectious coryza, avian infectious hepatitis, infectious synovitis, bluecomb, Newcastle disease, fowl pox, avian leukosis complex, coccidiosis, blackhead, infectious laryngotracheitis, infectious bronchitis and erysipelas.

42. The art of silk production is called sericulture that comprises cultivation of mulberry, silkworm rearing and post cocoon activities leading to production of silk yarn. Sericulture provides gainful employment, economic development and improvement in the quality of life to the people in rural area and therefore it plays an important role in anti poverty programme and prevents migration of rural people to urban area in search of employment.

43. The domesticated silkworm species, *Bombyx mori* L. evolved almost 4600 years ago from the wild species, *Bombyx mandarina* Moore, which is a native of China and Palaearctic region. The eggs of silkworm, *B. mori* were first introduced from China into Japan and Korea in the first century and subsequently into Middle Eastern and European countries and later into the neighboring countries around China in the sixth century.

44. India and China are the two main producers, together manufacturing more than 60% of the world production each year. Silkworm larvae are fed by mulberry leaves and, after the fourth moult, climb a twig placed near them and spin their silken cocoons.

45. Mulberry is a hardy plant capable of thriving under a variety of agroclimatic conditions. At the same time, it is also sensitive responding extremely well to optimum agricultural inputs but showing practically no growth when plant nutrients and moisture begin to operate as limiting factors.

46. Diseases are the behavioral and physiological changes induced by pathogens in an organism. All diseases have specific symptoms and characteristics. Similarly, silkworms are also affected by various types of diseases caused by protozoa, fungi, bacteria and viruses. Since they cause substantial financial loss to the industry, their prevention and control assumes utmost importance.

47. Apiculture is derived from the honeybee's Latin name *Apis mellifera*, meaning honey gatherer. Since bees do not collect honey but nectar from which honey is made, the scientific name should actually be *Apis mellifica* meaning honey maker. Although apiculture refers to the honeybee, the vital role all bees play in the pollination of crops and flowering plants has caused apiculture to also include the management and study of non-Apis bees such as bumblebees and leafcutter bees. Some 90 million years ago, flowering plants first appeared on earth.

48. Apiculture does not have to be a large scale project. Keeping a few hives can give families access to endless honey as well as related products like beeswax candles and fresh honeycombs.

49. Honey and beekeeping have a long history in India. Honey was the first sweet food tasted by the ancient Indian inhabiting rock shelters and forests. They hunted bee hives for this gift of God. India has some of the oldest records of beekeeping in the form of paintings by prehistoric man in the rock shelters.

50. The raw materials for the beekeeping industry are mainly pollen and nectar that come from flowering plants. Both the natural and cultivated vegetation in India constitute an immense potential for development of beekeeping.

51. Honey is a supersaturated sugar solution with approximately 17.1% water. Fructose is the predominant sugar at 38.5%, followed by glucose at 31%. Disaccharides, trisaccharides and oligosaccharides are present in much smaller quantities. Besides carbohydrates, honey contains small amounts of protein, (including enzymes), vitamins and minerals. Honey yields 64 calories per tablespoon, making it a more concentrated source of energy than other common sweeteners.

52. Lac culture is the cultivation of lac insects for the production of lac. The important lac producing countries are India and Thailand. The important centers in India are Bihar accounting 40 % of the country's total production, Madhya Pradesh, West Bengalorissa, Assam and Uttar Pradesh.

53. Lac is a resinous exudation from the body of female scale insect. Since Vedic period, it has been in use in India. Its earliest reference is found in *Atherva Veda*.

54. The major constituents of stick lac or crude lac are resin, sugar, protein, soluble salt, coloring matter, wax, volatile oils, sand, woody matters and insect bodies. The resin is always associated with an odoriferous principle, a wax and a mixture of three dyes.

55. India and Thailand are the two major producers of lac. The main lac producing states in India are Chhattisgarh, Jharkhand, Madhya Pradesh, West Bengal, Uttar Pradesh orissa, Maharashtra and Gujarat.

56. The lac insects thrive on the sap of certain plants called lac hosts. So far, over four hundred species of plants have been recorded as hosts of which those are of importance from the commercial stand point are Palas *(Butea monosperma)*, Kusum *(Schleichera oleosa)*, Ber *(Zizyphus mauritiana)*. Other important lac host plants are Khair *(Acacia catechu)*, Ghont *(Zizyphus zylopyra), Barh (Ficus bengalensis)*, Peepal *(Ficus religiosa)*, Arhar *(Cajanus cajan)*, Galwang *(Albizia lucida)* etc. There are other species of trees which are used in particular regions like *Crewia sp., Leea sp.* and *Cajanus cajan* in Brahmaputra valley, *Ficus sp.* in parts of Assam, U.P. and Punjab and *Shorea talura* in Karnataka and Salem area of Tamil Nadu.

57. Lac insect belongs to super family Coccoidea which includes all scale insects. Scale insect is a common name for about 2000 insect species found all over the world. Scale insects range from almost microscopic size to more than 2.5 cm.

58. Damage to lac crops may be due to both insects and causes other than insects, like monkeys, squirrels, rats, birds and lazards, adverse climatic conditions and bad pruning. The insect damage alone accounts for about 60 to 70% loss. There are many natural enemies of lac insects which include vertebrates, invertebrates (insect predators and parasites) and microbial flora.

59. Lac culture during rainy season is prone to fungal attack particularly when grown on Ber *(Ziziphus mauritiana)*, Kusum *(Schleichera oleosa)* due to their steady and spreading crown.

60. Application of fungicides, Bavistin (carbendazim 0.05%) and Dithane M-45 (mancozeb, 0.18%) by both dipping of brood lac before inoculation and spraying on standing crop gives significantly better yield of lac.

Chapter 4
Wild Life of India

4.1 Introduction

India is unique in the richness and diversity of its vegetation and wildlife. India is habitat to many National parks and Wildlife sanctuaries within diversity of its wildlife, much of its unique fauna and excels in the range. The major wildlife sanctuaries are Corbett National Park, Gir Wildlife Sanctury, Kaziranga National Park in Sikkim, Periyar Wildlife Sanctuary, Neyyar Sanctuary, Blackbuck National Park, Kutch Desert Wildlife Sanctuary and so on. The wildlife sanctuaries in India are home to around two thousand different species of birds, 3500 species of mammals, nearly 30000 different kinds of insects and more than 15000 varieties of plants. By 1970, India only had five national parks. In 1972, India enacted the Wildlife Protection Act and Project Tiger to safeguard the habitats of conservation reliant species. As of April 2012, there were 112 national parks. All national park lands then encompassed a total 39,919 km^2 (15,413 sq mi) km^2, comprising 1.21% of India's total surface area. A total of 166 national parks have been authorized by the ministry, plans are underway to establish the remaining scheduled parks. India has over 500 animal sanctuaries, referred to as Wildlife Sanctuaries. Among these, the 47 Tiger Reserves are governed by Project Tiger and are of special significance in the conservation of the tiger. The sanctuaries and forest reserves are home to several endangered species of animals and birds like Asiatic Elephant, Royal Bengal tiger, Snow Leopard and Siberian Crane. Many of the forest reserves and wildlife sanctuaries of India are famous for some particular species of animals. For instance, the Kaziranga in Assam is known for the Indian Rhinoceros, while Periyar in Kerala is famous for its elephants. The Jim Corbett National Park, which is located in the Himalayan foothills, is the first of its kind. The Dudhwa National Park is another park made famous by its huge swamp deer population. Tiger reserves are the best places to catch a glimpse of this big cat. The Kanha National Park in Madhya Pradesh is one of the largest tiger reserves of India. The wildlife sanctuaries of India also include the bird sanctuaries, like the one at Bharatpur in Rajasthan. The different species of birds that one can find over here is truly fascinating. The Great Indian bustard, Himalayan monal pheasant, lammergiers, choughs, white bellied sea eagle, white breasted swiftlet, fruit pigeons and griffon vultures are just some of the bird species.

North India: Naturally blessed this part of India is home to the vast Himalayas and the great Gangetic Plains. Due to its favorable climatic conditions and topographical diversity North India supports a rich mix of flora and fauna. North India provides shelter to some of the finest and the rarest wildlife and wildlife sanctuaries. Some of the species unique to this part of the country are blue sheep, Himalayan marmots, snow partridges, snow leopards, goats like ibex, Himalayan wolfs, makhor, etc. The list of most frequented wildlife sanctuaries in North India includes Corbett National Park, Ranthambore National Par and Bharatpur National Park.

East India: East India is home to some of the finest endangered species like Hispid Hare, Pigmy Hog, One-horned Rhinoceros and Wild Buffalos the wildlife in this part of the country is very different from the rest of India. The two most important wildlife sanctuaries in East India are Sundarbans and Kaziranga Wildlife Sanctuary.

South India: South India is popular all across the globe for its extraordinary, unusual and varied flora and fauna. Characterized with lush greeneries South India houses a fascinating wildlife that consists of about 500 species of mammals, 1225 varieties of Birds and1600 types of reptiles. Some of the famous wildlife sanctuaries in the southern part of India include Periyar Wildlife Sanctuary, Bandipur Wildlife Sanctuary and Dandeli Wildlife Sanctuary. The wildlife common to South India are; Bison, Malabar Trogon, Antelopes etc.

West India: Ideal for the wildlife enthusiasts the western part of India supports a prominent part of India's wildlife. Supporting the growth of a distinct flora and fauna this part of India resides more than 40 mammals' species and about 450 birds' species. Blessed in terms of topography and climate West India is home to some of the most popular wildlife sanctuaries in India. There are about 300 Asiatic Lions in the Sasan Gir Wildlife Sanctuary which is situated in Gujarat. The other important wildlife sanctuaries in West India include Dhangadhra Sanctuary, the Velavadar National Park, Marine National Park and Sanctuary and many more.

4.2 Wild Life Protection and Acts

The Government of India enacted Wild Life (Protection) Act 1972 with the objective of effectively protecting the wild life of this country and to control poaching, smuggling and illegal trade in wildlife and its derivatives. The Act was amended in January 2003 and punishment and penalty for offences under the Act have been made more stringent. The Ministry has proposed further amendments in the law by introducing more rigid measures to strengthen the Act. The objective is to provide protection to the listed endangered flora and fauna and ecologically important protected areas.

4.2.1 Wild Life (Protection) Act 1972

The wild life laws have a long history and are the carminative result of an increasing awareness of the compelling need to restore the catastrophic ecological imbalances introduced by the depredations inflicted on nature by human being. The earliest codified law can be traced to 3rd Century B.C. when Ashoka, the King of Maghadha, enacted a law in the matter of preservation of wild life and environment.

But, the first codified law in India which heralded the era of laws for the wild life and protection was enacted in the year 1887 by the British and was titled as the Wild Birds Protection Act, 1887 (10 of 1887). This Act enabled the Government to frame rules prohibiting the possession or sale of any kinds of specified wild birds, which have been killed or taken during the breeding season. Again the British Government in the year 1912 passed the Wild Birds and Animals Protection Act, 1912 (8 of 1912) as the Act of 1887 proved to be inadequate for the protection of wild birds and animals. The Act of 1912 was amended in the year 1935 by the Wild Birds and Animals Protection (Amendment) Act, 1935 (27 of 1935). After the Second World War the freedom struggle for India started taking its shape and wild life was relegated to the background. But after independence, the Constituent Assembly in the Draft Constitution placed "Protection of Wild Birds and Wild Animals" at entry No.20 in the State List and the State Legislature has been given power to legislate. It was not till late 1960's that the concern for the depleting wild finally stimulated.

Act 53 of 1972

The first comprehensive legislation relating to protection of wild life was passed by the Parliament and it was assented by the President on 9th September, 1972 and came to be known as The Wild Life (Protection) Act, 1972 (53 of 1972). An Act to provide for the protection of wild animals, birds and plants and for matters connected therewith or ancillary or incidental thereto.

List of Amending Acts

a)   The constitution (Forty-second Amendment) Act, 1976.

b)   The Wild Life (Protection) (Amendment) Act, 1982 (23 of 1982).

c)   The Wild Life (Protection) (Amendment) Act, 1986 (28 of 1986).

d)   The Wild Life (Protection) (Amendment) Act, 1991 (44 of 1991).

e)   The Wild Life (Protection) (Amendment) Act, 1993 (26 of 1993).

The Act provides for the protection of wild animals, birds and plants and for matters connected therewith or ancillary or incidental thereto. It extends to the whole of India, except the State of Jammu and Kashmir which has its own wildlife act. It has six schedules which give varying degrees of protection. Schedule I and part II of Schedule II provide absolute protection; offences under these are prescribed the highest penalties. Species listed in Schedule III and Schedule IV is also protected, but the penalties are much lower. Schedule V includes the animals which may be hunted. The plants in Schedule VI are prohibited from cultivation and planting. The hunting to the Enforcement authorities have the power to compound offences under this Schedule *i.e.* they impose fines on the offenders. Up to April 2010, there have been 16 convictions under this act relating to the death of tigers.

4.2.2 Wild Life (Protection) Act 1972 as amended in 1993

The Indian wildlife (Protection) act, 1972 as amended up to 1993 has seven chapters in it. Chapter I entitled Preliminary has short title, extent, commencement and definitions of various entities and objects which is used in this act. In the Chapter

II, the authorities to be appointed or constituted under the Act, appointment of Director and other officers, appointment of Chief Wildlife Warden and other officers, power to delegate, constitution of the Wildlife Advisory Board, procedure to be followed by the Board, duties of the Wildlife Advisory Board, etc has been discussed in detail. Chapter III discusses about hunting of Wild Animals, in which prohibition of hunting, maintenance of records of wild animals killed or captured, hunting of wild animals to be permitted in certain cases, grant of permit for special purposes, suspension or cancellation of license, appeals, hunting of young and female of wild animals, declaration of closed time and restrictions on hunting, etc. has been elaborated. Amendment has been added as Chapter IIIA for the protection of specified plants having prohibition of picking, uprooting of specified plants, grant of permit for special purposes, cultivation of specified plants without license prohibited, dealing in specified plants without license prohibited, declaration of stock, possession, etc. of plants by licensee, purchase etc., of specified plants, plants to be Government property. The Sanctuaries, National Parks and Closed Areas, Game Reserve, Sanctuaries or National Parks declared by Central Government are discussed in the chapter IV. Amendments in this chapter added as Chapter IVA for Central Zoo Authority and Recognition of Zoos. This declares about constitution of Central Zoo Authority, term of office and condition of service of chairperson and members etc., functions of the authority, Procedure to be regulated by the authority, grants and loans to authority and constitution of fund, annual report and audit report to be laid before parliament, recognition of zoos, acquisition of animals by a zoo, prohibition of teasing, etc. in a zoo. Chapter 5 of this act has Trade or Commerce in Wild Animals, Animal Articles and Trophies. An amendment has been added as chapter VA for Prohibition of trade or commerce in trophies, animal articles, etc. derived from certain animals. Chapter VI entitled prevention and detection of offences discussed about power of entry, search, arrest and detention, penalties, attempts and abetment, punishment for wrongful seizure, power to compound offences, cognizance of offences, operation of other laws not barred, presumption to be made in certain cases, offences by companies. The last chapter VII of this act has miscellaneous discussion such as officers to be public servants, protection of action taken in good faith, reward to persons, power to alter entries in schedules, declaration of certain wild animals to be vermin, power of central government to make rules, power of state government to make rules, rights of scheduled tribes to be protected, repeal and savings, etc. Animals are categorized in schedule I to VI and enlisted in the last of this act. The animal listed under Schedule I need special protection.

4.2.3 Wild Life (Protection) Amendment Act 2002

Wild Life (Protection) Amendment Act, 2002 is an Act of the Parliament of India amending the existing Wildlife Protection Act, 1972. The Wildlife Protection Act, 1972 was enacted with the objective of effectively controlling poaching and illegal trade in wildlife and its derivatives. The 2002 Amendment Act which came into force in January, 2003 have made punishment and penalty for offences under the Act more stringent. For offences relating to wild animals or their parts and products) included in schedule-I or part II of Schedule- II and those relating to hunting or altering the boundaries of a sanctuary or national park the punishment and penalty have been enhanced, the minimum imprisonment prescribed is three years which may extend to seven years, with a minimum fine of Rs. 10,000/-. For a subsequent offence of this nature, the term of imprisonment shall not be less than three years but may extend to seven years with a minimum fine of Rs. 25,000. Also a new section (51-A) has been inserted in the Act, making certain conditions applicable while granting bail; When any person accused of the commission of any offence relating to Schedule I or Part II of Schedule II or offences relating to hunting inside the boundaries of National Park or Wildlife Sanctuary or altering the boundaries of such parks and sanctuaries, is arrested under the provisions of the Act, then not withstanding anything contained in the Code of Criminal Procedure, 1973, no such person who had been previously convicted of an offence under this Act shall be released on bail unless:

(a) The Public Prosecutor has been given an opportunity of opposing the release on bail,

(b) Where the Public Prosecutor opposes the application, the Court is satisfied that there are reasonable grounds for believing that he is not guilty of such offences and that he is not likely to commit any offence while on bail.

In order to improve the intelligence gathering in wildlife crime, the existing provision for rewarding the informers has been increased from 20% of the fine and composition money respectively to 50% in each case. In addition to this, a reward up to Rs. 10,000/- is also proposed to be given to the informants and others who provide assistance in detection of crime and apprehension of the offender. At present, persons having ownership certificate in respect of Schedule I and Part II animals, can sell or gift such articles. This has been amended with a view to curb illegal trade and thus no person can now acquire Schedule I or Part II of Schedule II animals, articles or trophies except by way of inheritance (except live elephants). Stringent measures have also been proposed to forfeit the properties of hardcore criminals who have already been convicted in the past for heinous wildlife crimes. These provisions are similar to the provisions of Narcotic Drugs and Psychotropic Substances Act, 1985. Provisions have also been made empowering officials to evict encroachments from Protected Areas. Offences related to trade and commerce in trophies, animals articles etc. derived from certain animals (except chapter V A and section 38J) attracts a term of imprisonment up to three years and/or a fine up to Rs. 25,000/-.

4.2.4 Wild Life (Protection) Amendment Act 2006

The Wild Life (Protection) Amendment Act, 2006 (No. 39 of 2006) has come into force on 4th September 2006. The Act provides for creating the National Tiger Conservation Authority and the Tiger and Other Endangered Species Crime Control Bureau (Wildlife Crime Control Bureau). The implementation over the years has highlighted the need for a statutory authority with legal backing to ensure tiger conservation. On the basis of the recommendations of National Board for Wild Life, a Task Force was set up to look into the problems of tiger conservation in the country. The recommendations of the Task Force, inter alia include strengthening of Project Tiger by giving it statutory and administrative powers, apart from creating the Wildlife Crime Control Bureau. It has also recommended that an annual report should be submitted to the Central Government for laying in Parliament, so that commitment to

Project Tiger is reviewed from time to time, in addition to addressing the concerns of local people. The National Tiger Conservation Authority would facilitate MoU with States within federal set up for tiger conservation. It will provide for an oversight by Parliament as well. Further, it will address livelihood interests of local people in areas surrounding Tiger Reserves, apart from ensuring that the rights of Scheduled Tribes and such other people living nearby are not interfered or adversely affected. The core (critical) and buffer (peripheral) areas have been defined, while safeguarding the interests of Scheduled Tribes and such other forest dwellers.

The functions and powers of the Authority, inter-alia include approval of Tiger Conservation Plan prepared by States, laying down normative standards for tiger conservation, providing information on several aspects which include protection, tiger estimation, patrolling, etc. ensuring measures for addressing man-wild animal conflicts and fostering co-existence with local people, preparing annual report for laying before Parliament, constitution of Steering Committee by States, preparation of tiger protection and conservation plans by States, ensuring agricultural, livelihood interests of people living in and around Tiger Reserves, establishing the tiger conservation foundation by States for supporting their development.

The Notification of the National Tiger Conservation Authority has been issued on 4th September 2006, for a period of three years, with the Minister for Environment and Forests as its Chairperson and the Minister of State for Environment and Forests as the Vice-chairperson. The official members include Secretary, Ministry of Environment and Forests, Director General of Forests and Special Secretary, Ministry of Environment and Forests, Secretary, Ministry of Tribal Affairs, Secretary, Ministry of Social Justice and Empowerment, Chairperson, National Commission for the Scheduled Tribes, Chairperson National Commission for the Scheduled Castes, Secretary, Ministry of Panchayati Raj, Director, Wildlife Preservation, Ministry of Environment and Forests and six Chief Wildlife Wardens (in rotation from Tiger Reserve States) (Arunachal Pradesh, Madhya Pradesh, Orissa, Rajasthan, Tamil Nadu and Uttaranchal). Three Members of Parliament would be nominated by the Parliament.

The Ministry of Law and Justice would also be nominating an officer. The Ministry of Environment and Forests is in the process of selecting the eight non-official experts or professionals having prescribed qualifications and experience, of which at least two shall be from the field of tribal development. The Inspector General of Forests in charge of Project Tiger shall be the Member Secretary of the Authority. The Ministry is in the process of creating the Wildlife Crime Control Bureau, invoking the provisions created after the recent amendment. The Bureau would collate intelligence relating to wildlife crime, ensure coordination with State Governments and other Authorities through its set up, apart from developing infrastructure and capacity building for scientific and professional investigation into wildlife crimes and assist the State Governments in successful prosecution of such crimes. The penalty for an offence relating to the core area of a tiger reserve or hunting in the reserve has been increased. The first conviction in such offence shall be punishable with imprisonment not less than three years but may extend to seven years and also with fine not less than fifty thousand rupees but may extend to two lakh rupees. The second or subsequent conviction would lead to imprisonment not less than seven years and also with fine not less than five lakh rupees, which may extend to fifty lakh rupees.

4.2.5 Wildlife (Protection) Amendment Bill 2013

The Wild Life (Protection) Amendment Bill, 2013 was introduced in the Rajya Sabha on August 5, 2013. The Bill has been referred to the Standing Committee on Environment and Forests. The Bill seeks to amend the Wild Life (Protection) Act, 1972. This Act provides for the protection and conservation of wild animals, birds and plants. It also covers the management of their habitats and regulation and control of trade or commerce linked to wild life. According to the government, India is a party to the Convention on International Trade in Endangered Species of Wild Fauna and Flora (CITES) and amendments to the Act are necessary for India to fulfil its obligations under the CITES. The key amendments made by the Bill are:

- The manufacture, sale, transport or use of animal traps except for educational and scientific purposes (with permission) is prohibited.

- Under the Act, destruction, exploitation or removal of any wildlife including forest produce from a sanctuary is not permitted, except with a permit. The amendment allows certain activities such as grazing or movement of livestock, bona fide use of drinking and household water by local communities and hunting under a permit.

- Provisions to regulate international trade in endangered species of wild fauna and flora as per the CITES have been inserted. A schedule listing out flora and fauna for purposes of regulation of international trade under CITES has been added.

- The Tiger and Other Endangered Species Crime Control Bureau has been changed to the Wild life Crime Control Bureau.

- The term of punishment and fines for commission of offences under the Act have been increased.

- The Bill protects the hunting rights of Scheduled Tribes in the Andaman and Nicobar Islands.

4.3 Documentation of Wild Life

Species judged as threatened are listed by various agencies as well as by some private organizations. The most cited of this list is the Red Data Book. Red data book is a loose-leaf volume of information on the status of many kinds of species. Red, of course is symbolic of the danger that these species both plants and animals presently experience throughout the globe.

4.3.1 Conservation of Nature and Natural Resources (IUCN) and Red Data List

The IUCN Red List of Threatened Species (also known as the IUCN Red List or Red Data List), founded in 1964, is the world's most comprehensive inventory of the global conservation status of biological species. The International Union for the Conservation of Nature (IUCN) is the world's main authority on the conservation status of species. A series of Regional Red Lists are produced by countries or organizations, which assess the risk of extinction to species within a political management unit. The IUCN Red List is set upon precise criteria to evaluate the extinction risk of thousands of species and subspecies. These criteria are relevant to all species and all regions of the world. The aim is to convey the urgency of conservation issues to the public and policy makers, as well as help the international community to try to reduce species extinction. According to IUCN (1996), the formally stated goals of the Red List are (1) to provide scientifically based information on the status of species and subspecies at a global level, (2) to draw attention to the magnitude and importance of threatened biodiversity, (3) to influence national and international policy and decision-making and (4) to provide information to guide actions to conserve biological diversity.

Major species assessors include BirdLife International, the Institute of Zoology (research division of Zoological Society of London), the World Conservation Monitoring Centre and many Specialist Groups within the IUCN Species Survival Commission (SSC). Collectively, assessments by these organizations and groups account for nearly half the species on the Red List. The IUCN aims to have the category of every species re-evaluated every five years if possible or at least every ten years. This is done in a peer reviewed manner through IUCN Species Survival Commission (SSC) Specialist Groups, which are Red List Authorities responsible for a species, group of species or specific geographic area or in the case of BirdLife International, an entire class (Aves).

The International Union for the Conservation of Nature and Natural Resources (IUCN) developed the first established approach in dealing with the presentation of information on rare and threatened species. The Red Data Book was first issued in 1966 by the IUCN's Special Survival Commission as a guide for formulation, preservation and management of species listed. In this Book, information for endangered mammals and birds is more extensive than other groups of animals and plants, coverage is also given to less prominent organisms facing extinction. The pink pages in this publication include the critically endangered species. As the status of the animal's changes, new pages are sent to the subscribers. Green pages are used for those species that were formerly endangered, but have now recovered to a point where they are no longer threatened. With passing time, the number of pink pages continues to increase. There are pitifully few green pages. A Red Data Book contains lists of species whose continued existence is threatened. Species are classified into different categories of perceived risk. Each Red Data Book usually deals with a specific group of animals or plants *i.e.* reptiles, insects and mosses. They are now being published in many different countries and provide useful information on the threat status of the species.

The red-listing assessment is a simple logical process to determine the status of threat to a species based on available information. More formal IUCN Red List Categories and Criteria were developed in the early nineties to further objectively assess and priorities species for conservation purposes at a global scale. A review of these categories and criteria was completed in 1998 and 1999 and the current version the IUCN Red list categories and criteria (Version 3.1) is now widely used around the world for species assessments. The IUCN also produce regularly updated guidelines for using the categories and criteria and have produced guidelines for applying the criteria at a regional level.

The Red list has listed 132 species of plants and animals as Critically Endangered, the most threatened category from India in 2012. Plants seemed to be the most threatened life form with 60 species being listed as Critically Endangered and 141 as Endangered. The Critically Endangered list included 18 species of amphibians, 14 fishes and 10 mammals. There are also 15 bird species in the category. The agency listed 310 species as endangered ones, including 69 fishes, 38 mammals and 32 amphibians. Two plant species were reported to be extinct in the wild, including the Euphorbia mayuranthanii of Kerala. A leaf frog species and six plants were recorded as extinct, according to the latest assessment. Of the total 63,837 species globally assessed, the IUCN classified 3,947 as Critically Endangered, 81 as Extinct, 63 as Extinct in the Wild. In the lower risk categories, there were 5766 species in Endangered, 10,104 in Vulnerable and 4,467 in Near Threatened categories. Scientific data regarding 10,497 species was not available and hence classified as Data Deficient. The threat level of as many as seven Indian bird species had increased in the last one year. According to the latest figures, 15 species of Indian birds, including the great Indian bustard, Siberian crane and sociable lapwing are there in the list of Critically Endangered birds. In the lower risk categories, the agency included 14 bird species as Endangered and 51 as vulnerable ones. Four fish species from Kerala, including the Pookode Lake Barb and Nilgiri Mystus, are included in the Critically Endangered fishes of India. The agency listed 39 species from Kerala as endangered, including the Periyar Latia, Nilgiri Danio, Cardamom Garra, Periyar Garra and Anamalai Sucker Catfish. The Imperial White Collared Yellow Catfish, Santhampara Loach, Nilgiri Barb, Hump Backed Mahseer, Periyar Barb and Peninsular Hill Trout are among the endangered fish species of Kerala. The number of Critically Endangered species from Kerala has dropped to four from seven of last year whereas the endangered list had gone up to 39 from the 37 of the previous assessment.

4.3.2 Convention on International Trade in Endangered Species of Wild Fauna and Flora (CITES) 1975

CITES (Convention on International Trade in Endangered Species of Wild Fauna and Flora) is an international agreement between governments. CITES was drafted as a result of a resolution adopted in 1963 at a meeting of members of IUCN (The World Conservation Union). The text of the Convention was finally agreed at a meeting of representatives of 80 countries in Washington, D.C. USA. The convention was opened for signature in 3rd March 1973 and CITES entered into force on 1 July 1975. Its aim is to ensure that international trade in specimens of wild animals and plants does not threaten their survival. Widespread information nowadays about the endangered status of many prominent species, such as the tiger and elephants, might make the need for such a convention seem obvious. But at the time when the ideas for CITES were first formed, in the 1960s, international discussion of the regulation of wildlife trade for conservation purposes was something relatively new. With hindsight, the need for CITES is clear. Annually, international wildlife trade is estimated to be worth billions of dollars and to include hundreds of millions of plant and animal specimens. The trade is diverse, ranging from live animals and plants to a vast array of wildlife products derived from them, including food products, exotic leather goods, wooden musical instruments, timber, tourist curios and medicines. Levels of exploitation of some animal and plant species are high and the trade in them, together with other factors, such as habitat loss, is capable of heavily depleting their populations and even bringing some species close to extinction. Many wildlife species in trade are not endangered, but the existence of an agreement to ensure the sustainability of the trade is important in order to safeguard these resources for the future. Because the trade in wild animals and plants crosses borders between countries, the effort to regulate it requires international cooperation to safeguard certain species from over-exploitation. CITES was conceived in the spirit of such cooperation. Today, it accords varying degrees of protection to more than 35,000 species of animals and plants, whether they are traded as live specimens, fur coats or dried herbs. The original of the Convention was deposited with the Depositary Government in Chinese, English, French, Russian and Spanish languages, each version being equally authentic. CITES is an international agreement to which States (countries) adhere voluntarily. States that have agreed to be bound by the Convention are known as Parties. Although CITES is legally binding on the Parties, in other words they have to implement the Convention, it does not take the place of national laws. Rather it provides a framework to be respected by each Party, which has to adopt its own domestic legislation to ensure that CITES is implemented at the national level. For many years CITES has been among the conservation agreements with the largest membership, with now 180 Parties. CITES places species into three appendices based on their conservation status and risk from trade.

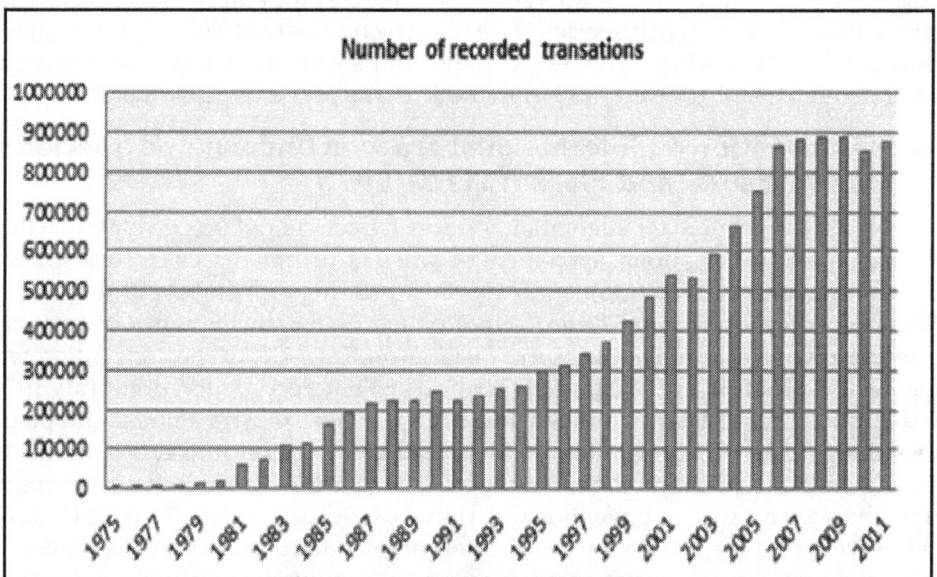

Figure 4.1 Records of CITES

Operation

CITES is one of the largest and oldest conservation and sustainable use agreements in existence. Participation is voluntary and countries that have Funding for the activities of the Secretariat and Conference of the Parties (CoP) meetings comes from a Trust Fund derived from Party contributions. Trust Fund money is not available to Parties to improve implementation or compliance. These activities and all those outside Secretariat activities (training, species specific programmes such as Monitoring the Illegal Killing of Elephants- MIKE) must find external funding, mostly from donor countries and regional organizations such as the European Union. Although the Convention itself does not provide for arbitration or dispute in the case of noncompliance, 36 years of CITES in practice has resulted in several strategies to deal with infractions by Parties. The Secretariat, when informed of an infraction by a Party, will notify all other parties. The Secretariat will give the Party time to respond to the allegations and may provide technical assistance to prevent further infractions. Other actions the Convention itself does not provide for but that derive from subsequent COP resolutions may be taken against the offending Party. These include:

- Mandatory confirmation of all permits by the Secretariat,

- Suspension of cooperation from the Secretariat,

- A formal warning,

- A visit by the Secretariat to verify capacity,

- Recommendations to all Parties to suspend CITES related trade with the offending party,

- Dictation of corrective measures to be taken by the offending Party before the Secretariat will resume cooperation or recommend resumption of trade.

Bilateral sanctions have been imposed on the basis of national legislation *e.g.* USA used certification under the Pelly Amendment to get Japan to revoke its reservation to hawksbill turtle products in 1991, thus reducing the volume of its exports. Infractions may include negligence with respect to permit issuing, excessive trade, lax enforcement and failing to produce annual reports. Originally, CITES addressed depletion resulting from demand for luxury goods such as furs in Western countries, but with the rising wealth of Asia, particularly in China, the focus changed to products demanded there, particularly those used for luxury goods such as ivory or shark fins or for superstitious purposes such as rhinoceros horn. As of 2013 the demand was massive and had expanded to include thousands of species previously considered unremarkable and in no danger of extinction such as manta rays or pangolins.

Reservations

Any Party (member State) of CITES may make a reservation to the Convention. A reservation is a unilateral statement that the Party will not be bound by the provisions of the Convention relating to trade in a particular species listed in the Appendices. For species included in Appendix I or II, there are restrictions on when a reservation may be entered. They may be entered either when a State becomes a Party to the Convention or within 90 days after the adoption of an amendment to the Appendices. For example, if the Conference of the Parties agrees at a meeting to transfer a species from Appendix II to Appendix I, reservations against the Appendix-I listing have to be entered within 90 days after the end of the meeting. This is allowable under Article XV, paragraph 3 and Article XXIII of the Convention. For species included in Appendix III, a State may enter a reservation at the time of becoming a Party or at any time thereafter. This is allowable under Article XVI and Article XXIII of the Convention. A Party that has entered a reservation may withdraw it at any time. However, while the reservation is in effect, the Party is formally treated as a non-Party with respect to trade in the species or specimen concerned.

Conservation Impacts

After four decades, CITES remains one of the cornerstones of international conservation with 175 member countries and trade regulated in more than 34,000 species. Representatives of CITES nations meet every two to three years at a Conference of the Parties where progress is reviewed and adjustments are made to the list of protected species, which is grouped into three categories with different levels of protection:

CITES Appendix I: Appendix I contain species threatened with extinction. Trade in these specimens is usually prohibited (occurs only in very exceptional circumstances) or is limited to pre-CITES specimens (specimens harvested before the date of listing on CITES). Appendix I species includes (but is not limited to) great apes, lemurs, the giant panda, many South American monkeys, great whales, cheetah, leopards, tiger, elephants (Australian stricter domestic measure applies), rhinoceroses, many birds of prey, cranes, pheasants and parrots, all sea turtles, some crocodiles and lizards, giant salamanders and some mussels orchids, cycads and cacti. If we want to trade in Pre-CITES specimens, we will need a pre-CITES certificate issued by the CITES management authority in the country of export.

CITES Appendix II: Appendix II contains species that, although not threatened with extinction now, might become so unless trade in them is strictly regulated. Australia has chosen to list some Appendix II species as Appendix I via stricter domestic measures. If one want to trade in Appendix II species to/from Australia, it will generally need both a CITES export and import permit issued by CITES management authorities. Some Appendix II specimens carried as personal effects will not require permit. Appendix II also includes some non-threatened species, to prevent threatened species from being traded under the guise of non-threatened species that are similar in appearance. These are referred to as lookalike species.

CITES Appendix III: Appendix III contains species that are protected in at least one country that has asked other CITES parties for help in controlling trade. If we are importing or exporting an Appendix III specimen to/from Australia from the listing country, it is treated like an Appendix II specimen and we will need both an export and an import permit. If the Appendix III specimen comes from any other country *i.e.* not the listing country, a CITES certificate of origin must be obtained. CITES also brings together law enforcement officers from wildlife authorities, national parks, customs and police agencies to collaborate on efforts to combat wildlife crime targeted at animals such as elephants and rhinos.

Action in Bangkok

The WWF urges governments to recognize the serious nature of wildlife crime and take strong action at the 16th Conference of the Parties hosted in the Thai capital city of Bangkok from 3-24 March 2013. As poaching of rhinos and elephants reaches crisis levels, parties should be prepared to assess countries' compliance with rhino and elephant resolutions and to recommend a suspension of trade in CITES listed species for countries where progress is not made. WWF is urging governments to support all proposals relating to sharks and manta rays. These species take a long time to reach maturity and produce relatively few young in their lifetime so they are extremely vulnerable to overfishing. WWF supports the regulation of trade in Madagascar's ebony and rosewood species, which have been massively impacted by illegal logging. WWF and TRAFFIC provide important scientific and technical support to CITES and work with member countries to implement legislation and regulations on CITES and to ensure that those laws are effectively enforced.

Importance of CITES: The Convention on International Trade of Endangered Species of Wild Fauna and Flora (CITES) is the only treaty that regulates international trade in wildlife. CITES has three lists (Appendices) that offer different levels of regulation. The Appendix I list prohibits commercial international trade, Appendix II allows international trade with regulations and scientific analysis for issuing the permits and Appendix III offers help to individual countries to keep track of trade in their species. Altogether, CITES lists around 37,000 species of wild animals and plants. Defenders of Wildlife participates in CITES by helping countries make proposals to list species or increase the level of protection that need better conservation measures at the international level and to ensure that the necessary tools and implementation policies are in place for the survival of the listed species. Defenders' work with CITES has resulted in several important wins for wildlife, including making it illegal to trade parrots and other birds, preventing a proposal to roll back protections for the hawksbill sea turtle and most recently in 2010, increasing protections for the Kaiser's spotted newt, prohibiting trade of this critically endangered amphibian.

As CITES has expanded greatly through the inclusion of many more species and entire taxa on its Appendices, enforcement has become increasingly difficult worldwide. The United States has long been considered a leader in biological conservation efforts and has some of the best national laws in place; yet it maintains only about 100 qualified wildlife inspectors for all of its air and sea ports nationally and is still the largest importer of many animal and plant products. With so many listed species and differing permit requirements for those listed on CITES appendices, proper identification of specimens becomes increasingly difficult. This has resulted in legal shipments being held in quarantine for very long time periods and many more illegal shipments having cleared through inspection or having passed through undetected. Corruption in developing countries is also very widespread for species protected by CITES. Cases have come to light, of forged Appendix II export permits having been issued from one country, when the specimens were in fact from a neighboring country that banned trade under Appendix III. In other cases, Appendix I specimens from the wild have been misrepresented as having been raised in captivity, permitting their trade when it should have been prohibited under CITES. The worldwide TRAFFIC network that works in conjunction with the World Wide Fund for Nature and IUCN-The World Conservation Union, as well as the CITES Secretariat, regularly publishes bulletins concerning enforcement in trade in endangered species and is the best single source of information on CITES enforcement. Most people in international conservation agree that while the Convention itself articulates a strong and progressive legal framework and structure, much greater strides in enforcement are needed worldwide. Advances have been made to identify specimens or parts using molecular techniques and great strides have been made in many countries to infiltrate illegal smugglers of wildlife products, but ever greater problems have emerged with the expansion of CITES and the ever growing demand for species and specimens of species in many countries.

4.3.3 World Conservation Monitoring Centre (WCMC)

The loss of biodiversity and associated degradation of ecosystems has serious consequences for society, including the businesses that depend on and often impact upon, the range of services that ecosystems provide. With increasing attention at the national and international levels from investors and regulators, license to operate, access to finance and insurance and protection of a businesses' reputation are now intrinsically linked to the management of biodiversity and ecosystem services. Understanding the global policy context, having access to data and the right tools to make decisions and support to interpret and make use of data are priorities for businesses to facilitate the transition from policy to performance. The UNEP World Conservation Monitoring Centre was established in 2000 as the world biodiversity information and assessment centre of the United Nations Environment Programme. The Centre's roots go back to 1979 when IUCN established a Cambridge office to monitor endangered species.

In 1988, the independent, non-profit World Conservation Monitoring Centre was founded jointly by IUCN, WWF and UNEP. The UNEP World Conservation Monitoring Centre (UNEP-WCMC) is the specialist biodiversity assessment arm of the United Nations Environment Programme, the world's foremost intergovernmental environmental organization. The Centre delivers scientific analyses to the UN, multilateral environmental agreements, national governments organizations and companies to use in the development and implementation of their policies and decisions. UNEP-WCMC is the biodiversity assessment and policy implementation arm of the United Nations Environment Programme (UNEP), the world's foremost intergovernmental environmental organization. The centre has been in operation since 1989, combining scientific research with practical policy advice. UNEP-WCMC provides objective, scientifically rigorous products and services to help decision makers recognize the value of biodiversity and apply this knowledge to all that they do. Its core business is managing data about ecosystems and biodiversity, interpreting and analyzing that data to provide assessments and policy analysis and making the results available to international decision makers and businesses. UNEP-WCMC provides objective, science-based products and services that include ecosystem and species assessments, support for implementation of environmental agreements, regional and global biodiversity information, research on threats and impacts and development of indicators and future scenarios for the living world. The main objectives is to provide early warning and assessment of emerging challenges in biodiversity conservation and sustainable management, to support the development and implementation of multilateral environmental agreements (MEAs) and programmes that promote biodiversity conservation and sustainable management and to enhance access to expertise, tools, techniques and information for public awareness, education, capacity-building and cross-sectoral cooperation.

The activities of UNEP-WCMC include biodiversity assessment, support to international conventions such as the Convention on Biological Diversity (CBD) and the Convention on International Trade in Endangered Species of Wild Fauna and Flora (CITES), capacity building and management of both aspatial and spatial data on species and habitats of conservation concern. UNEP-WCMC has a mandate to facilitate the delivery of the global indicators under the CBD's 2010 Biodiversity Target on the rate of loss of biological diversity and works alongside the CITES Secretariat producing a range of reports and databases. It also manages the World Database of Protected Areas in collaboration with the IUCN World Commission on Protected Areas. A series of world atlases on biodiversity topics have been published by UNEP-WCMC through University of California Press. UNEP-WCMC itself is composed of multiple Programmes that are concerned with different conservation sectors such as Biodiversity Informatics, Business and Biodiversity, Climate Change, Ecosystem Assessment Food Security, Biomass and Biodiversity, Marine Decision and Support, Protected Areas and Species.

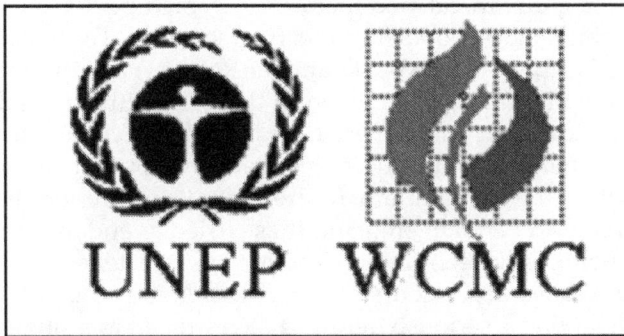

Figure 4.2 Logo of WCMC

4.3.4 Networked Organisms and Habitats (NOAH)

Project Noah is a powerful tool for learning about nature and a leading technology platform for crowd sourcing ecological data. Noah stands for networked organisms and habitats. Project Noah was adopted by National Geographic since 2010. Project Noah has set out to mobilize a new generation of nature explorers. The ultimate goal is to build the go-to platform for documenting all the world's organisms. By helping the mobile masses document their encounters with nature, building a powerful force for data collection and an important educational tool for wildlife awareness and preservation. Project Noah is an award-winning software platform designed to help people reconnect with the natural world. Launched out of NYU's Interactive Telecommunications Program in early 2010, the project began as an experiment to mobilize citizen scientists and build a digital butterfly net for the 21st century. Backed by National Geographic, Project Noah is mobilizing a new generation of nature explorers and helping people from around the world appreciate their local wildlife. The community is harnessing the power and popularity of new mobile technologies to collect important ecological data and help preserve global biodiversity.

4.4 Rare, Endangered and Endemic species

India is uniquely blessed with wildlife diversity. One of eighteen mega diverse countries, it is home to 7.6% of all mammalian, 12.6% of all avian, 6.2% of all reptilian, 4.4% of all amphibian, 11.7% of all fish and 6.0% of all flowering plant species. This diversity becomes even more remarkable given that our country, with only 2.4% of the total land area of the world, contributes 8 per cent to the known global biological diversity, while also being the second largest populous nation in the world, with over 1.2 billion people.

India has been identified as one of the top 12 mega-diversity countries of the world. Among the 18 hot spots recognized in the world, two are in India-Eastern Himalayas and Western Ghats. The Western Ghats, which is one of the nine biogeographic regions of India possess various types of tropical forests, ranging from wet evergreen to dry deciduous. Nearly 63% of the tree species of the low and the medium elevation evergreen forests of Western Ghats are endemic. This high level of diversity and endemism in the Western Ghats has conferred on them the hot spot status. In order to categorize threatened species, IUCN has updated the categories on the basis of geographical range, population and fragmentation. The threatened species categories now used in the Red Data Books and the Red List are critically endangered (facing an extremely high risk of extinction in the wild in the immediate future), endangered (not critical, but facing a very high risk of extinction in the wild in the near future) and vulnerable (not critical or endangered but facing a high risk of extinction in the wild in the medium-term future). Taxa listed as critically endangered qualify for vulnerable and endangered and those listed as endangered qualify for vulnerable. Together these categories are described as threatened. A rare species is one that occurs in widely separated small sub-population so that inter-breeding between sub-populations is seriously reduced or restricted to a single population. They are not at present endangered or vulnerable but face a high risk of being so and usually localized within restricted geographical areas or habitats or are thinly scattered over a more extensive range. A hypothetical rare species is one with narrow habitat range, low climate tolerance, specialized adaptation requiring an outside agency for pollination, poor dispersal strategies, few seeds per fruit and poor viability of seeds. The spatial distribution of plants and location, their degree of habitat niche specialization and the spatial distribution of sensitive habitats are some of the major aspects to be analyzed. It is relatively straightforward to classify species by their distribution among habitats defined by fixed topographic or edaphic features of the plot. Most of the endemic species with a small geographic range end up as rare species and later threatened species unless their habitat is protected. Rarity rests on a specific species being represented by a small number of organisms worldwide, usually fewer than 10,000. However, a species having a very narrow endemic range or fragmented habitat also influences the concept. The Red list of 2012 is out on 18th February 2012 at Rio +20 Earth Summit. Red List has listed 132 species of plants and animals as Critically Endangered from India.

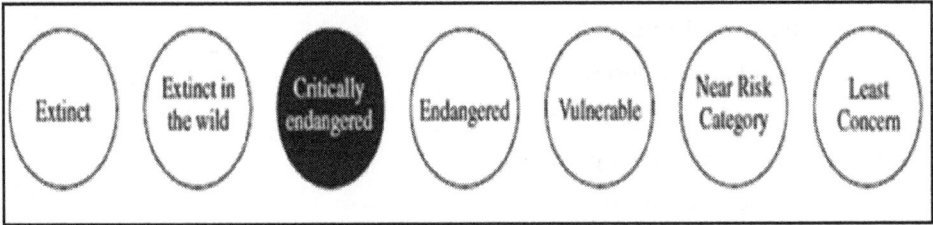

Figure 4.3 Risk Category

4.4.1 Endangered Species of India

A plant, animal or microorganism that is in immediate risk of biological extinction is called endangered species or threatened species. In India, 450 plant species have been identified as endangered species. The 100 mammals and 150 birds are estimated to be endangered. India's biodiversity is threatened primarily due to:

a) Habitat destruction,

b) Degradation,

c) Over exploitation of resources.

The Red-data book contains a list of endangered species of plants and animals. It contains a list of species of that are endangered but might become extinct in the near future if not protected. Some of the rarest animals found in India are:

i. Asiatic cheetah,

ii. Asiatic Lion,

iii. Asiatic Wild Ass,

iv. Bengal Fox,

v. Gaur,

vi. Indian Elephant,

vii. Indian Rhinocerous,

viii. Marbled Cat,

ix. Markhor.

Extinct species is no longer found in the world. Endangered or threatened species is one whose number has been reduced to a critical number. Unless it is protected and conserved, it is in immediate danger of extinction. Vulnerable species is one whose population is facing continuous decline due to habitat destruction or over exploitation. However, it is still abundant.

Rare species is localized within a restricted area or is thinly scattered over an extensive area. Such species are not endangered or vulnerable. A few endangered species in the world are listed below:

i.   West Virginia Spring Salamander (U.S.A)

ii.   Giant Panda (China)

iii. Golden Lion Tamarin (Brazil)

iv.   Siberian Tiger (Siberia)

v.   Mountain Gorilla (Africa)

vi.   Pine Barrens Tree Frog (Male)

vii. Arabian Oryx (Middle East)

viii. African Elephant (Africa)

Other important endangered species are:

i.   Tortoise, Green sea Turtle, Gharial, Python (Reptiles),

ii.   Peacock, Siberian White Crane, Pelican, Indian Bustard (Birds),

iii. Hoolock gibbin, Lion-tailed Macaque, Capped mokey, Golden monkey (Primates),

iv.   Rauvol fia serpentina (medicinal plant), Sandal wood tree, etc.

Factors affecting Endangered Species

a) Human beings dispose wastes indiscriminately in nature thereby polluting the air, land and water. These pollutants enter the food chain and accumulate in living creatures resulting in death.

b) Over-exploitation of natural resources and poaching of wild animals also leads to their extinction.

c) Climate change brought about by accumulation of green houses gases in the atmosphere. Climate change threatens organisms and ecosystems and they cannot adjust to the changing environmental conditions leading to their death and extinction.

An international treaty to help protect endangered wildlife is, Convention on International Trade in Endangered Species 1975 (CITES). This treaty is now signed by 160 countries.

• CITES lists 900 species that cannot be commercially traded as live specimens or wildlife products as they are in danger of extinction.

• CITES restricts trade of 2900 other species as they are endangered.

Drawbacks of CITES:

i.   This treaty is limited as enforcement is difficult and convicted violators get away by paying only a small fine.

ii.   Member countries can exempt themselves from protecting any listed species.

4.4.2 Endemic species of India

Species that are found only in a particular region are known as endemic species. Almost 60% the endemic species in India are found in Himalayas and the Western Ghats. Endemic species are mainly concentrated in:

i.   North-East India,

ii.   North-West Himalayas,

iii.   Western Ghats,

iv.   Andaman and Nicobar Islands.

Examples of endemic Flora species are

i.   Sapria Himalayana,

ii.   Ovaria Lurida,

iii.   Nepenthis khasiana etc.

Endemic fauna of significance in the Western Ghats are:

i.   Lion tailed macaque,

ii.   Nilgiri langur,

iii.   Brown palm civet,

iv.   Nilgiri tahr.

Factors affecting Endemic Species:

i.   Habitat loss and fragmentation due to draining and filling of inland wetlands.

ii.   Pollution also plays an important role.

Examples:

a)   Frog eggs, tadpoles and adults are extremely sensitive to pollutants especially pesticides.

b)   Over-hunting.

c)   Populations can be adversely affected by introduction of non active predators and competitors. Disease producing organisms also play an important adversary in reducing populations of endemic species.

4.4.3 Extinct species of India

There was a time when India was home for some of the most beautiful wild animals, due to excessive hunting and poaching for sport and body parts by man, these wild animals have become extinct. Some of the wild species are on the brink of extinction and some of them are already extinction such as Dangs Giant Squirrel and

Aldabra banded snail. Critically endangered species in India are the Great cats, one Horne rhinoceros, Ganges river dolphins, Purple frog, birds species such as Himalayan Quail, Great Indian Bustard and Indian Horn-bill and many small mammals. The Indian government is planning a re-wilding project for Cheetahs.

Indian Cheetah: Indian Cheetah also known as Asiatic Cheetah has been known to exist in India for a very long time. Due to access hunting, deforestation and habitat loss, the fastest land animal on earth become extinct in India. The Asiatic Cheetah is a rare and critically endangered species of Big Cats family, now found today only in Iran so also known as the Iranian Cheetah, world's last few are occasional sightings in neighbor countries of India. Indian Cheetah was found in semi-desert area of Rajasthan and Gujarat and other open habitats where prey is available.

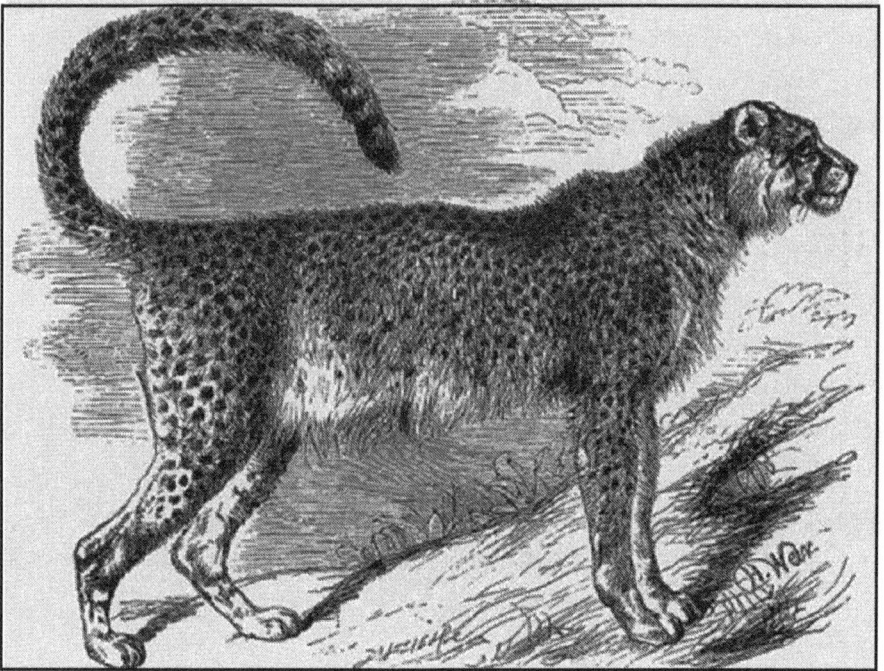

Indian Aurochs: The Indian Aurochs once lived in the hot and dry areas of India. The huge wild cattle were larger than most modern domestic cattle with height of 6.6 fit and weight of 1,000 kilograms. The Indian bison or the gaur is the largest species of wild cattle found in India. Zebu and gaur are the Indian cattle, which are quite similar to the extinct wild Indian Aurochs. Extinct type of cattle was the most challenging hunting wild animal like the wild water buffalo and wild boar.

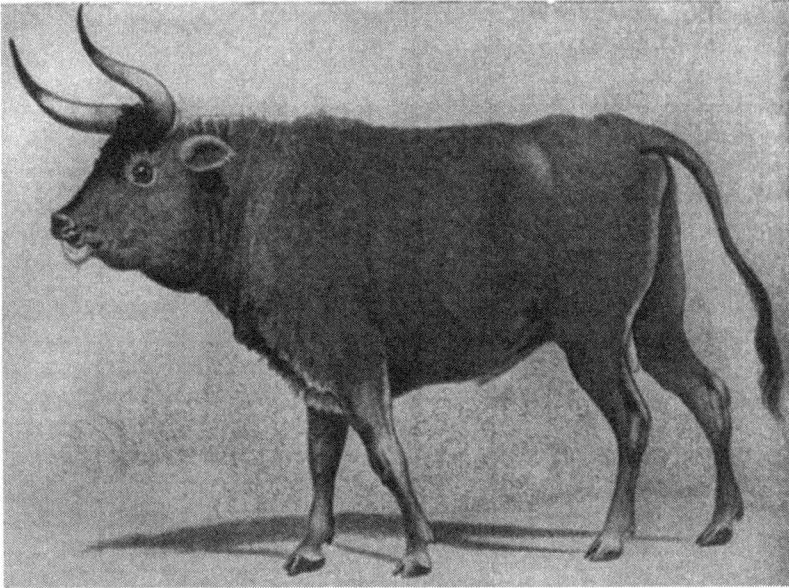

Sivatherium: Sivatherium was a very large approximately 7 fit tall extinct animal found in India. The giant beast was first discovered in India, where it was called as Sivatherium due to the Hindu God Lord Shiva. The Sivatheres were the tallest and fastest monsters found in India ever.

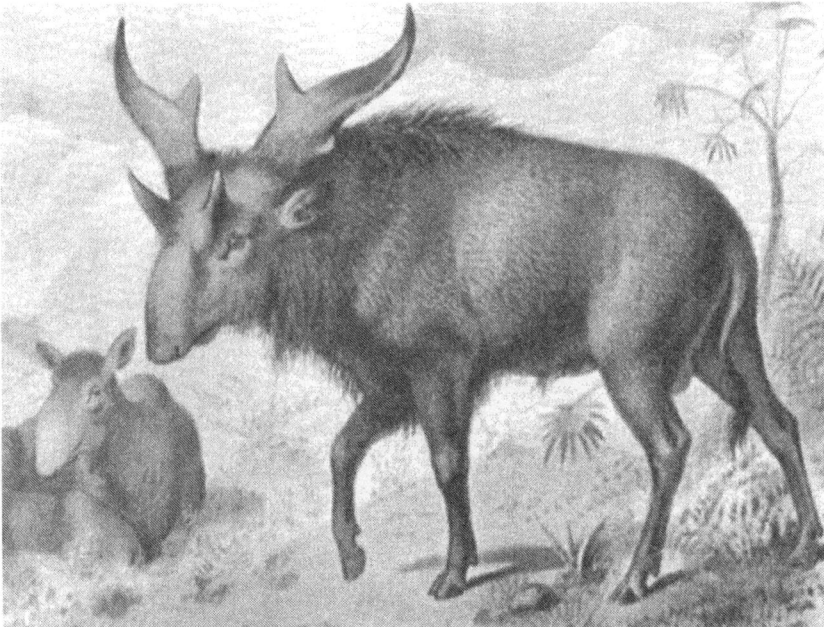

Sumatran Rhinoceros: The Sumatran Rhinoceros has been declared as one of the extinct animal in India. The sumatran rhinoceros is the smallest rhinoceros with two horns and only extant species of the genus Dicerorhinus. The extinct sumatran rhinoceros once roamed and inhabited rainforests of India and neighbor north East Asian countries.

They are now critically endangered species and estimated to number fewer than 275 only and found in neighbor countries of India.

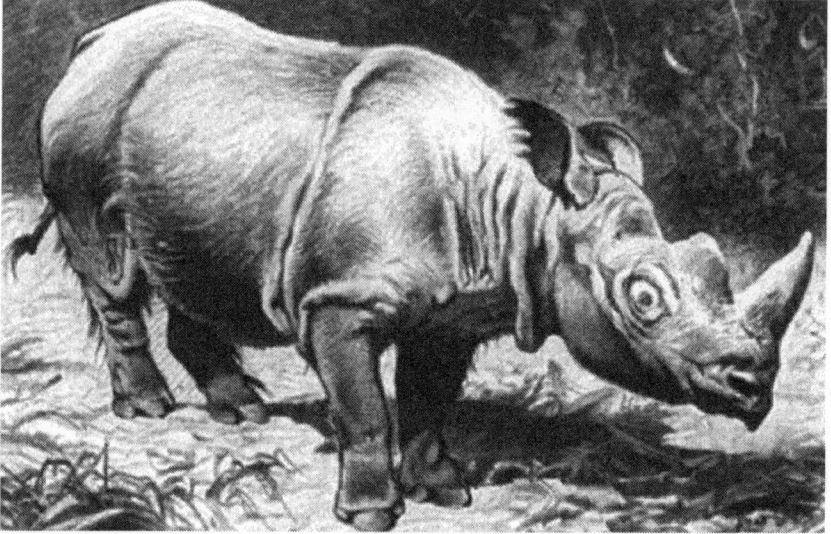

Pink-Headed Duck: Pink-headed Duck was a large diving blackish-brown duck; it was one of the most beautiful birds in India. The long-necked duck once found in throughout India, but it's beautiful appearance made it most hunted birds in India, Due to access of hunting this beautiful bird is fall in the category of extinct birds in India. There is hope that the critically endangered species could still survive in some part of India our neighbor countries.

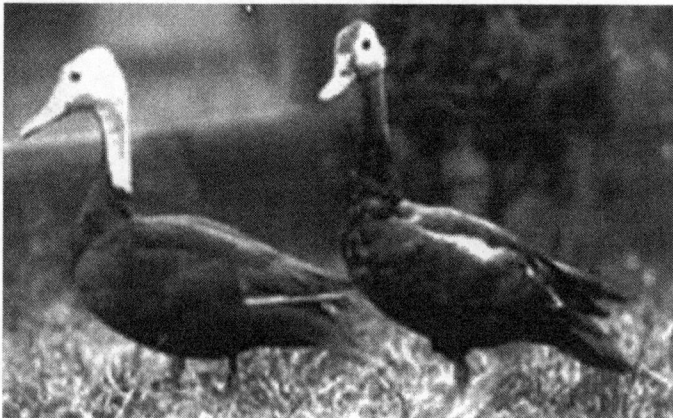

Table 4.1: Extinct species as per IUCN

S.No.	Name	Description	Figure
1.	Japanese eel	The Japanese eel a popular dish in the Japanese cuisine is listed as endangered in the 2014 IUCN Red List.	
2.	Spoon-billed Sandpiper	The Spoon-billed Sandpiper (*Eurynorhynchus pygmeus*) is a critically endangered wader from Russia and Southeast Asia with possibly less than 1000 individuals left.	
3.	Black Stilts	Total 91 captive reared young Black Stilts were released into the wild in September 2013.	
4.	Whooping Crane	Once nearly extinct the population of the Whooping Crane raised from 21 in 1941 to 437 in 2011.	
5.	Mauritius Parakeet	Thanks to a breeding program by the Mauritian Wildlife Foundation and the Gerald Durrell Endemic Wildlife Sanctuary the entire population of the Mauritius Parakeet raised from roughly 10 in the 1980s to 300 in 2007.	

Contd...

Table 4.1: Contd...

S.No.	Name	Description	Figure
6.	Black Stilts	Total 91 captive reared young Black Stilts were released into the wild in September 2013.	
7.	Whooping Crane	Once nearly extinct the population of the Whooping Crane raised from 21 in 1941 to 437 in 2011.	
8.	Mauritius Parakeet	Thanks to a breeding program by the Mauritian Wildlife Foundation and the Gerald Durrell Endemic Wildlife Sanctuary the entire population of the Mauritius Parakeet raised from roughly 10 in the 1980s to 300 in 2007.	
9.	Whooping Crane	Once nearly extinct the population of the Whooping Crane raised from 21 in 1941 to 437 in 2011.	
10.	Night Heron	The last individual of the Bonin Nankeen Night Heron was shot in 1889.	

Contd...

Table 4.1: Contd...

S.No.	Name	Description	Figure
11.	Painted frog	One of the first photographs of a living Hula painted frog which was rediscovered in November 2011 after it was thought to be extinct since 1955.	
12.	Large Copper	The British Large Copper (*Lycaena dispar dispar*) was an endemic subspecies of the Large Copper from the British Isles. It was last seen in 1851.	
13.	Alaotra Grebe	The Alaotra Grebe was officially declared extinct in 2010 after its last confirmed sighting in the 1980s.	
14.	Lesser Stick-nest	The last living Lesser Stick-nest Rat was seen in 1933. The last fresh stick-nest of this species was found in 1970.	
15.	White-footed Rabbit-rat	The White-footed Rabbit-rat was last seen in 1845.	

Contd...

Table 4.1: Contd...

S.No.	Name	Description	Figure
16.	Kioea	The Kioea from the likewise extinct Hawaiian bird family Mohoidae became extinct around 1858.	
17.	Bulldog Rat	The Bulldog Rat was endemic to Christmas Island and became extinct by 1903.	
18.	Galapagos damsel	The Galapagos damsel was last seen in the early 1980s. It disappeared after the El Niño-Southern Oscillation had turned off the plankton production in the Eastern Pacific.	
19.	Hawai	The last sighting of the Hawai was in 1934.	
20.	Auckland Islands Merganser	The last pair of the Auckland Islands Merganser was shot in 1902.	
21.	Syrian Wild Ass	The last Syrian Wild Ass died in captivity in 1928.	

Contd...

Table 4.1: Contd...

S.No.	Name	Description	Figure
22.	Megatherium	The Megatherium was a large ground sloth of the South American megafauna.	
23.	Schomburgk's Deer	The last known Schomburgk's Deer was killed in 1938.	
24.	Woolly Mammoth	The Woolly Mammoth was a well-known elephant like mammal of the Ice Age.	
25.	Aurochs	The last purebred Aurochs was beaten to death in 1627.	
26.	Sloane's Urania	*Urania sloanus* is an extinct butterfly from Jamaica which was last collected in the 1890s.	

Contd...

Table 4.1: Contd...

S.No.	Name	Description	Figure
27.	Newton's Parakeet	The Newton's Parakeet was last seen in 1875.	
28.	Beelze bufo	Beelze bufo is one of the largest known frogs. It died out in the Cretaceous period.	
29.	Bubal Hartebeest	The last known Bubal Hartebeest died in captivity in 1923.	
30.	Seychelles Parakeet	The last Seychelles Parakeet died in captivity in 1883	
31.	New Zealand Quail	The New Zealand Quail have been extinct in 1875.	

Contd...

Table 4.1: Contd...

S.No.	Name	Description	Figure
32.	Portuguese Ibex	The Portuguese Ibex became extinct in the late 19th century.	
33.	Cuban Red Macaw	The Cuban Red Macaw is an extinct parrot species from Cuba.	
34.	Dusky Seaside Sparrow	Orange Band, the last Dusky Seaside Sparrow died in 1987 in a captive facility in the Walt DisnSparrowey World Resort.	
35.	Huia (New Zealand Wattlebird)	The Huia, (*Heteralocha acutirostris*), was a species of New Zealand Wattlebird endemic to the North Island of New Zealand. This species became extinct in the early 20th century, primarily as a result of massive over hunting and widespread habitat destruction. The last accepted sighting was made by one W.W. Smith who saw three birds in the Tararua Ranges on 28 December 1907 but quite credible reports of further sightings were made as late as 1922.	

Contd...

Table 4.1: Contd...

S.No.	Name	Description	Figure
36.	Bush Wren	The Bush Wren (*Xenicus longipes*) or Matuhituhi in Maori, is a very small and almost flightless bird endemic to New Zealand. It grows to about 9 cm long and 16 g in weight. It feeds mostly on invertebrates which it captures by running along the branches of trees. It nests on or near the ground.	
37.	Falkland Island Fox	The Falkland Island Fox (*Dusicyon australis*, formerly named *Canis antarcticus*), also known as the Warrah and occasionally as the Falkland Island Wolf or Antarctic Wolf, was the only native land mammal of the Falkland Islands.	
38.	Thylacine	The last known Thylacine photographed at Hobart Zoo in 1933.	
39.	Imperial Woodpecker	The Imperial Woodpecker (*Campephilus imperialis*), is a possible extinct woodpecker species from Mexico. It was the largest woodpecker in the world.	
40.	Quagga	The Quagga (*Equus quagga quagga*), is an extinct zebra species.	

4.5 Protected Area Network

India is unique in having immense natural beauty is its different lions and in possessing a rich and diverse wild life fauna Indian wild life is incomparable in its variety for example, the tiger, the lion and the leopard room about in the same country elephants and the one horned rhinoceros are found here in abundance. India has more types of the graceful deer and cats than any other country in the world. In facts, India includes more than 120 families of terrestrial vertebrates. It has been estimated that there are more than 400 species of mammals, 1200 species of Birds, more than 350 Species of Reptiles and more that 29,70,000 species of insects in India. A National Board for Wildlife (NBWL), chaired by the Prime Minister of India provides for policy framework for wildlife conservation in the country. The National Wildlife Action Plan (2002-2016) was adopted in 2002, emphasizing the people's participation and their support for wildlife conservation. India's conservation planning is based on the philosophy of identifying and protecting representative wild habitats across all the ecosystems. The Indian Constitution entails the subject of forests and wildlife in the Concurrent list. The Federal Ministry acts as a guiding torch dealing with the policies and planning on wildlife conservation, while the provincial Forest Departments are vested with the responsibility of implementation of national policies and plans.

The Ministry of Environment & Forests (MoEF) is the nodal agency in the Central Government for overseeing the implementation of India's environment and forest policies and programmes relating to conservation of the country's natural resources including lakes and rivers, its biodiversity, forests and wildlife, ensuring the welfare of animals and prevention and abatement of pollution. While implementing these policies and programmes, the Ministry is guided by the principle of sustainable development.

Authorization of the Ministry of Environment and Forests (MOEFCC)

- Environment and Ecology, including environment in coastal waters, in mangroves and coral reefs but excluding marine environment on the high seas.

- Survey and Exploration of Natural Resources for Forest, Flora, Fauna, Ecosystems etc.

- Bio-diversity Conservation including that of lakes and wetlands.

- Conservation, development, management and abatement of pollution of rivers include National River Conservation Directorate.

- Environmental Impact Assessment.

- Environment research and development, education, training, information and awareness.

- Environmental Health.
- Forest Development Agency and Joint Forest Management Programme for conservation, management and afforestation.
- Wildlife conservation, preservation, protection planning, research, education, training and awareness including Project Tiger and Project Elephant.
- International co-operation on issues concerning Environment, Forestry and Wildlife.
- Botanical Survey of India and Botanical Gardens.
- Zoological Survey of India.
- National Museum of Natural History.
- Biosphere Reserve Programme.
- National Forest Policy and Forestry Development including Social Forestry.
- All matters relating to Forest and Forest Administration in the Andaman and Nicobar Islands.
- Indian Forest Service.
- Wild Life Preservation and protection of wild birds and animals.
- Fundamental and applied research and training including higher education in forestry.
- Padmaja Naidu Himalayan Zoological Park.
- National Assistance to Forestry
- Indian Plywood Industries Research and Training Institute, Bangalore.
- National Afforestation and Eco-Development Board.
- Desert and Desertification.
- Forest Survey of India.
- Indian Institute of Bio-diversity, Itanagar.
- Central Pollution Control Board.
- G.B. Pant Institute of Himalayan Environment & Development.
- Wildlife Institute of India and Indian Board for Wildlife.
- Indian Institute of Forest Management.
- Central Zoo Authority including National Zoological Park.
- Indian Council of Forestry Research & Education.

- Andaman and Nicobar Islands Forest and Plantation Development Corporation Limited.

- Prevention of Cruelty to Animals.

- Matters relating to pounds and cattle trespass.

- Gau-shalas and Gau-sadans.

- The Prevention of Cruelty to Animals Act, 1960 (59 of 1960).

- The National Environment Tribunal Act, 1995 (27 of 1995).

- The National Environment Appellate Authority Act, 1997 (22 of 1997).

- The Water Prevention and Control of Pollution Act, 1974 (6 of 1974).

- The Water (Prevention and Control of Pollution) Cess Act, 1977 (36 of 1977).

- The Air (Prevention and Control of Pollution) Act, 1981 (14 of 1981).

- The Indian Forest Act, 1927 (16 of 1927).

- The Wildlife (Protection) Act, 1972 (53 of 1972).

- The Forest (Conservation) Act, 1980 (69 of 1980).

- The Environment (Protection), Act, 1986 (29 of 1986).

- The Public Liability Insurance Act, 1991 (6 of 1991).

As per MoEF (2013); a network of 668 Protected Areas (PAs) has been established, extending over 1,61,221.57 sq. kms. (4.90% of total geographic area), comprising 102 National Parks, 515 Wildlife Sanctuaries, 47 Conservation Reserves and 4 Community Reserves. The State/Union Territory wise details of PAs in the country with year of notification and area is given at Annexure-I. 39 Tiger Reserves and 28 Elephant Reserves have been designated for species specific management of tiger and elephant habitats. UNESCO has designated 5 Protected Areas as World Heritage Sites. As the ecosystems and species do not recognize political borders, the concept of Transboundary Protected Areas has been initiated for coordinated conservation of ecological units and corridors with bilateral and/or multilateral cooperation of the neighboring nations. There are 4 categories of the Protected Areas *viz*. National Parks, Sanctuaries, Conservation Reserves and Community Reserves.

4.5.1 Sanctuaries

Sanctuary is an area which is of adequate ecological, faunal, floral, geomorphological, natural or zoological significance. The Sanctuary is declared for the purpose of protecting, propagating or developing wildlife or its environment. Certain rights of people living inside the Sanctuary could be permitted. Further, during the settlement of claims, before finally notifying the Sanctuary, the Collector may, in consultation with the Chief Wildlife Warden, allow the continuation of any right of any person in or over any land within the limits of the Sanctuary.

4.5.2 National Park

National Park is an area having adequate ecological, faunal, floral, geo-morphological, natural or zoological significance. The National Park is declared for the purpose of protecting, propagating or developing wildlife or its environment, like that of a Sanctuary. The difference between a Sanctuary and a National Park mainly lies in the vesting of rights of people living inside. Unlike a Sanctuary, where certain rights can be allowed, in a National Park, no rights are allowed. No grazing of any livestock shall also be permitted inside a National Park while in a Sanctuary; the Chief Wildlife Warden may regulate, control or prohibit it. In addition, while any removal or exploitation of wildlife or forest produce from a Sanctuary requires the recommendation of the State Board for Wildlife, removal etc. from a National Park requires recommendation of the National Board for Wildlife. However, as per orders of Hon'ble Supreme Court dated 9th May 2002 in Writ Petition (Civil) No. 337 of 1995, such removal/ exploitation from a Sanctuary also require recommendation of the Standing Committee of National Board for Wildlife.

4.5.3 Conservation Reserves

Conservation Reserves can be declared by the State Governments in any area owned by the Government, particularly the areas adjacent to National Parks and Sanctuaries and those areas which link one Protected Area with another. Such declaration should be made after having consultations with the local communities. Conservation Reserves are declared for the purpose of protecting landscapes, seascapes, flora and fauna and their habitat. The rights of people living inside a Conservation Reserve are not affected.

4.5.4 Community Reserves

Community Reserves can be declared by the State Government in any private or community land, not comprised within a National Park, Sanctuary or a Conservation Reserve, where an individual or a community has volunteered to conserve wildlife and its habitat. Community Reserves are declared for the purpose of protecting fauna, flora and traditional or cultural conservation values and practices. As in the case of a Conservation Reserve, the rights of people living inside a Community Reserve are not affected.

The PAs are constituted and governed under the provisions of the Wild Life (Protection) Act, 1972, which has been amended from time to time, with the changing ground realities concerning wildlife crime control and PAs management. Implementation of this Act is further complemented by other Acts viz. Indian Forest Act, 1927, Forest (Conservation) Act, 1980, Environment (Protection) Act, 1986 and Biological Diversity Act, 2002 and the Scheduled Tribes and Other Traditional Forest Dwellers (Recognition of Forest Rights) Act, 2006. The Wildlife Crime Control Bureau of the Central Government supplements the efforts of provincial governments in wildlife crime control through enforcement of CITES and control of wildlife crimes having cross-border, interstate and international ramifications.

Table 4.2: State-wise details of Protected Area Network

S.No.	State/UT	No.of National Parks	No.of Wildlife Sanctuaries	No.of Conservation Reserves	No.of Community Reserves
1.	Andhra Pradesh	6	21	0	0
2.	Arunachal Pradesh	2	11	0	0
3.	Assam	5	18	0	0
4.	Bihar	1	12	0	0
5.	Chhatisgarh	3	11	0	0
6.	Goa	1	6	0	0
7.	Gujarat	4	23	1	0
8.	Haryana	2	8	2	0
9.	Himachal Pradesh	5	32	0	0
10.	Jammu &Kashmir	4	15	34	0
11.	Jharkhand	1	11	0	0
12.	Karnataka	5	22	2	1
13.	Kerala	6	16	0	1
14.	Madhya Pradesh	9	25	0	0
15.	Maharashtra	6	35	1	0
16.	Manipur	1	1	0	0
17.	Meghalaya	2	3	0	0
18.	Mizoram	2	8	0	0
19.	Nagaland	1	3	0	0
20.	Orissa	2	18	0	0
21.	Punjab	0	12	1	2
22.	Rajasthan	5	25	3	0
23.	Sikkim	1	7	0	0
24.	Tamil Nadu	5	21	1	0
25.	Tripura	2	4	0	0
26.	Uttar Pradesh	1	23	0	0
27.	Uttaranchal	6	6	2	0
28.	West Bengal	5	15	0	0
29.	Andaman &Nicobar	9	96	0	0
30.	Chandigarh	0	2	0	0
31.	Dadar & NagarHaweli	0	1	0	0
32.	Lakshadweep	0	1	0	0
33.	Daman & Diu	0	1	0	0
34.	Delhi	0	1	0	0
35.	Pondicherry	0	1	0	0
	Total	102	515	47	4

In order to strengthen and synergise global wildlife conservation efforts, India is a party to major international conventions viz. Convention on International Trade in Endangered Species of wild fauna and flora (CITES), International Union for Conservation of Nature (IUCN), International Convention for the Regulation of Whaling, UNESCO-World Heritage Committee and Convention on Migratory Species (CMS).

4.6 Conservation of Wild Life

The conservation of wildlife is the practice of protecting endangered plant and wild animal species and their habitats. Among the goals of wildlife conservation are to ensure that nature will be around for future generations to enjoy and to recognize the importance of wildlife and wilderness lands to humans. Many nations have government agencies dedicated to wildlife conservation, which help to implement policies designed to protect wildlife. Numerous independent non-profit organizations also promote various wildlife conservation causes. Wildlife conservation has become an increasingly important practice due to the negative effects of human activity on wildlife. The science of extinction is called dirology. An endangered species is defined as a population of a living being that is at the danger of becoming extinct because of several reasons. Either they are few in number or are threatened by the varying environmental or prepositional parameters.

4.6.1 Major Threats to Wildlife

Fewer natural wildlife habitat areas remain each year. Moreover, the habitat that remains has often been degraded to bear little resemblance to the wild areas which existed in the past. Habitat loss due to destruction, fragmentation or degradation of habitat is the primary threat to the survival of wildlife. When an ecosystem has been dramatically changed by human activities such as agriculture, oil and gas exploration, commercial development or water diversion, it may no longer be able to provide the food, water, cover and places to raise young. Every day there are fewer places left that wildlife can call home. There are three major kinds of habitat loss:

- *Habitat destruction*: A bulldozer pushing down trees is the iconic image of habitat destruction. Other ways that people are directly destroying habitat, include filling in wetlands, dredging rivers, mowing fields and cutting down trees.

- *Habitat fragmentation:* Much of the remaining terrestrial wildlife habitat in the U.S. has been cut up into fragments by roads and development. Aquatic species' habitat has been fragmented by dams and water diversions. These fragments of habitat may not be large or connected enough to support species that need a large territory in which to find mates and food. The loss and fragmentation of habitat make it difficult for migratory species to find places to rest and feed along their migration routes.

- *Habitat degradation:* Pollution, invasive species and disruption of ecosystem processes (such as changing the intensity of fires in an ecosystem) are some of the ways habitats can become so degraded that they no longer support native wildlife.

There are some others threats to wildlife.

- *Climate change*: Global warming is making hot days hotter, rainfall and flooding heavier, hurricanes stronger and droughts more severe. This intensification of weather and climate extremes will be the most visible impact of global warming in our everyday lives. It is also causing dangerous changes to the landscape of our world, adding stress to wildlife species and their habitat. Since many types of plants and animals have specific habitat requirements, climate change could cause disastrous loss of wildlife species. A slight drop or rise in average rainfall will translate into large seasonal changes. Hibernating mammals, reptiles, amphibians and insects are harmed and disturbed. Plants and wildlife are sensitive to moisture change so, they will be harmed by any change in moisture level. Natural phenomena like floods, earthquakes, volcanoes, lightning, forest fires.

- *Unregulated Hunting and poaching*: Unregulated hunting and poaching causes a major threat to wildlife. Along with this, mismanagement of forest department and forest guards triggers this problem.

- *Pollution:* Pollutants released into the environment are ingested by a wide variety of organisms. Pesticides and toxic chemical being widely used, making the environment toxic to certain plants, insects and rodents.

Perhaps the largest threat is the extreme growing indifference of the public to wildlife, conservation and environmental issues in general. Over-exploitation of resources *i.e.* exploitation of wild populations for food has resulted in population crashes *e.g.* over-fishing and over-grazing. Over exploitation is the over use of wildlife and plant species by people for food, clothing, pets, medicine, sport and many other purposes. People have always depended on wildlife and plants for food, clothing, medicine, shelter and many other needs. But today we are taking more than the natural world can supply. The danger is that if we take too many individuals of a species from their natural environment, the species may no longer be able to survive. The loss of one species can affect many other species in an ecosystem. The hunting, trapping, collecting and fishing of wildlife at unsustainable levels is not something new. The passenger pigeon was hunted to extinction early in the last century and over-hunting nearly caused the extinction of the American bison and several species of whales.

The Convention on International Trade in Endangered Species of Fauna and Flora (CITES) works to prevent the global trade of wildlife. But there are many species that are not protected from being illegally traded or over-harvested. In order of the sexual lifestyle to continue it is needed to come about with everything that we need especially if a currency of the conservation is initially under consecration and wildlife. The Wildlife Conservation Act was enacted by the Government of India in 1972. Soon after the trend of policy makers enacting regulations on conservation a strategy was developed to allow actors, both government and non-government, to follow a detailed framework to successful conservation. The World Conservation Strategy was developed in 1980 by the "International Union for Conservation of Nature and Natural Resources (IUCN) with advice, cooperation and financial assistance of the United Nations Environment Programme (UNEP) and the World Wildlife Fund and in collaboration with the Food and Agriculture Organization of the United Nations (FAO) and the United Nations Educational, Scientific and Cultural Organization (UNESCO). The strategy aims to provide an intellectual framework and practical guidance for conservation actions. This thorough guidebook covers everything from the intended users of the strategy to its very priorities. It even includes a map section containing areas that have large seafood consumption and are therefore endangered by over fishing.

4.6.2 Species Recovery Programme

The development and implementation of species recovery plans and programmes provide integrated conservation strategies for wildlife. These often involve a combination of *in situ* assessment of natural plant populations, monitoring of their status and the current or past causes of their decline and the determination of future priorities, therefore enabling their recovery. Recovery measures include land protection, habitat management and/or restoration, *ex situ* cultivation and reintroduction and public education programmes. Out of 16 species identified for the species recovery programme, financial assistance has been provided for nine species by Ministry of Forest and Environment (MoEF). The amount provided to the State/ Union Territory in respect of these species is as below:

i. Project Snow Leopard -(J&K– Rs.169.20 lakh, Uttarakhand–Rs.86.40 lakh, Himachal Pradesh- Rs.164.696 lakh and Rs. 3.20 lakhs to Arunachal Pradesh).

ii. Project Hangul- (J&K- Rs.268.56 lakh).

iii. Project Vulture-(Haryana- Rs.43.60 lakh, Punjab- 18.40 lakh, Gujarat-Rs.12.30 lakh).

iv. Project Sanghai Deer- (Manipur- Rs.33.96 lakh).

v. Project Edible nest swiftlet- (A&N Islands- Rs.106.192 lakh).

vi. Project Nilgiri Tahr- (Tamil Nadu- Rs. 4.80 lakh).

vii. Project Dugong (A&N Islands-Rs. 55.54 lakh).

viii. Project Lion (Gujarat-Rs. 1350.40 lakh).

ix. Project Wild Buffalo (Chhattisgarh-Rs. 108.92 lakh).

Financial assistance has also been provided by MoEF to the States for relocation of communities from within PAs to areas outside. Details of such assistance area as follows:

x. Rs. 540.00 lakhs has been released to Chhattisgarh for relocation of 135 families from villages in Barnawapara Sanctuary during 2009-10.

xi. Rs. 550.00 lakh for voluntary relocation of 55 families during 2011-12 and Rs. 784.00 lakh for voluntary relocation of 98 eligible families during 2012-13 from Wayanad Sanctuary has been released.

xii. Rs.488.00 lakh has been released to Mizoram for relocation of 61 families from Dumpui 'S' village in Thorangtlang Sanctuary 2010-11.

xiii. Rs. 30.00 lakh has been released to Kerala for relocation of 3 families from Malabar Wildlife Sanctuary during 2011-12.

4.6.3 Human-Animal Conflict

In India, human-animal conflict is seen across the country in a variety of forms, including monkey menace in the urban centers, crop raiding by ungulates and wild pigs, depredation by elephants, cattle lifting and human death and injury by tigers, leopards and other wild animals. Human-animal conflict occurs both inside Protected Areas as well as outside Protected Areas. The intensity of the conflict is generally more in areas outside Protected Area network than inside. Recently the incident of human-animal conflict has increased considerably. The increase is due to various reasons. Important among them are increase in wild animal population, fragmentation of habitats, non availability of food and water in the habitat due to degradation, disturbance in the corridors due to developmental activities, change in cropping pattern, increase in human populations etc. Various other reasons include adaptability of certain animals like leopard, monkey, nilgai, bear etc which allow them to live successfully close to human habitation. The human-animal conflict is an important part of wildlife management as the co-operation of local population depends largely on winning their support by reducing loss to them by wild animals among many others. In order to mitigate the human animal conflict, a national workshop on 'Developing Strategies for Mitigation of Human wildlife conflict' was held on 20.8.2013 at New Delhi wherein the matter was discussed and several mitigating measures were suggested. The Division is pursuing to have a separate component under the scheme for managing human-animals conflict.

4.6.4 Organizations for Conservation of Wildlife

i. World Wildlife Fund (WWF)

The WWF works with multilateral and bilateral agencies to promote sustainable development in the world's poorest countries. Its aims are threefold, to protect natural areas and wild populations, to minimize pollution and to promote efficient, sustainable use of natural resources. The WWF focuses their efforts at multiple levels, starting with wildlife, habitats and local communities and expanding up through governments and global networks. The WWF views the planet as a single, complex web of relationships between species, the environment and human institutions such as government and global markets.

ii. National Development and Reform Commission (NDRC)

The NRDC is an environmental action organization that consists of 350 lawyers, scientists and other professionals and commands a membership of about 1.3 million people. The NRDC uses the law, science and their wide network of members and activists to protect wildlife and habitats around the globe. The issues the NRDC focuses on include curbing global warming, creating clean energy, preserving wild lands, restoring ocean habitats, stopping the spread of toxic chemicals and working towards greener living in China.

iii. Nature Conservancy

The Nature Conservancy works with local communities, businesses and individuals to protect over 100 million acres of land around the world. In doing so, The Nature Conservancy preserves entire wildlife communities and the rich species diversity that inhabits those lands. It's a wholistic approach, one that I feel is vital to the health of our planet. Among The Nature Conservancy's more innovative conservation approaches is the debt-for-nature swaps. Such transactions ensure biodiversity conservation in exchange for debt owed by a developing country. Such debt-for-nature programs have been successful in many countries including Panama, Peru and Guatamala.

iv. International Crane Foundation (ICF)

The International Crane Foundation (ICF) was established by founders George Archibald and Ron Sauey in 1973 on a horse farm in Baraboo, Wisconsin. The ICF works around the world to protect cranes and the habitats on which they depend. Although they focus on cranes, their work is valuable on a wider scale, giving insights into endangered species management, wetland ecology, habitat restoration and the critical need for international cooperation. The ICF provides education about cranes on three levels, local, national and international. In addition to educating people about cranes, the ICF also conducts captive breeding and reintroduction of cranes into the wild.

v. Friends of Haleakala National Park

The Friends of Haleakala National Park conservation organization is a personal favorite of mine because they support a wide range of conservation projects to protect Hawaii's unique Haleakala National Park. Their efforts include educational activities, cultural projects, research and service projects. The Friends of Haleakala National Park strives to preserve the ecosystems of Haleakala National Park, to protect the Native Hawaiian cultural and to preserve the area's scenic character. Haleakala National Park is located atop Maui's Haleakala volcano and is home to more threatened and endangered species than any other national park in the United States. Among the park's endangered species is the Hawaiian state bird, the Nene. The Friends of Haleakala National Park offers an adopt-a-nene program that raises funds to protect the endangered nene goose from a range of threats including invasive predators such as mongooses, feral cats and rats.

vi. Wildlife Conservation Society (WCS)

The Wildlife Conservation Society (WCS) is another superb group working for the protection of animals and wildlife. The WCS supports zoos and aquariums while promoting environmental education and conservation of wild populations and their habitats. They also offer educational resources and a wide variety of conservation programs. Their efforts are focused on a select group of animals including bears, big cats, elephants, great apes, hoofed mammals, cetaceans and carnivores. Their conservation projects stretch around the globe and are at work in regions including Africa, Asia, Latin America, the Caribbean, North America and throughout the world's Oceans. The Wildlife Conservation Society was established in 1895 as the New York Zoological Society. Its mission was and is, to promote wildlife protection, foster the study of zoology and create a top-notch zoo. Today not one but five Wildlife Conservation Zoos exist in the State of New York, the Bronx Zoo, Central Park Zoo, Queens Zoo, Prospect Park Zoo and the New York Aquarium.

vii. Royal Society for the Protection of Birds (RSPB)

The Royal Society for the Protection of Birds (RSPB) began in 1889 as an organization that opposed the inhumane use of exotic feathers in the fashion industry, particularly the use of exotic plumes to adorn the women's hats that were so much in vogue at the time. The RSPB's rules were straightforward-to discourage the mindless destruction of birds, to promote the protection of birds and to refrain from wearing feathers of any bird. Today, the RSPB has over 1 million members with a network of 12,200 volunteers all devoted to the protection of birds. The RSPB protects and restores habitat for birds and other wildlife, conducts recovery projects, researches problems facing bird populations, works with landowners and farmers to protect birds and manages 200 nature reserves. Each year, the RSPB conducts the Big Garden Birdwatch survey, which is a great way for people in the UK to participate in a nation-wide bird count.

viii. Conservation International

Conservation International employs scientists and policy experts to balance healthy ecosystems with sustainable human use. Conservation International aims to help stabilize global climate, protect fresh water and ensure human well being. To achieve their goals they work with indigenous peoples and non-governmental organization. Conservation International's primary initiatives include climate, fresh water, food, health, culture and biodiversity. Of all the significant initiatives Conservation International has achieved, its Biodiversity Hotspots project is the most impressive. This project identifies and protects biological hotspots, places that exhibit the richest diversity and most threatened collections of plants and animals on our planet.

4.6.5 Project Tiger

In the beginning of the 1970s, once tiger hunting had officially been banned in India, a tiger count was done across the entire country. This lead to the astonishing discovery that only 1800 specimens of this magnificent animal were left. This jolted the concerned authorities and some serious thought went into devising plans to save the tiger. The result was the launch of "Project Tiger" in 1972 at the Dhikala Forest Rest House in Corbett National Park. The main idea behind the project was to provide safe havens for tigers where they could flourish as a species and hopefully reverse the startling decline in their population. The project initially had 9 parks that were chosen for its implementation. This number has slowly risen and a total of 19 parks are now attached to the project. The project was begun in association with and still receives its main funding from the WWF. Although the experts affirm that the project has its shortcomings, the increase in the populations of the tiger is clearly evident to even the common man. Many experts had predicted that the tiger would be extinct by the turn of the century, but the tiger has proudly proved them wrong. Tiger population may not still be in thrilling numbers and poaching still may be quite rampant but a lot more effort is being put into saving this beautiful animal. This is good news for the entire natural treasure of the country because if the tiger flourishes, so will the jungle and vice-versa. Tiger sightings have become quite rare these days in India, reason being the Tiger killings because of its multitude of medicinal or magical properties that is why tiger trade is very profitable. Genuinely the tiger skin is not fashionable but the smuggling of Tiger fur coats and rugs are not difficult for the impoverished hunters. Tiger in India Even after the bans made by the government warning not to gather even wood from the former hunting grounds, poaching of tigers continue. Still efforts are continuously made to preserve these magnificent predators from extinction. Till 1970, the hunting of tigers was legal in India and this majestic animal was hunted by the erstwhile royals and elites for pleasure and its beautiful skin. According to various estimates, during the 1950s and early 1960s, over 3,000 tigers lost their lives to trophy hunters. In the beginning of the 1970s, the tiger population in India was estimated to be around 1,800, shocking and jolting the concerned authorities to formulate an immediate plan to save Indian tigers and the result was the launch of Project Tiger in 1972.

The Government of India has taken a pioneering initiative for conserving its national animal, the tiger, by launching the Project Tiger in 1972-73. From 9 tiger reserves since its formative years, the Project Tiger coverage has increased to 44 at present, spread out in 17 of our tiger range states. This amounts to around 2.08 per cent of the geographical area of our country. The tiger reserves are constituted on a core/buffer strategy. The core areas have the legal status of a national park or a sanctuary, whereas the buffer or peripheral areas are a mix of forest and non-forest land, managed as a multiple use area. The Project Tiger aims to foster an exclusive tiger agenda in the core areas of tiger reserves, with an inclusive people oriented agenda in the buffer. Project Tiger is an ongoing Centrally Sponsored Scheme of the Ministry of Environment and Forests, providing central assistance to the tiger States for tiger conservation in designated tiger reserves. The National Tiger Conservation Authority (NTCA) is a statutory body of the Ministry, with an overarching supervisory / coordination role, performing functions as provided in the Wildlife (Protection) Act, 1972. The Regional Offices of the NTCA have been recently established at Bangalore, Guwahati and Nagpur, each headed by an IGF and assisted by an AIG. The allocation for Project Tiger during the XII Plan is Rs 1245 Crore. The expenditure during 2012-13 and 2013-14 are Rs 163.87 Crore and 169.48 Crore respectively. Due to concerted efforts under Project Tiger, at present India has the distinction of having the maximum number of tigers in the world (1706) as per 2010 assessment, when compared to the 13 tiger range countries. The 2010 country level tiger assessment has also shown a 20% increase of tigers in the country (from 1411 in 2006 to 1706 in 2010). However, there is a decline in tiger occupancy (12.6%) in other areas of tiger States. The tiger corridors for gene flow have been mapped in the GIS domain.

Project Tiger Scheme

Project Tiger Scheme has been under implementation since 1973 as a Centrally Sponsored Scheme of Government of India. The aim of Project Tiger is to ensure a viable population of tiger in India for economic, aesthetic, cultural and ecological values and to preserve areas of biological importance as natural heritage. Project tiger scheme includes wildlife management, protection measures and site specific eco development to reduce the dependency on tiger reserve resources. At the turn of the century, the estimated tiger population in India was placed at 40,000 but the first ever all India tiger census in 1972 shockingly revealed the existence of only 1827 tigers. Before that a ban on tiger hunting was imposed in the year 1970 and in 1972 the Wildlife Protection Act came into force. Thereafter a Task Force was set up to formulate a project for tiger conservation. With the launch of Project tiger in 1973, various tiger reserves were created in different parts of the country on a core-buffer strategy. Under this strategy, the core areas were freed from all human activities and the buffer areas were to have 'conservation oriented land use'. Initially, 9 tiger reserves were established in different States during the period 1973-74. These nine Tiger reserves were Manas (Assam), Palamau (Bihar), Similipal (Orissa), Corbett (U.P.), Kanha (M.P.), Melghat (Maharashtra), Bandipur (Karnataka), Ranthambore (Rajasthan) and Sunderbans (West Bengal). The main achievements of this project are excellent recovery of the habitat and consequent increase in the tiger population in the reserve areas, from a mere 268 in 9 reserves in 1972 to 1576 in 27 reserves in 2003.

The main objective of Project Tiger is to ensure a viable population of tiger in India for scientific, economic, aesthetic, cultural and ecological values and to preserve for all time, areas of biological importance as a natural heritage for the benefit, education and enjoyment of the people. Main objectives under the scheme include wildlife management, protection measures and site specific eco-development to reduce the dependency of local communities on tiger reserve resources. Initially, the Project started with 9 tiger reserves, covering an area of 16,339 sq.km, with a population of 268 tigers. At present there are 27 tiger reserves covering an area of 37761 sq.Km, with a population of 1498 tigers. This amounts to almost 1.14% of the total geographical area of the country. The selection of reserves was guided by representation of ecotypical wilderness areas across the biogeographic range of tiger distribution in the country. Project Tiger is undisputedly a custodian of major gene pool. It is also a repository of some of the most valuable ecosystem and habitats for wildlife. Tiger Reserves are constituted on a core-buffer strategy. The core area is kept free of biotic disturbances and forestry operations, where collection of minor forest produce, grazing, human disturbances are not allowed within. However, the buffer zone is managed as a 'multiple use area' with twin objectives of providing habitat supplement to the spillover population of wild animals from the core conservation unit and to provide site specific ecodevelopmental inputs to surrounding villages for relieving their impact on the core. Except for the National Parks portion if contained within, normally no relocation of villages is visualised in the buffer area and forestry operations, NTFP collection and other rights and concessions to the local people are permitted in a regulated manner to complement the initiatives in the core unit.

Table 4.3: List of Tiger Reserves in India with Year of creation and Area

S.No.	Year of Creation	Name of Tiger Reserve	State	Total area of the Core/Critical Tiger habitat (Sq. Kms.)
1.	1973-74	Bandipur	Karnataka	872.24
2.	1973-74	Corbett	Uttarakhand	821.99
3.	1973-74	Kanha	Madhya Pradesh	917.43
4.	1973-74	Manas	Assam	840.04
5.	1973-74	Melghat	Maharashtra	1500.49
6.	1973-74	Palamau	Jharkhand	414.08
7.	1973-74	Ranthambhore	Rajasthan	1113.364
8.	1973-74	Similipal	Orissa	1194.74
9.	1973-74	Sunderbans	West Bengal	1699.62
10.	1978-79	Periyar	Kerala	881
11.	1978-79	Sariska	Rajasthan	681.1124
12.	1982-83	Buxa	West Bengal	390.5813
13.	1982-83	Indravati	Chhattisgarh	1258.37
14.	1982-83	Nagarjunsagar	Andhra Pradesh	2527
15.	1982.83	Namdapha	Arunachal Pradesh	1807.82
16.	1987-88	Dudhwa	Uttar Pradesh	1093.79*
17.	1988-89	Kalakad-Mundanthurai	Tamil Nadu	895
18.	1989-90	Valmiki	Bihar	840.00*
19.	1992-93	Pench	Madhya Pradesh	411.33
20.	1993-94	Tadoba Andheri	Maharashtra	625.82
21.	1993-94	Bandhavgarh	Madhya Pradesh	716.903
22.	1994-95	Panna	Madhya Pradesh	576.13
23.	1994-95	Dampa	Mizoram	500
24.	1998-99	Bhadra	Karnataka	492.46
25.	1998-99	Pench	Maharashtra	257.26
26.	1999-2000	Pakke	Arunachal Pradesh	683.45
27.	1999-2000	Nameri	Assam	200
28.	1999-2000	Satpura	Madhya Pradesh	1339.264
29.	2008-09	Anamalai	Tamil Nadu	958
30.	2008-09	Udanti-Sitanadi	Chhattisgarh	851.09
31.	2008-09	Satkosia	Orissa	523.61
32.	2008-09	Kaziranga	Assam	625.58
33.	2008-09	Achanakmar	Chhattisgarh	626.195
34.	2008-09	Dandeli-Anshi	Karnataka	814.884
35.	2008-09	Sanjay-Dubri	Madhya Pradesh	831.25*
36.	2008-09	Mudumalai	Tamil Nadu	321
37.	2008-09	Nagarhole	Karnataka	643.35
38.	2008-09	Parambikulam	Kerala	390.89
39.	2009-10	Sahyadri	Maharashtra	Notification Awaited
		Total		**32137.14**

Project Tiger has put the tiger on an assured course of recovery from the brink of extinction and has resurrected the floral and faunal genetic diversity in some of our unique and endangered wilderness ecosystem. The population of tigers in the country has increased significantly to about 4000 from less than 2000 at the time of launch of the project. The effective protection and concerted conservation measures inside the reserves have brought about considerable intangible achievements also, *viz.* arresting erosion, enrichment of water regime thereby improving the water table and overall habitat resurrection. Labour intensive activities in tiger reserves have helped in poverty alleviation amongst the most backward sections and their dependence on forests has also reduced. The project has been instrumental in mustering local support for conservation programme in general.

4.6.6 Project Elephant

Elephant (*Elephas maximus*) is the largest terrestrial mammal of India placed in schedule-I under Willife (Protection) Act 1972. Elephant being wide ranging animal requires large areas. As per our mythology, elephant took birth from celestial waters and thus are closely associated with rains /water because of the belief. The requirement of food and water for elephants are very high and therefore their population can be supported only by forests that are under optimal conditions.

The status of elephant can be the best indicator of the status of the forests. Asian elephants were believed to be widely distributed from Tigris, Euphrates in West Asia eastward through Persia into the Indian sub-continent, South and Southeast Asia including Sri Lanka, Java, Sumatra, Borneo and up to North China. However currently they are confined to Indian Subcontinent, South East Asia and some Asian Islands - Sri Lanka, Indonesia and Malaysia. About half of the Asian elephant population is in India. Old literatures indicate that even during the Moghul period, elephants were found all over India including many part of Central India like Marwar, Chanderi, Satwas, Bijagarh and Panna. However current distribution of wild elephant in India is confined to South India; North East including North West Bengal; Central Indian states of Orissa, South WB and Jharkhand and North West India in Uttarakhand and UP. Project Elephant (PE) was launched by the Government of India in the year 1992 as a Centrally Sponsored Scheme with following objectives:

(a) To protect elephants, their habitat and corridors,

(b) To address issues of man-animal conflict,

(c) Welfare of domesticated elephants.

Financial and Technical support are being provided to major elephant bearing States in the country. The Project is being mainly implemented in 13 States / UTs *viz.* Andhra Pradesh, Arunachal Pradesh, Assam, Jharkhand, Karnataka, Kerala, Meghalaya, Nagaland Orissa, Tamil Nadu, Uttarakhand, Uttar Pradesh and West Bengal. Small support is also being given to Maharashtra and Chhattisgarh. Main activities under the Project are as follows:

i. Ecological restoration of existing natural habitats and migratory routes of elephants,

ii. Development of scientific and planned management for conservation of elephant habitats and viable population of Wild Asiatic elephants in India,

iii. Promotion of measures for mitigation of man elephant conflict in crucial habitats and moderating pressures of human and domestic stock activities in crucial elephant habitats,

iv. Strengthening of measures for protection of Wild elephants form poachers and unnatural causes of death,

v. Research on Elephant management related issues,

vi. Public education and awareness programmes,

vii. Eco-development,

viii. Veterinary care.

Elephant Reserves: There are only 17 states in which elephants exist in the wild state. Project Elephant has declared 24 elephant reserves in 12 states to protect elephant populations in the wild and develop their habitat. It was launched in the year 1991-92 as a sequel to a series of efforts to conserve this magnificent species covering primarily twelve states of India, namely Assam, Arunachal Pradesh, Bihar andhra Pradesh, Karnataka, Kerala, Meghalaya, Nagaland Orissa, Tamilnadu, Uttar Pradesh and West Bengal. Till now 26 Elephant Reserves (ERs) extending over about 60,000 sq. km. has been formally notified by various State Governments. Consent for establishment 6 more ERs- Baitarini ER and South Orissa ER in Orissa, Lemru and Badalkhod in Chhattisgarh and Ganga-Jamuna (Shiwalik) ER in U.P, Khasi ER in Meghalaya has been accorded by MoEF. The concerned State Governments are yet to notify these ERs.

Monitoring of Illegal Killing of Elephants (Mike) Sites: Project Elephant has been formally implementing MIKE (Monitoring of Illegal Killing of Elephants) programme of CITES in 10 ERs since 01.04.2004. These include Shiwalik (Uttarakhand); Eastern Dooars (West Bengal); Mayurbhanj (Odisha); Ripu-Chirang and Dehing-Patkai (Assam); Garo Hills (Meghalaya); Deomali (Arunchal Pradesh); Wayanad (Kerala), Mysore (Karnataka) and Nilgiri (Tamil Nadu).

Table 4.4: Elephant (*Elephas maximus*) population estimates for 2007 and 2012

S.No.	States	Elephant	Population
		2007	2012
1.	Arunachal Pradesh	1690	1690*
2.	Assam	5281	5281*
3.	Meghalaya	1811	1811*
4.	Nagaland	152	212
5.	Tripura	59	59*
6.	West Bengal	325-350	325-350*
7.	Jharkhand	624	688

Contd...

Table. 4.4: Contd..

S.No.	States	Elephant	Population
		2007	2012
8.	Odisha	1862	1930
9.	Chattisgarh	122	215
10.	Uttarakhand	1346	1346*
11.	Uttar Pradesh	380	380
12.	Tamil Nadu	3867	3726
13.	Karnataka	4035	3900-7458**
14.	Kerala	6068	6177
15.	Andhra Pradesh	28	41
16.	Maharshtra	7	4
		27657-27682	27785-31368

*Census figure as per 2007. The census report of 2012 is still awaited from the States
**3900-7458 (Confidence Limits)

Table 4.5: Elephant Reserves in India

S.No.	Elephant Range	Elephant Reserve	State Area	Total In ER	P.A. (Sq. km)
I.		1. MayurjharnaER (24.10.2002)	West Bengal	414	-
		2. Singhbhum ER(26.9.2001)	Jharkhand	4530	193
		3. Mayurbhanj ER(29.9.2001)	Orissa	3214	1309
		4. Mahanadi ER(20.7.2002)§	Orissa	1038	964
		5. Sambalpur ER(27.3.2002)§	Orissa	427	427
		6. Baitarni ER#	Orissa	1755	-
		7. South Orissa ER#	Orissa	4216	750
		8. Lemru #	Chattisgarh	450	-
		9.Badalkhol-Tamorpingla #	Chattisgarh	1048.3	1154.93
II.	North Brahamputra	10. Kameng ER (19.6.2002)	Arunachal	1892	748
	(Arunachal-Assam)	11. Sonitpur ER (6.3.2003)	Assam	1420	420
III.	South Brahamputra	12. Dihing-Patkai ER(17.4.2003)	Assam	937	345
	(Assam- Arunachal)	13. South Arunachal ER (29.2.2008)	Arunachal	1957.5	378.13
IV.	Kaziranga(Assam-Nagaland)	14. Kaziranga-KarbiAnglong ER (17.4.2003)	Assam	3270	1073
		15. Dhansiri-LungdingER (19.4.2003)	Assam	2740	
		16. Intanki ER (28.2.2005)	Nagaland	202	202
V.	Eastern Dooars	17. Chirang-Ripu ER(7.3.2003)	Assam	2600	526+

Contd...

Table. 4.5: Contd..

S.No.	Elephant Range	Elephant Reserve	State Area	Total In ER	P.A. (Sq. Km)
	(Assam- W.Bengal)	18. Eastern Dooars ER (28.8.2002)	W.Bengal	978	484
VI.	E. Himalayas	19 Garo Hills ER(31.10.2001)	Meghalaya	3,500	402
	(Meghalaya)	20. Khasi Hills ER#	Meghalaya	1331	-
VII.	Nilgiri –EasternGhat	21. Mysore ER (25.11.2002)	Karnataka,	6724	3103
	(Karnataka- Kerala-	22. Wayanad ER (2.4.2002)	Kerala	1200	394
	Tamilnadu-Andhra)				
	(Karnataka- Kerala-	23. Nilgiri ER (19.9.2003)	Tamilnadu	4663	716
	Tamilnadu-Andhra)	24. Rayala ER (9.12.2003)	Andhra	766	525
VIII.	South Nilgiri	25. Nilambur ER (2.4.2002)	Kerala	1419	90
	(Kerala-Tamilnadu)	26. Coimbatore ER (19.9.2003)	Tamilnadu	566	482
IX.	Western Ghat	27. Anamalai ER(19.9.2003)	Tamilnadu	1457	300
	(Tamilnadu-Kerala)	28. Anamudi ER (2.4.2002)	Kerala	3728	780
X.	Periyar	29. Periyar (2.4.2002)	Kerala	3742	1058
	(Kerala-Tamilnadu)	30. SrivilliputturER(19.9.03)	Tamilnadu	1249	568
XI.	Northern India	31. Shivalik ER(28.10.2002)	Uttarakhand	5405	1340
	(Uttarakhand-U.P.)	32. Uttar Pradesh ER(09.09.2009)	U.P.	744	-
	Total		69582.80	18732.06	

Approved by Govt. of India, but not yet notified by the State Government.

§ Proposal for extension approved by GOI, but not yet notified by the State.

*** Statistical lower / upper limits could not be ascertained owing to small size of the population.

Source: Elephant Task Force Report of MoEF

4.7 *In-situ* and *Ex-situ* conservation

Conservation of Wildlife along with their natural habitats is the demand of the time and the only way to mitigate the self-destruction processes initiated by the mankind since the inception of human civilization. Among the two conservation measures in vogue, *viz. ex-situ* (outside natural habitat) and *in-situ* (within natural habitat), the first one is the older practice since ancient times. Due to huge hue and cry made by the naturalists and the scientists from various disciplines regarding the climate change accusing the gross outrage over the natural ecosystem for last five decades or so, the latter has got prominence and the outcome is the establishment / declaration of different conservation systems. Zoo is a common example of ex-situ conservation and Protected Areas (PA) like National Park, Sanctuary, Conservation Reserve, Biosphere Reserve; Community Reserve etc. are examples of *in-situ* conservation. *In situ* conservation means that the conservation activities occur where the species naturally occurs in the wild. *Ex situ* conservation means that actions are taking place that involve removing the species from its natural setting. Although viable populations of some organisms can be maintained *ex-situ* either under cultivation or in captivity, these methods are far less effective than *in-situ* methods and, generally, they are extremely costly. Likewise, although *ex-situ* methods are important under a number of conditions, *in-situ* methods are generally recognized as being more secure and financially efficient.

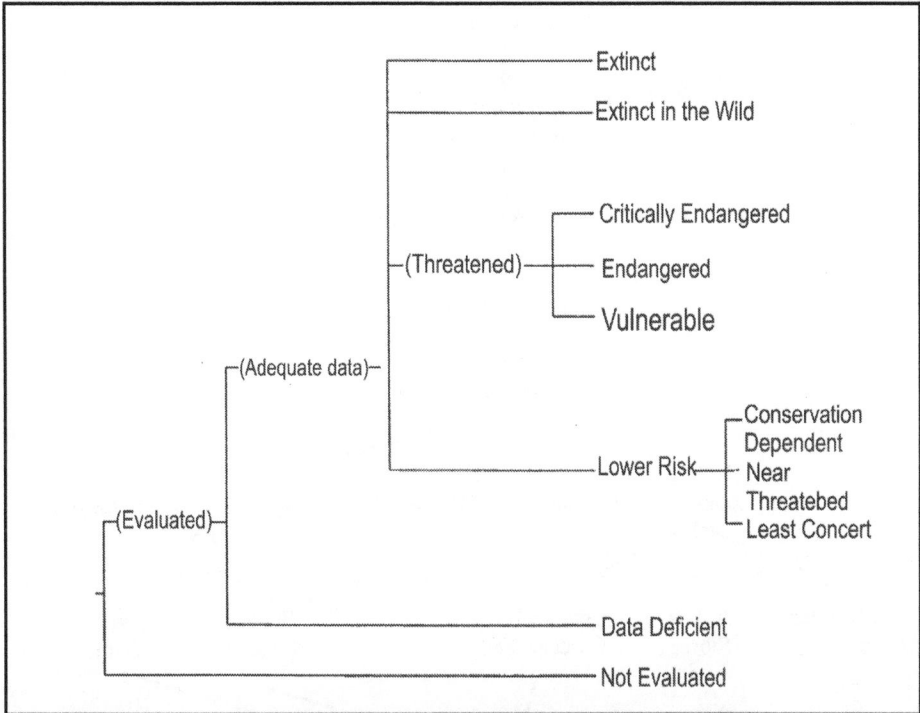

Figure 4.4: Structure of IUCN category of threat

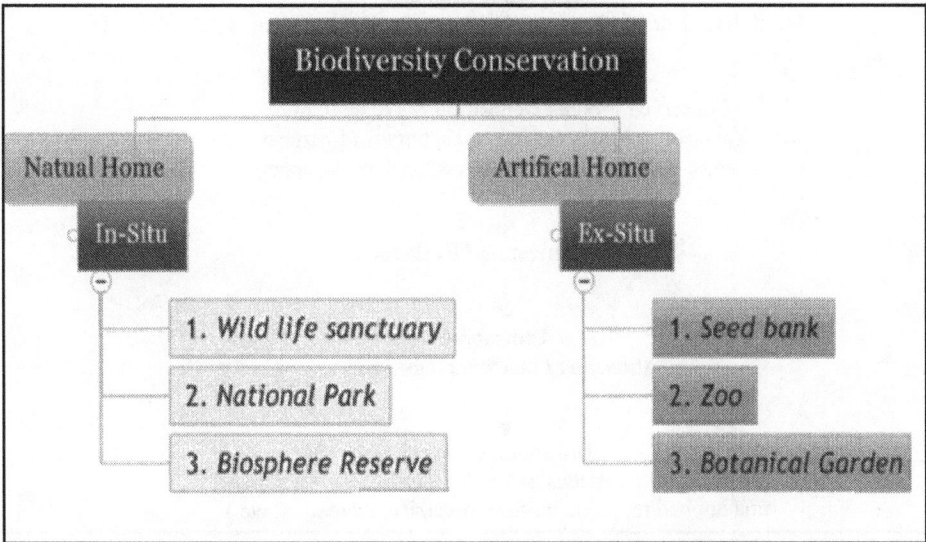

Figure 4.5: Concept of Biodiversity conservation

Selection of Target Taxa

↓

Project Commission

↓

Ecogeographic Survey /
Preliminary survey Mission

↓

Conservation Objectives

↓

Field Exploration

↓

Conservation Strategies

Ex Situ
(Sampling, transfer and storage)

In Situ
(Designation, management and monitoring)

Seed / Semen /
Ovule Storage

In Vitro
Storage

Botanical
Garden / Zoo

Genetic
Reserve

On-
farm

Conservation Products
(seed, live & dried plants, *in vitro* explants, DNA, pollen, data)

↓

Conserved Product Deposition & Dissemination
(gene or semen banks, reserves, botanical gardens,
zoos, conservation laboratories, on-farm systems)

↓

Characterization / Evaluation

↓

Utilisation
(breeding / biotechnology / etc)

↓

Utilisation Products
(breeding new varieties and crops, pharmaceuticals, pure
and applied research, on-farm diversity, recreation, etc.)

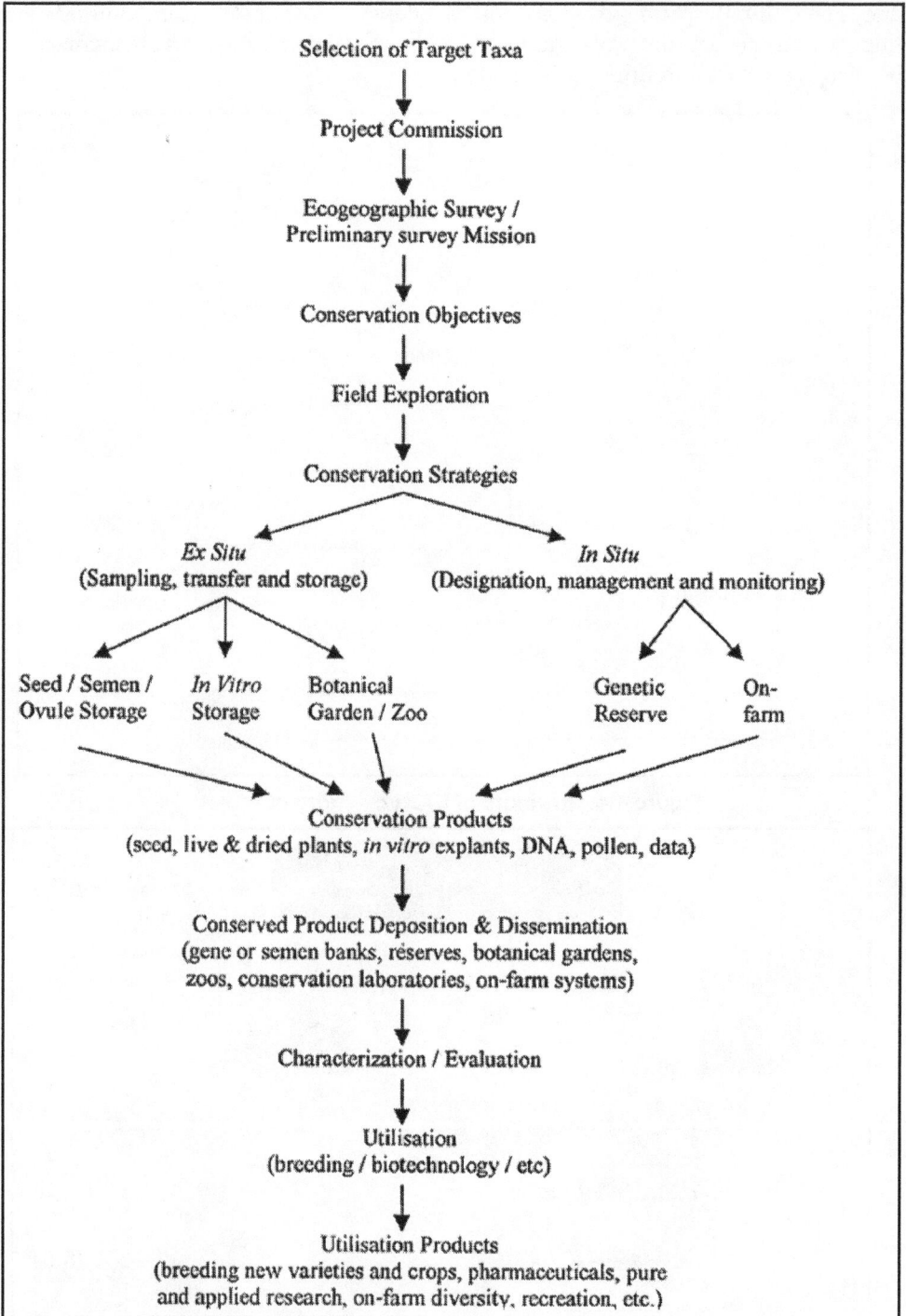

Figure 4.6: Model of Biodiversity Conservation (adopted from Maxted et al., 1997)

The challenge in using *in-situ* methods is to expand our vision of protected areas to include multiple use and extractive reserves and to develop new models for conservation including such innovative proposals as using damaged ecosystems to preserve rare, endangered and threatened species. The biological diversity to be sustained which is the essence of life having variety and variability of life forms along with the ecological functions and processes interacting together as envisaged by Decker *et al*. 1991.

4.7.1 *In-situ* Conservation

Conserving the areas where populations of species exist naturally is an underlying condition for the conservation of biodiversity. That's why protected areas form a central element of any national strategy to conserve biodiversity. Until recent times, human being tried to establish his own command over other animals to get food and shelter. There was indiscriminate felling of trees, hunting of the damages already done to the nature. It also felt necessary to conserve the habitat which is an outcome of evolutionary processes and susceptible to random environmental, demographic and genetic events. Among these, impacts caused by human activities are also to be considered. By that time many plant and animal species had become extinct or on the way of extinction. National Parks, Sanctuaries and other Protected Areas had been established to conserve the bio-diversity of the locality and even re-introduction of species either directly or through *ex-situ* conservation method. So many species had been declared as Endangered or Rare and ameliorating measures are being taken for successful rehabilitation, though mangrove forest of Sundarban is very dynamic and potential ecosystem in the earth. In Indian Sundarban 31 major species of mammals are found. The mammalian species that once existed in Sundarban and have become extinct today are Javan Rhinoceros (Rhinoceros sondaicus), Wild Buffalo (*Bubalis arnee*), Swamp deer (*Cervus duvaucelii*), Barking deer (*Muntiacus muntjac*) and Hog deer (*Hyelaphus porcinus*). The Royal Bengal Tiger (*Panthera tigris tigris*) had its uniqueness for adaptation in the mangrove habitat having distribution in the Gangetic delta of West Bengal and Bangladesh. Due to indiscriminate hunting for its valuable body parts and regular encroachment into its natural habitat, there is continuous man-animal conflict which eventually resulted in declining of tiger population in Sundarban areas of both the countries. It is a flagship species also as an indicator of health of forests and ecosystems. It has be considered as globally endangered and a conservation dependent species listed under Schedule-I of Wildlife (Protection) Act, 1972 in India and Appendix- I of the CITES. Considering the importance and impact, Sundarban Tiger Reserve had been established for in-situ conservation of Royal Bengal Tiger and other indigenous species of that locality in the year 1973. Protected Areas (PA) viz., National Park, Wildlife Sanctuary, Conservation Reserve, Community Reserve, Biosphere Reserve etc. have been declared since the last quarter of the last Century with the aim to conserve wildlife and its natural habitat.

i. Genetic Reserve Conservation

Conservation of wild species in a genetic reserve involves the location, designation, management and monitoring of genetic diversity in a particular natural location. This technique is the most appropriate for the bulk of wild species, because it can, when the management regime is minimal, be relatively inexpensive. Whether dealing with plants or animals, the objective is to contain the minimum number of individuals that can maintain genetic diversity within the species. If too few individuals are protected, genetic diversity will decline over time and if too many are protected, resources may be wasted in managing the large population. To guide such efforts, conservationists will need to estimate the effective population size (Ne) *i.e.* the number of conserved individuals that would undergo the same amount of random genetic drift as the actual population. Genetic reserves are appropriate for animals as well as for orthodox and non-orthodox seeded plant species, because numerous taxa can be protected in a single reserve that allows the continued evolution of species. However, the disadvantages are that the conserved material is not immediately available for human exploitation and, if the management regime is minimal, little characterization or evaluation data may be available. In the latter case, the reserve manager may even be unaware of the complete specific composition of the reserve that he or she is managing.

ii. On-Farm Conservation

Farmer-based conservation involves the maintenance of traditional crop or animal breeds or cultivation systems by farmers within traditional agricultural systems. On traditional farms, what are generally known as land-races of plants are sown and harvested and each season the farmers keep a proportion of harvested seed for re-sowing. Traditional breeds of domestic animal are maintained by inter-breeding within and between local village stocks. Thus the land-race or breed is highly adapted to the local environment and is likely to contain locally adapted alleles that may prove useful for specific breeding programs. Home garden plant conservation is a closely related variant of on-farm conservation of landraces but on a smaller scale. It involves the cultivation of more species-diverse material in home, kitchen, backyard or door-yard gardens. These home gardens focus on medicinal, flavoring and vegetable species *e.g.* tomatoes, peppers, digitalis, mint, thyme, parsley. The overall advantage of the on-farm technique is that it ensures the maintenance of highly adapted landraces and breeds and those wild species that traditional agriculture often depends on. However, these landraces or traditional breeds may yield less than their modern counterparts and so traditional farmers may require some subsidy and possibly monitoring to ensure continued farming. It should be noted that contemporary economic forces tend to act against the continued farming of ancient land-races and breeds, which are currently suffering rapid genetic erosion; many face imminent extinction.

Table 4.6: Difference between National park, Wildlife Sanctuary and Biosphere reserve

National Park	No human activity or settlement allowed. Villagers cannot graze their animals, extremely strict rules about jungle produce collection (Tendu leaves, Honey etc.)
Wildlife Sanctuary	People are not allowed to live (some exceptions) but some human activities are allowed, such as grazing, firewood collection. Tourism is permitted.A Sanctuary can be upgraded as a National Park. However a National Park cannot be downgraded as a Sanctuary.
Biosphere reserve	People are allowed to live, own private land and carry on their traditional activities in the outer-zone.

Ex-situ conservation is the preservation of components of biological diversity outside their natural habitats. This involves conservation of genetic resources, as well as wild and cultivated or species and draws on a diverse body of techniques and facilities. Some of these include:

- Gene banks *e.g.* seed banks, sperm and ova banks, field banks,

- In vitro plant tissue and microbial culture collections,

- Captive breeding of animals and artificial propagation of plants, with possible reintroduction into the wild,

- Collecting living organisms for zoos, aquaria and botanic gardens for research and public awareness.

At prehistoric times human being acted as gatherer, hunter, farmer, conqueror and eventually on today modified his own environment as a consequence of his own misdeeds. From the beginning, his attitude towards the animals was contradictory; the animals were worshipped, domesticated, hunted and decimated. Human relations with animals date back more than ten thousand years. As back as 2500 BC in Egypt in zoo type collection the pet animals like monkeys, antelopes, mongooses etc. were found. At about 1100 BC Chinese Emperor Wen Wang built his Garden of Intelligence in an area of 1500 acres to house his animal collection including Giant Panda. Several Emperors from Greek, Roman and Mughal dynasty established their Menagerie to house their animal collections. The first recognized Zoo in the world was established in 1759 in Schonbrunn near Vienna by the Emperor Francis I. The Zoo is still operating at the same site and more than 500 species have found their home at this Zoo. In India, the first private Zoo was established in 1854 at Marble Palace of Kolkata by Raja Rajendra Mullick Bahadur. The Zoo is commonly known as Marble Palace Zoo. Like Schonbrunn zoo, the Marble Palace Zoo is still operating at the same site. Since then Madras Zoo (1855) which was shifted later on in 1980 at Vandalur, Chennai and presently known as Arignar Anna Zoological Park, Trivandrum Zoo (1857), Mumbai Zoo (1863), Alipore Zoo (1875) and other Zoos in India gradually came into being. Presently, there are 71 major Zoos which include 7 large, 16 medium, 48 small Zoos, 86 mini Zoos,18 rescue centres and 23 circuses (According to the Inventory of Animals in Indian Zoos, 2010-2011 published by Central Zoo Authority).

Historically Zoos were established to meet the curiosity of the people in respect of animal and to entertain them as well. Conservation of wild animals did not get any attention to the managers of the Zoos in those days. Probably as animals were abundant at nature in those days and the threat of extinction of wild animals was not that acute as it is today, people were not serious about conservation of wild animals. With the establishment of Zoological Society of London in 1826, utility of Zoos was realized. In 1907, Carl Hegenback developed the concept of bar-less moated enclosures and this concept of display of animals influenced the managers of the Zoos around the world. In place of smaller cages, spacious enclosures came into being that also helped in maintaining biological and psychological need of the captive animals, but even then animals were continued to be kept in cages for part time *i.e.* during night time and adverse climatic conditions. With the tremendous growth of human population and development of infrastructure like roads, buildings etc. as a support system of growing human population, exploitation of natural resources started leading to depletion of forests. As a consequence, animal populations day by day became fragmented leading to loss of genetic variability and ultimately animal populations enter into extinction vortex. Species extinction caused primarily by indiscriminate poaching of animals and deforestation, may eliminate between 20% and 50% of wild species within the next decades. Under the circumstances, the role of Zoos has also dramatically changed. The Menagerie of 19th Century developed into Zoological Park in 20th Century and ultimately the same developed into Conservation Centre in 21st Century. Over the period of time, the objectives of establishing a Zoo have changed from mere exhibitionism, entertainment and amusement into research, education and ex-situ conservation to complement *in-situ* conservation.

Ex-situ conservation measures can be complementary to in-situ methods as they provide an insurance policy against extinction. These measures also have a valuable role to play in recovery programmes for endangered species. The Kew Seed Bank in England has 1.5% of the world's flora about 4,000 species-on deposits. In agriculture, *ex-situ* conservation measures maintain domesticated plants which cannot survive in nature unaided. *Ex-situ* conservation provides excellent research opportunities on the components of biological diversity. Some of these institutions also play a central role in public education and awareness rising by bringing members of the public into contact with plants and animals they may not normally come in contact with. It is estimated that worldwide, over 600 million people visit zoos every year. *Ex situ* conservation measures should support *in-situ* conservation measures (*in-situ* conservation should be the primary objective). The World Conservation Union (IUCN) has a key role in promoting the establishment of protected areas throughout the world. Since 1948, IUCN has developed standards and guidelines for PA management. Protected areas have been established following the categories defined by the IUCN.

- **Category I** *Strict Protection*: Sometimes called strict nature reserve/wilderness areas. Protected areas managed mainly for science or wilderness protection. Generally smaller areas where the preservation of important natural values with minimum human disturbance are emphasized.

- **Category II** *Ecosystem Conservation and Tourism:* Sometimes called national parks. Generally larger areas with a range of outstanding features and ecosystems that people may visit for education, recreation and inspiration as long as they do not threaten the area's values.

- **Category III** *Conservation of Natural Features*: Sometimes called natural monuments. Similar to National Parks, but usually smaller areas protecting a single spectacular natural feature or historic site.

- **Category IV** *Conservation through Active Management:* Sometimes called habitat and wildlife (species) management areas. Areas managed to protect and utilize wildlife species.

- **Category V** *Landscape/Seascape Conservation and Recreation*: Sometimes called protected landscapes/seascapes.

- **Category VI** *Sustainable Use of Natural Ecosystems*: Sometimes called managed resource protected areas. Protected areas managed mainly for the sustainable use of natural ecosystems.

In the past, it was assumed that the best way to preserve biodiversity was to conserve it through protected areas by reducing human activities or completely excluding humans. Population growth and poverty were seen as main causes of environmental degradation; people were regarded as a problem from which the environment needed protecting. Accordingly, protected areas and parks were fenced off from local people, traditional practices were prohibited and people were held under penalties of fines or imprisonments for utilising park resources. However, there are very controversial scientific and social problems with this approach, which was characterized by serious conflicts between local communities and the state.

4.7.2 *Ex situ* Conservation Techniques

(a) **Captive Breeding:** When a wild population falls below a viable state, one of the measures that can be undertaken to assist its survival is to take individuals from the wild or from a pre-existing captive population and instigate a breeding program. The young can either be held to increase the captive population or they can be re-introduced back into the wild. Captive breeding provides the opportunity for conservationists to selectively breed individuals from a small population in order to maximize heterozygosity, in addition to producing more clutches and lower mortality rate than in wild scenarios. Increased genetic diversity results in increased resilience and can contribute to a healthier and sustainable population.

(b) **Seed/Embryo Storage Conservation:** *Ex situ* seed/embryo collection and storage is the most convenient and widely used method of genetic conservation. Seeds and embryos are the natural dispersal, storage or generative organs for the majority of species. This technique involves collecting samples from individuals or populations and then transferring them to a gene bank for storage, usually at sub-zero temperatures. The procedure used for the bulk of orthodox-seeded plant species is to dry the seeds or embryos to a suitable moisture content (5–6%) before freezing at -20°C, but this method is only suitable for species that can be dried and stored at low temperature without losing viability. The advantages of this technique are that it is efficient and reproducible and feasible for short, medium and long-term secure storage. However, the disadvantages are that there are problems in storing recalcitrant-seeded plant species. The latter species cannot be dried and frozen in the way used for orthodox seeds, because they rarely produce seed or are normally clonally propagated.

(c) **Botanical/Zoological Garden Conservation:** Historically, botanical or zoological gardens were often associated with physic or medicinal gardens or displays of single specimens of zoological curiosities and as such they did not attempt to reflect the genetic diversity of the species. These gardens now hold living collections of species that were collected in a particular location and moved to the garden to be conserved. The advantage of this method is that gardens do not have the same constraints as many other conservation agencies; they have the freedom to focus on wild species that may otherwise not be given sufficient priority for conservation. Yet there are two disadvantages to this technique. The first is that the number of species that can be genetically conserved in a botanical or zoological garden will always be limited because of the available space. The majority of these gardens are located in urban areas in temperate countries and at their present sites most expansion would be prohibitively expensive. The majority of botanical and animal diversity is located in tropical climates, yet because most botanical and zoological gardens are in temperate countries, the collections must be kept in expensive greenhouses or other facilities, which also limits the space available. The second disadvantage is related to the first, namely, very few individuals of each species can be held and this severely restricts the range of genetic diversity found in the wild that is protected. However, if the target species is very near extinction and only one or two specimens remain extant, this objection of course does not hold.

(d) *In vitro* **Conservation:** *In vitro* conservation involves the maintenance of explants in a sterile, pathogen-free environment and it is widely used for vegetative propagated and recalcitrant-seeded species. This method offers an alternative to field gene banks. It involves the establishment of tissue cultures of accessions on nutrient agar and their storage under controlled conditions of either slow or suspended growth. The main advantage is that it offers a solution to the long term conservation problems of recalcitrant, sterile or clonally propagated species. The main disadvantages are the risk of somaclonal variation, the need to develop individual maintenance protocols for the majority of species and the relatively high level technology and high cost required. The best answer for cheap, long-term *in vitro* conservation in the future may be cryopreservation *i.e.* the storage of frozen tissue cultures at very low temperatures *e.g.* in liquid nitrogen at -196°C. If this technique can be perfected to reduce the damage caused by freezing and thawing, it may be possible to preserve materials indefinitely.

(e) **Field Gene Bank/Livestock Park Conservation:** The conservation of germplasm in field gene banks or livestock parks involves the collecting of plant or animal specimens from one location and the transfer and conservation at a second site. It has traditionally been the method for recalcitrant whose seeds cannot be dried and frozen without loss of viability or sterile-seeded plant species or for those species for which it is preferable to store clonal material. Field gene banks are commonly used for species such as cocoa, rubber, coconut, mango, coffee, banana, cassava, sweet potato and yam. Livestock parks or rare breed centers, as distinct from zoos, emphasize captive breeding programs and therefore genetic conservation. The advantages of field gene banks and livestock parks are that the species are easily accessible for utilization and evaluation can be undertaken while the material is being conserved. The disadvantages are that the material is restricted in terms of genetic diversity, is susceptible to pests, disease and vandalism and may require large areas of land.

(f) **Pollen/Semen/Ovule/DNA Conservation:** The storage of pollen grains is possible under appropriate conditions that allow their subsequent use for crossing with living plant material. It may also be possible in the future to regenerate haploid plants routinely from pollen cultures, but no generalized protocols have been developed yet. The development of artificial insemination techniques in recent years has made semen and ovule storage routine, especially for domesticated animals. The storage of DNA under prescribed conditions can easily and inexpensively be achieved given the appropriate level of technology, but the regeneration of entire organisms from DNA cannot be envisaged at present, although single or small numbers of genes could subsequently be utilized. The advantage of pollen storage is that it is low cost and simple, but the disadvantage is that only paternal material would be conserved and with DNA storage there are problems with subsequent gene isolation, cloning and transfer.

Case Study: Wild buffalo conservation plan for Central India in Limbo

The *ex-situ* conservation plan to establish 200 genetically acceptable wild buffaloes in Central India in five years has been in limbo owing to the poor numbers of the third biggest mammal on land only after elephants and rhinos. *Ex-situ* conservation means literally off-site conservation. It is the process of protecting an endangered species of plant or animal outside its natural habitat. Wild buffaloes are listed under Schedule I of the Wildlife Protection Act (WPA) 1972. The critically endangered species is facing extinction. In November 2012, a three-day international-level workshop in Nagpur by the Maharashtra forest department in coordination with International Union for Conservation and Nature (IUCN), Satpuda Foundation and Wildlife Trust of India (WTI), had set a goal to establish genetically pure wild buffaloes. However, even after two years, there is no progress and no one is either ready to come clear on the issue. On December 3, 2013, a meeting was held on conservation plan and decision was taken to finalize it in a month by taking views of Assam, Madhya Pradesh and Chhattisgarh forest departments and ministry of environment and forests (MoEF). The global wild buffalo population is estimated to be around 3,400 of which 3,100 (91%) is in India, mostly in Assam. Few numbers are reported in Udanti-Sitanadi in Chhattisgarh and Kolamarka in Maharashtra. In Kolamarka, already steps are taken to conserve the mammals by forming a nine-member monitoring team. Plans are happening to develop grassy meadows. Camera traps are deployed where evidence found. Besides, information about direct and indirect evidence is being gathered with the help of locals.

Summary

1. In 1972, India enacted the Wildlife Protection Act and Project Tiger to safeguard the habitats of conservation reliant species. As of April 2012, there were 112 national parks. All national park lands then encompassed a total 39,919 km^2 (15,413 sq mi) km^2, comprising 1.21% of India's total surface area. A total of 166 national parks have been authorized by the ministry, plans are underway to establish the remaining scheduled parks. India has over 500 animal sanctuaries, referred to as Wildlife Sanctuaries. Among these, the 47 Tiger Reserves are governed by Project Tiger and are of special significance in the conservation of the tiger.

2. The Government of India enacted Wild Life (Protection) Act 1972 with the objective of effectively protecting the wild life of this country and to control poaching, smuggling and illegal trade in wildlife and its derivatives. The Act was amended in January 2003 and punishment and penalty for offences under the Act have been made more stringent.

3. The wild life laws have a long history and are the carminative result of an increasing awareness of the compelling need to restore the catastrophic ecological imbalances introduced by the depredations inflicted on nature by human being.

4. The first comprehensive legislation relating to protection of wild life was passed by the Parliament and it was assented by the President on 9th September, 1972 and came to be known as The Wild Life (Protection) Act, 1972 (53 of 1972). An Act to provide for the protection of wild animals, birds and plants and for matters connected therewith or ancillary or incidental thereto.

5. The Indian wildlife (Protection) act, 1972 as amended up to 1993 has seven chapters in it.

6. Wild Life (Protection) Amendment Act, 2002 is an Act of the Parliament of India amending the existing Wildlife Protection Act, 1972. The Wildlife Protection Act, 1972 was enacted with the objective of effectively controlling poaching and illegal trade in wildlife and its derivatives.

7. The Wild Life (Protection) Amendment Act, 2006 (No. 39 of 2006) has come into force on 4th September 2006. The Act provides for creating the National

Tiger Conservation Authority and the Tiger and Other Endangered Species Crime Control Bureau (Wildlife Crime Control Bureau). The implementation over the years has highlighted the need for a statutory authority with legal backing to ensure tiger conservation.

8. The Wild Life (Protection) Amendment Bill, 2013 was introduced in the Rajya Sabha on August 5, 2013. The Bill has been referred to the Standing Committee on Environment and Forests. The Bill seeks to amend the Wild Life (Protection) Act, 1972. This Act provides for the protection and conservation of wild animals, birds and plants.

9. Species judged as threatened are listed by various agencies as well as by some private organizations. The most cited of this list is the Red Data Book. Red data book is a loose-leaf volume of information on the status of many kinds of species. Red, of course is symbolic of the danger that these species both plants and animals presently experience throughout the globe.

10. The IUCN Red List is set upon precise criteria to evaluate the extinction risk of thousands of species and subspecies.

11. The International Union for the Conservation of Nature and Natural Resources (IUCN) developed the first established approach in dealing with the presentation of information on rare and threatened species.

12. The Red list has listed 132 species of plants and animals as Critically Endangered, the most threatened category from India in 2012. Plants seemed to be the most threatened life form with 60 species being listed as Critically Endangered and 141 as Endangered.

13. CITES (Convention on International Trade in Endangered Species of Wild Fauna and Flora) is an international agreement between governments. CITES was drafted as a result of a resolution adopted in 1963 at a meeting of members of IUCN (The World Conservation Union).

14. CITES is one of the largest and oldest conservation and sustainable use agreements in existence. Participation is voluntary and countries that have Funding for the activities of the Secretariat and Conference of the Parties (CoP) meetings comes from a Trust Fund derived from Party contributions.

15. The UNEP World Conservation Monitoring Centre was established in 2000 as the world biodiversity information and assessment centre of the United Nations Environment Programme. The Centre's roots go back to 1979 when IUCN established a Cambridge office to monitor endangered species. In 1988 the independent, non-profit World Conservation Monitoring Centre was founded jointly by IUCN, WWF and UNEP.

16. The activities of UNEP-WCMC include biodiversity assessment, support to international conventions such as the Convention on Biological Diversity (CBD) and the Convention on International Trade in Endangered Species of Wild Fauna and Flora (CITES), capacity building and management of both aspatial and spatial data on species and habitats of conservation concern.

17. Project Noah is a powerful tool for learning about nature and a leading technology platform for crowd sourcing ecological data. Noah stands for networked organisms and habitats. Project Noah was adopted by National Geographic since 2010. Project Noah has set out to mobilize a new generation of nature explorers.

18. India is uniquely blessed with wildlife diversity. One of eighteen mega diverse countries, it is home to 7.6 per cent of all mammalian, 12.6 per cent of all avian, 6.2 per cent of all reptilian, 4.4 per cent of all amphibian, 11.7 per cent of all fish and 6.0 per cent of all flowering plant species.

19. India has been identified as one of the top 12 mega-diversity countries of the world. Among the 18 hot spots recognized in the world, two are in India-Eastern Himalayas and Western Ghats.

20. A plant, animal or microorganism that is in immediate risk of biological extinction is called endangered species or threatened species. In India, 450 plant species have been identified as endangered species. The 100 mammals and 150 birds are estimated to be endangered.

21. Species that are found only in a particular region are known as endemic species. Almost 60 per cent the endemic species in India are found in Himalayas and the Western Ghats.

22. There was a time when India was home for some of the most beautiful wild animals, due to excessive hunting and poaching for sport and body parts by man, these wild animals have become extinct.

23. Indian biodiversity includes more than 120 families of terrestrial vertebrates. It has been estimated that there are more than 400 species of mammals, 1200 species of Birds, more than 350 Species of Reptiles and more that 29,70,000 species of insects in India.

24. Sanctuary is an area which is of adequate ecological, faunal, floral, geomorphological, natural or zoological significance. The Sanctuary is declared for the purpose of protecting, propagating or developing wildlife or its environment. Certain rights of people living inside the Sanctuary could be permitted.

25. National Park is an area having adequate ecological, faunal, floral, geo-morphological, natural or zoological significance. The National Park is declared for the purpose of protecting, propagating or developing wildlife or its environment, like that of a Sanctuary.

26. Conservation Reserves can be declared by the State Governments in any area owned by the Government, particularly the areas adjacent to National Parks and Sanctuaries and those areas which link one Protected Area with another.

27. Community Reserves can be declared by the State Government in any private or community land, not comprised within a National Park, Sanctuary or a Conservation Reserve, where an individual or a community has volunteered to conserve wildlife and its habitat.

28. Fewer natural wildlife habitat areas remain each year. Moreover, the habitat that remains has often been degraded to bear little resemblance to the wild areas which existed in the past. Habitat loss due to destruction, fragmentation or degradation of habitat is the primary threat to the survival of wildlife.

29. The development and implementation of species recovery plans and programmes provide integrated conservation strategies for wildlife. These often involve a combination of *in situ* assessment of natural plant populations, monitoring of their status and the current or past causes of their decline and the determination of future priorities, therefore enabling their recovery.

30. In India, human-animal conflict is seen across the country in a variety of forms, including monkey menace in the urban centers, crop raiding by ungulates and wild pigs, depredation by elephants, cattle lifting and human death and injury by tigers, leopards and other wild animals.

31. In the beginning of the 1970s, once tiger hunting had officially been banned in India, a tiger count was done across the entire country. This lead to the astonishing discovery that only 1800 specimens of this magnificent animal were left. This jolted the concerned authorities and some serious thought went into devising plans to save the tiger. The result was the launch of "Project Tiger" in 1972 at the Dhikala Forest Rest House in Corbett National Park.

32. Project Tiger Scheme has been under implementation since 1973 as a Centrally Sponsored Scheme of Government of India.

33. Elephant (*Elephas maximus*) is the largest terrestrial mammal of India placed in schedule-I under Willife (Protection) Act 1972. Elephant being wide ranging animal requires large areas. As per our mythology, elephant took birth from celestial waters and thus are closely associated with rains / water because of the belief.

34. There are only 17 states in which elephants exist in the wild state. Project Elephant has declared 24 elephant reserves in 12 states to protect elephant populations in the wild and develop their habitat.

35. Project Elephant has been formally implementing MIKE (Monitoring of Illegal Killing of Elephants) programme of CITES in 10 ERs since 01.04.2004. These include Shiwalik (Uttaranchal); Eastern Dooars (West Bengal); Mayurbhanj (Orissa); Ripu-Chirang and Dehing-Patkai (Assam); Garo Hills (Meghalaya); Deomali (Arunchal Pradesh); Wayanad (Kerala), Mysore (Karnataka) and Nilgiri (Tamilnadu).

36. Conservation of Wildlife along with their natural habitats is the demand of the time and the only way to mitigate the self-destruction processes initiated by the mankind since the inception of human civilization. Among the two conservation measures in vogue, *viz. ex-situ* (outside natural habitat) and *in-situ* (within natural habitat), the first one is the older practice since ancient times.

37. Conserving the areas where populations of species exist naturally is an underlying condition for the conservation of biodiversity. That's why

protected areas form a central element of any national strategy to conserve biodiversity.

38. Conservation of wild species in a genetic reserve involves the location, designation, management and monitoring of genetic diversity in a particular natural location. This technique is the most appropriate for the bulk of wild species, because it can, when the management regime is minimal, be relatively inexpensive.

39. Farmer-based conservation involves the maintenance of traditional crop or animal breeds or cultivation systems by farmers within traditional agricultural systems. On traditional farms, what are generally known as land-races of plants are sown and harvested and each season the farmers keep a proportion of harvested seed for re-sowing.

40. *Ex-situ* conservation is the preservation of components of biological diversity outside their natural habitats. This involves conservation of genetic resources, as well as wild and cultivated or species and draws on a diverse body of techniques and facilities.

41. *Ex-situ* conservation measures can be complementary to *in-situ* methods as they provide an insurance policy against extinction. These measures also have a valuable role to play in recovery programmes for endangered species.

Glossary

Abundance: How commonly a taxon or group of taxons occurs. Usually used without units. More precise terms are distribution, prevalence and density.

Adaptation: Process by which populations undergo modification so as to function better than their immediate ancestors in a given environment.

Additive genetic variance: Part of the phenotypic variance of quantitative traits, such as body size or age at maturity. The additive genetic variance is proportional to the expected change attributable to selection and is used to calculate the heritability.

Allozyme: Gene product of one of several alleles that have the same function but differ in their amino acid sequence and therefore in their physio-chemical properties so that they migrate different distances in an electrophoretic assay. They are used as genetic markers to identify a genotype.

Ameba: A single celled organism which has no rigid body structure. Amebas move about and take in food by extending *pseudopods*. Examples of parasitic amoebae include *Entamoeba histolytica* (cause of amebic dysentery) and *Naegleria* sp. and *Acanthameba* sp. (causes of eosinophilic meningitis).

Apomixis: Form of asexual reproduction. Offspring is formed without meiosis and fertilization. Daughters are genetically identical to their mothers.

Arachnid: A group of arthropods normally featuring 4 pairs of legs and two major body segments (cephalothorax and abdomen). Parasitic arachnids include mites and ticks. The group also includes the spiders and scorpions.

Arthropod: A group of organisms comprising a whole phylum to themselves (Phylum Arthropoda). These organisms are characterized by having a number of jointed legs, numerous body segments which may be fused or unfused and a hard outer covering or exoskeleton made of chitin. Phylum Arthropoda contains the following Classes: Insecta (insects), Arachnida (spiders, mites, ticks, scorpions, etc), Chilopoda (centipedes), Diplopoda (millipedes), and Crustacea (crabs, shrimp, lobsters, water fleas, etc. Related groups include the Onychophora (*Peripatus*, etc), the Tardigrades (water bears, etc) and the Pentastomids (tongue worms).

Biodiversity: (Greek. bios, life) Refers to aspects of variety in the living world; used to describe the number of species, the amount of genetic variation or the number of community types present in the area.

Biogeochemical Cycle: The movement of chemical elements between organisms and non-living compartments of the atmosphere, lithosphere and hydrosphere.

Biogeography: The study of the geographical distribution of organisms; it largely depends on abiotic factors, resources, community interaction, mobility of organisms (whether large or small), topography, geohistorical factors (continental drift, island formation, etc.) e.g. small island hosts fewer species, fewer resources, fewer habitats than a larger one; the species on an island are balanced by the death and immigration rate of organisms but is less stable compared to a larger island or even continent applies for natural reserves as well.

Biosphere: The zone of air, land and water at the surface of the earth that is occupied by organisms.

Canopy: (Greek. canopion, net) The dense roof-forming vegetation, typically represented by the crowns of the trees; kelps, brown algae, can also form dense forest-like canopies.

Cilia: Small beating hairs on the outside of cells. In complex organisms like humans, these cilia may be found on cells lining the respiratory passages, where they help the flow of mucus. In simpler organisms they may aid in movement. Single celled organisms which use cilia to move around are called ciliates.

Cladocera: Order of the Entomostraca. They have a bivalve shell covering the body but not the head, four to six pairs of legs, and two pairs of antennae used for swimming. They mostly inhabit fresh water.

Coevolution: Changes in the genotypes of two or more species that are a direct consequence of the species' interaction with one another. Coevolution can occur among mutualists and host—parasite pairs, as well as among entire groups of interacting organisms (e.g., pollinator—plant systems).

Coexistance: The living together of two species or organisms in the same habitat, such as that neither tends to be eliminated by the other.

Commensal: A commensal organism is one which lives within the body of another but does not normally cause any harm. In times of stress, commensals may turn into pathogens.

Competition: Interaction between members of the same population or of two or more populations to obtain a resource that both require and which is available in limited supply, hence, limiting overall fitness (survival, growth, reproduction of an organism).

Consumer: An organism within an ecosystem, plant or animal that derives its food from another organism.

Crustacea: Aquatic arthropods characterized by the presence of biramous appendages and two sets of antennae. Examples include crabs, lobsters, copepods, barnacles, shrimps, and waterfleas.

Cyclical parthenogenesis: Mode of reproduction in which phases of parthenogenetic (asexual) and sexual reproduction alternate. Several asexual generations may follow a sexual generation.

Cyst: The term cyst may have two meanings. Firstly, a cyst may be the resistant dormant stage of a single celled organism which is passed out and encourages the propagation of the species. Alternatively, cyst may refer to the intermediate stage of some tapeworms *e.g.* hydatid cysts. This cyst must be eaten by the definitive host for it to be infected.

Decomposer: Organisms (bacteria, fungi, heterotrophic protists) in ecosystems that break down complex organic material into smaller inorganic molecules that then are recirculated.

Definitive Host: The definitive host is the organism which houses the mature or sexually reproducing stage of the parasite. For example, the dog is the definitive host of the hydatid tapeworm, while the mosquito is the definitive host of the malarial parasite.

Denitrification: The conversion of nitrate to gaseous nitrogen; carried out by a few genera of free living soil bacteria.

Density dependence: Indicates that the intensity of a process depends on the density of a population. When fecundity or individual survival in a population is negatively dependent on density *e.g.* parasite-induced host mortality, the process could potentially regulate population density. Transmission of horizontally transmitted parasites is usually host density dependent.

Depth selection behavior: Behavior by which the zooplankton maintains a particular vertical distribution in relation to the stratification of the water (light, temperature, food, predation pressure).

Diarrhea: Frequency of bowel movements or stool often associated with a loose consistency.

Diel vertical migration (DVM): Special case of depth selection behavior in which the preferred depth changes in a diel (daily) pattern.

Dioecious: Having two sexes as opposed to hermaphroditic.

Dose effect: A change in response to exposure to some agent attributable to a change in that agent's concentration. For example, the increase in virulence or infection risk for hosts during exposure to increasing parasite spore doses.

Dysentery: Diarrhea with associated blood and mucus discharge.

Endoparasite: Symbionts located within the body of the host. They may be intra- or extracellular.

Epibiont: Organism that lives attached to the body surface of another organism. Sometimes regarded as ecto-parasites. In zooplankton, epibionts are often ciliates, algae, bacteria, and fungi.

Epidemic: Sudden, rapid spread or increase in the prevalence or intensity of an infection. Compare Endemic.

Epidemiology: Study of infectious diseases and disease-causing agents on the population level in a parasitological context. It seeks to characterize the disease's patterns of distribution and prevalence and the factors responsible for these patterns. In a more applied context, it also strives to identify and test prevention and treatment measures.

Evolution: Changes in allele frequencies over time.

Experimental epidemiology: Study of epidemiology in replicated experimental populations.

Experimental evolution: Study of evolutionary change in replicated experimental populations.

Filarial Worm: A group of long, hair-like nematodes in which the adults live in the blood or tissues of vertebrates. In some species, the larvae may be found in the blood. Examples of diseases caused by filarial worms include Elephantiasis and River Blindness.

Fitness: Extent to which an individual contributes its genes to future generations in relation to the contribution of other genotypes in the same population at the same time.

Flagellum: A long beating hair found on a cell which normally aids in movement. Human sperm cells have a flagellum. Single celled organisms which move about using flagella are called Flagellates.

Flatworms: A group of organisms comprising a whole phylum (Phylum Platyhelminths). Flatworms have flat bodies (as the name suggests) and are normally hermaphroditic. Phylum Platyhelminths consists of three classes: Class Trematoda (flukes), Class Cestoda (tapeworms) and Class Tubellaria (free-living flatworms *e.g.* Planarians and ribbon worms).

Flukes: A group of organisms characterized by having a flat, unsegmented body and complex multi-stage life cycles. Flukes (comprising Class Trematoda) are members of the Phylum Platyhelminths, or the flatworms, which also includes the Tapeworms and the non-parasitic Turbellarians *e.g.* Planarians. Flukes are entirely parasitic, and are hermaphroditic, save for some groups *e.g.* Schistosomes. Examples of flukes include the liver fluke and the schistosomes.

Food: Organic compounds used in the synthesis of new biomolecules and as fuel in the production of cellular energy *i.e.* carbohydrates (glucose), starch (amylose, amylopectic), proteins (from aminoacids), fatty acids, vitamins, trace elements.

Genetic polymorphism: Occurrence of two or more genotypes in a population.

Genetic variation: Degree to which members of a population differ at certain loci.

Gigantism: Phenomenon describing increased growth (or large body size) of certain members of a population. Sometimes parasitized hosts show gigantism compared with non-parasitized conspecifics. In this case, gigantism is often associated with parasite-induced host castration.

Habitat: The living place of a population, characterized by its physical, chemical, and/or biotic properties.

Helminth: Wormy parasite. Helminths are not a taxonomic group.

Horizontal transmission: Parasite transmission between infected and susceptible individuals or between disease vectors and susceptible.

Imago: The last stage of development of an insect, after the last ecdysis (molt) of an incomplete metamorphosis, or after emergence from pupation where the metamorphosis is complete. As this is the only stage which is sexually mature, and has functional wings in winged species, the imago is often referred to as the adult stage. The Latin plural of imago is imagines, and this is the term generally used by entomologists, however imagos or imagoes are also acceptable spellings.

Insect: A group of organisms comprising the Class Insecta of Phylum Arthropoda. Insects are characterized by having 3 pairs of legs and three major body segments (head, thorax and abdomen). Some species have wings. Parasitic insects include the fleas and lice. Other groups, such as flies, mosquitoes and some beetles, are important vectors of parasitic disease or intermediate hosts.

Instar: Discrete stages of development in insects and crustaceans, whose growth is accomplished by molting.

Intermediate host: The organism which houses the immature or non-sexually reproducing stage of a parasite. For example, the sheep is the normal intermediate host for the hydatid tapeworm, while humans are the intermediate host for the malarial parasite.

Isotherms: Virtual lines of identical temperature patterns across a given area in which similar species and communities can prosper, they are more numerous in the equatorial regions (more numerous predatorprey communities, a larger primary production etc.) than near the poles.

Kairomone: Chemical cues released from predators and recognized by the prey. Kairomones from several different predators have been reported to lead to adaptive morphological and life history changes in *Daphnia*.

Keystone Species: Top predator affecting the prosperity of organisms lower in trophic level.

Larva: An immature stage of an organism which bears no structural resemblance to the mature stage. For example, a maggot is the larva of a fly, a caterpillar is the larva of a moth or butterfly.

Life table: A summary of the age or stage-related survivorship of individuals in a population based on natality and mortality rates.

Local adaptation: Genetic differentiation attributable to selective forces specific to the local environment. Local adaptation is best demonstrated by showing that immigrant genotypes are inferior to resident genotypes. Locally adapted parasites usually show higher levels of damage and have higher levels of transmission stage production in their local hosts.

Local species: Tendency of a community to return to its original state when subject to small perturbations.

Macroparasite: Parasite that usually does not multiply within its definitive hosts but instead produces transmission stages (eggs and larvae) that pass into the external environment or to vectors. Macroparasites are typically parasitic helminths and arthropods. The key epidemiological measurement is generally the number of parasites per host.

Melanin: Substance used by invertebrates to (among other functions) encapsulate parasites.

Metapopulation: Group of partially isolated populations belonging to the same species. Migration among subpopulations is important for the ecological and evolutionary dynamics of a metapopulation.

Microparasite: Parasite that undergoes direct multiplication within its definitive hosts (e.g., viruses, bacteria, fungi, and protozoa). Microparasites are characterized by small size and short generation times. The key epidemiological variable, by contrast with macroparasites, is whether the individual host is infected.

Microsatellite locus: Place in the genome where a short string of nucleotides, usually two to five bases long, is repeated in tandem. The number of repeats at any given locus is usually highly variable (many alleles) in a population and can be used for DNA fingerprinting.

Morbidity: State of ill-health produced by a disease. Includes aspects of reduced fecundity, lethargy, and other signs of disease.

Multiple infections: Infection in which an individual is infected by parasites of more than one species or more than one genotype of the same species.

Nematode: A group of organisms also known as the Roundworms. Nematodes have what can only be described as a typical worm shape-long, tapered at the ends and round in cross-section (think of the shape of an earthworm, but earthworms are not nematodes). They have an internal body cavity, with recognizable digestive and reproductive tracts. Nematodes are generally dioecious. They reproduce by laying eggs, or larvae which hatch from their eggs inside the body of the female worm. They are among the most common multicellular parasite of humans in the world, although the majority of nematodes are not parasitic, living in the soil. Examples of parasitic roundworms include Human Roundworm (*Ascaris*), Pinworm/Threadworm, Whipworm, Hookworm and Filarial Worms.

Nymph: An immature stage of an organism which largely resembles the adult stage, save for some minor differences. For example, cockroach nymphs can be differentiated from the adults by the fact that the nymphs do not have wings.

Obligate parasite: A parasite which cannot survive or reproduce outside the body of its host organism.

Opportunistic pathogen: An organism which is normally harmless (Commensal), but which may turn nasty if given the opportunity. For example, one of the dangers for people in the last stages of HIV infection is infection by any number of organisms which pose no threat to individuals with fully functioning immune systems.

Parasite: 1. Disease-causing organism. 2. Organism exhibiting an obligatory, detrimental dependence on another organism (its host). Conceptually, parasite and pathogen are the same. Endoparasites live in the host's interior. They may be intra- or extracellular. Ectoparasites live on the surface of the host.

Pathogen: Disease-causing microorganism, such as viruses, bacteria, and protozoa. In the context of this book, equivalent to parasite.

Population dynamics: Changes in the population size through time. Also used to describe change in the demographic structure of the population (sex ratio, age and size structure, etc.).

Population growth rate (Malthusian growth rate, *r*): Measure of population growth. The instantaneous rate of increase of a population or genotype. It is used as a measure of fitness.

Population: Group of interbreeding individuals and their offspring. In asexual species, this definition cannot be applied; in this case, a population is a group of phenotypically matching individuals living in the same area.

Predator: An animal that kills its victim, the prey item, and then feeds on it to subsist until the next kill.

Predator-induced defense: Defense reaction of prey triggered by the presence or action of a predator so as to reduce the expected damage of the predator.

Prepatent phase: In helminthes infections, time period from infection until a female starts to produce eggs. It is equivalent to the latent period in microparasitic infections.

Prevalence: Proportion of host individuals infected with a particular parasite. Often expressed as a percentage. A measure of how widespread an infection or disease in a host population is. Sometimes used to indicate the proportion of infected hosts in a sample with any parasite species. In many studies, prevalence is measured only in a certain fraction of hosts. In zooplankton studies, often only adult hosts or adult females are considered. Prevalence is usually underestimated in field samples because new infections may escape detection by the investigator.

Primipare: Female producing offspring or eggs for the first time.

Protozoa: A subgroup of the Kingdom Protista, or the single celled organisms. The name Protozoa is a carry-over from an old system of classification and is generally used to describe those single celled organisms which show more animal than plant characteristics. Naturally, such a distinction is meaningless, as animals and plants belong to completely different kingdoms, but in general, Protozoa refers to those organisms which do not carry out photosynthesis. Parasitic protozoa comprise a number of subgroups: The Sarcomastigophora (amebas and flagellates), The Ciliates (ciliated organisms), the Sporozoa (malaria, *Toxoplasma*, *Cryptosporidium* and allies), and Microsporidia.

Pupa: The dormant stage in the life cycle of some insects where the larva changes into the adult or imago.

Red Queen hypothesis: Hypothesis that states that the adaptive importance of genetic recombination is to create genetic variation among the offspring, which is important in confrontation with coevolving parasites.

Resistance: Reduction in host susceptibility to infection. Resting period during unfavorable conditions *e.g.* during winter freezing or during draughts.

Richness: Number of parasite species per host individual or the mean number of parasite species within members of the host population.

Ringworm: A commonly mistaken term. Ringworm is the common name given to skin infections by certain fungi. The correct term is Tinea. The condition is not caused by a worm at all, and the name dates from a time where all ailments were blamed on worms of some description.

Selection: Process by which certain phenotypes are favored over other phenotypes. Selection leads to adaptation. Clonal selection is found when clones differ in their lifetime reproductive success and is usually seen in the form of genotype frequency changes.

Sex allocation: Allocation of resources into male and female functions. For *Daphnia*, which reproduce asexually for most of the life cycle and thus produce mostly daughters, sex allocation refers to the extent to which males and resting eggs are produced.

Shell gland: Organ found in *Daphnia* that may have a role in excretion and/or osmo-regulation.

Species Diversity: Community diversity that takes into account both species richness and the relative abundance of species = diversity index (D) minus number of species (N) plus relative abundance.

Species Richness: The total number of species in a community depends on bio-geographical conditions.

Species: In taxonomy, a group of organisms whose members have the same structural traits and who can interbreed with each other.

Specificity: Describes the observation that only a subset of hosts is susceptible to infection. A high specificity refers to the observation that only a few host lines can be infected by a given parasite.

Spore bank: Spores resting in soil or sediments.

Spore load: Number of spores or sporophorous vesicles of a parasite (e.g., microsporidium, bacterial) in a host individual. It is a measure of parasite infection intensity and may be used to calculate parasite multiplication rate within the host.

Spore: In a parasitological context, transmission stage.

Sporozoan A group of single celled organisms which are characterized by having a sexual and an asexual generation in their life cycle. Examples of parasitic Sporozoans include the malarial parasites, *Toxoplasma* and *Cryptosporidium*.

Succession: The orderly progression of changes in a community composition that occurs during development of vegetation in any area; from initial colonization to the attainment of the climax typical of a particular geographic area.

Susceptible: Accessible to or liable to infection by a particular parasite.

Symbiont: Organism living together with another organism. This includes mutualists, parasites, and commensals.

Tapeworm*:*   Name for the parasitic flatworms forming the class Cestoda. All tapeworms spend the adult phase of their lives as parasites in the gut of a vertebrate animal (called the primary host). Most tapeworms spend part of their life cycle in the tissues of one or more other animals (called intermediate hosts), which may be vertebrates or arthropods.

Transmission stage: Life stage of a parasite that is able to cause a new infection.

Transmission: The process by which a parasite passes from a source of infection to a new host. Horizontal transmission is transmission by direct contact between infected and susceptible individuals or between disease vectors and susceptible individuals. Vertical transmission occurs when a parent conveys an infection to its unborn offspring, as in HIV in humans.

Trophozoite*:*   The active or feeding stage of a single-celled organism.

Vertical transmission: Parasite transmission from parent to offspring.

Virulence: Morbidity and mortality of a host that is caused by parasites and pathogens. More specifically, it is the fitness component of the parasite that is associated with the harm done to the host.

Wolbachia: Intracellular bacteria that commonly infect a variety of arthropod species and induce various changes in its hosts' life history, sex allocation, and sex ratio.

Worm*:* A multicellular organism which is generally longer than it is wide or deep. The scientific name for worms is *Helminth*. In human parasitic terms there are three major groups of organisms which are properly called worms: The Nematodes, the Flukes and the Tapeworms. These and other sorts of worms may parasitize other organisms *e.g.* Acanthacephalans (thorny headed worms) and Gordians (horsehair worms). Other sorts of worms are free living *e.g.* free living nematodes, Annelids *e.g.* earthworms, polychaetes, leeches, etc. Planarians and other Turbellarians.

Zoonosis*:* An infection of a human by an organism which is usually parasitic in other hosts. For example, since hydatid tapeworms are usually found in dogs and sheep, hydatid disease is usually considered to be a zoonosis in humans.

Zooplankton: Animal component of small aquatic organisms that mainly drift with water movements. They include protozoans, small crustaceans, and in early summer, the larval stages of many larger organisms.

Bibliography

Alongi, D.M., (1996). The dynamics of benthic nutrient pools and fluxes in tropical mangrove forests. *J. Mar Res*, 54: 123-148.

Anderson, J.H. (1975). Reproductive efficiency of beef and dairy cows under beef management. Ames, Iowa State University Library. (Thesis)

Armstrong, D.T., Michalska, A., Ashman, R.J., Bessoudo, E., Seamark, R.F., Vize, P. and Wells, J.R.E. (1987). Gene transfer in goats: methodologies and potential applications. Int. Conf. on Goats, Brasilia, 1987.

Bateman N. (1974). Growth in mice after selection on maize-milk diets. *Anim. Prod.*, 19:233.

Bell, A.E. and Burris, M.J. (1973). Simultaneous selection for two correlated traits in Tribolium. *Genet. Res.*, 21:29.

Bereskin, B., Hetzer, H.D., Peters, W.H. and Norton, H.W. (1974). Genetic and maternal effects in pre-weaning traits in crosses of high and low-fat lines of swine. *J. Anim. Sci.*, 39: 1.

Biery, K.A., Bondioli, K.R. and de Mayo, F.J. (1988). Gene transfer by pronuclear injection in the bovine. *Theriogenology*, 29: 2-24.

Block, S.S. (Ed.). (2001). Disinfection, Sterilization, and Preservation (5ᵗʰ ed.). Philidelphia: Lippincott Williams & Wilkins.

Bockarie M.J., Taylor, M. J., Gyapong, J. O. (2009). Current practices in the management of lymphatic filariasis. *Expert Review of Anti-Infective Therapy*, 7 (5), 595-605.

Bohren, B.B. (1975). Designing artificial selection experiments for specific objectives. *Genetics*, 80: 205.

Bradford, G.E., Taylor, St. C. S., Quirke, J.F. and Hart, H. (1974). An egg transfer study of litter size, birth weight, and lamb survival. *Anim. Prod.*, 18: 249.

Brem, G. (1986). Inter- and intra-species DNA transfer. Expert Consultation on Biotechnology for Livestock Production and Health. Rome, FAO. October 1986.

Brem, G., Brenig, B., Goodman, H.M., Selden, R.C., Graf, F., Kruff, B., Springmann, K., Hondele, J., Meyer, J., Winnacker, E.L. and Kräusslich, H. (1985). Production of transgenic mice, rabbits and pigs by microinjection into pronuclei. *Zuchthygiene*, 20: 251-252.

Brem, G., Brenig, B., Kräusslich, H., Müller, M., Springmann, K. and Winnacker, E.L. (1988). Gene transfer by DNA microinjection of growth hormone genes in pigs.Eleventh International Congress on Animal Reproduction and Artificial Insemination. Dublin. June 1988.

Brinster, R.L., Sandgren, E.P., Behringer, R.R. and Palmiter, R.D. (1989). No simple solution for making transgenic mice. *Cell*, 59: 239-241.

Brown, C.J., Brown, J.E. and Butis, W.T. (1974). Evaluating relationships among immature measures of size, shape and performance of beef bulls. IV. Regression models for predicting postweaning performance of young Hereford and Angus bulls using preweaning measures of size and shape. *J. Anim. Sci.*, 38: 12.

Bryan, C., Caldwell, J. and Weseli, D.F. (1975). Analysis of the cattle histocompatibility system. *J. Anim. Sci.*, 41: 247.

Cairns, J. Jr. (1987). Disturbed Ecosystems as Opportunities for Research in Restoration Ecology. In: William Jordan et al. (eds.), Restoration Ecology: A Synthetic Approach to Ecological Research. New York. Cambridge University Press, pp. 307-319.

Cartwright, T.C., Fitzhugh, H.A. Jr. and Long, C.R. (1975). Systems analysis of sources of genetic and environmental variation in efficiency of beef production: mating plans. *J. Anim. Sci.*, 40: 433.

Ceballos, G., Ehrlich, P.R., Soberon, J., Salazar, I. and Fay, J.P., (2005). Global Mammal Conservation: what must we manage? *Science*, 309: 603-607.

Chowdhuri A.B. and A. Chowdhury (1994). Mangroves of the Sundarbans. Vol. - I: India. World Conservation, *Gland.* : 247

Christian L.L. (1972). A review of the role of genetics in animal stress susceptibility and meat quality. The Proceedings of the Pork Quality Symposium, ed. by R. Cassera, F. Grisler and Q. Kolb. University of Wisconsin Extension (Publ.) 72–0.

Church, R.B. (1987). Embryo manipulation and gene transfer in domestic animals. *TibTech*, 5: 13- 19.

Church R.B., McRae A. and McWhir J. (1986). Embryo manipulation and gene transfer in livestock production. Proc. 3rd World Congr. *Genetics Appl. Livestock Prod. Lincoln*, Nebraska. July 1986.

Clark A.J., Simons P., Wilmut I. and Lathe R. (1987). Pharmaceuticals from transgenic livestock. TibTech, 5: 20-24.

Cone R.D. and Mulligan R.C. (1984). High-efficiency gene transfer into mammalian cells: generation of helper-free recombinant retrovirus with broad mammalian host range. *Proc. Nat. Acad. Sci.*, USA, 81: 6349-6353.

Dickerson G.E. (1947). Composition of hog carcasses as influenced by heritable differences in the rate and efficiency of gain. Ames, Iowa Agricultural Experiment Station. Research Bulletin 354.

Dickerson G.E., Kunzi N., Cundiff L.V., Koch R.M., Arthaud V.H. and Gregory K.E. (1974). Selection criteria for efficient beef production. *J. Anim. Sci.*, 39: 659.

Donelson J. (2003). Antigenic variation and the African trypanosome genome Acta Tropica. Volume 85 p.391-404

Dreyer G., Noroes, J., Figueredo-Silva, J., Piessens, W. F. (2000). Pathogenesis of lymphatic disease in bancroftian filariasis: a clinical perspective. *Parasitology Today* (Personal Ed.), 16 (12), 544-548.

Drucker, Peter F. (1994). The Theory of Business. Harvard Business Review, vol. 72, no. 5. pp. 95-104.

Eisner Thomas. (1990). Prospecting for Nature's Chemical Riches. *Issues in Science and Technology*, vol. 6. pp. 31-34.

Eisner Thomas. (1992). Chemical Prospecting: A Proposal for Action. In F.H. Bormann and S.R. Kellert (eds.), Ecology, Economics, and Ethics: The Broken Circle.New Haven. Yale University Press, pp. 196-202.

Fabricant J.D., Nuti L.C., Minhas B.S., Baker W.C., Capehart L.S., Marrack P., Chalmers, J.H., Bradbury M.W. and Womack J. E. (1987). Gene transfer in goats. Theriogenology, 27: 229.

Falconer, D.S. (1973). Replicated selection for body weight in mice. *Genet. Res.*, 22: 291.

Fenn, K. Matthews, K.R. (2007). The cell biology of Trypanosoma brucei differentiation. *Current Opinion in Microbiology* Volume 10 p.539-546

Fitzhugh H.A. Jr. and Taylor St. C.S. (1971). Genetic analysis of degree of maturity. *J. Anim. Sci.*, 33: 717.

Fitzhugh H.A. Jr., Long, C.R. and Cartwright, T.C. (1975). Systems analysis of sources of genetic and environmental variation in efficiency of beef production: heterosis and complementarity. J. Anim. Sci., 40: 421.

Fleming D.O., Richardson, J.H., Tulis J.J., Vesley D. (Eds.) (1995). Laboratory Safety Principles and Practices (2nd ed.). Washington: American Society for Microbiology.

Frahm R.R. and Brown, M.A. (1975). Selection for increased preweaning and postweaning weight gain in mice. *J. Anim. Sci.*, 41: 33.

Fraser S. and Burnell D. (1970). Computer models in genetics. New York, McGraw-Hill.

Freeman, A.E. 1973. A quarter century of artificial insemination of dairy cattle: are changes and new approaches indicated? *J. Anim. Sci.*, 37: 658.

Gandolfi F., Lavitrano M., Camaioni A., Spadafora C., Siracusa G. and Lauria A. (1989). The use of sperm-mediated gene transfer for the generation of transgenic pigs. *J. Reprod. Fert.*, Abstract Series, 4: 10.

Gordon J.W., Scangos G.A., Plotkin D.J., Barbosa A. and Ruddle F.H. (1980). Genetic transformation of mouse embryos by microinjection. *Proc. Nat. Acad. Sci.* USA, 77: 7380-7384.

Gordon K., Lee, E., Vitale J.A., Smith A.E., Westphal H. and Hennighausen L. (1987). Production of human tissue plasminogen activator in transgenic mouse milk. *Biotechnology*, 5: 1183-1187.

Hammer R.E., Pursel, V.G., Caird, E., Rexroad, J., Wall, R.J., Bolt, D.J., Palmiter, R.D. and Brinster R.L. (1986). Genetic engineering of mammalian embryos. *Anim. Sci.*, 63: 269-278.

Hammer R.E., Pursel, V.G., Rexroad, C.E., Wall, R.J., Bolt, D.J., Ebert, K.M., Palmiter, R.D. and Brinster, R.L. (1985). Production of transgenic rabbits, sheep and pigs by microinjection. *Nature*, 315: 680-683.

Hanrahan J.P. and Eisen, E.J. (1974). Genetic variation in litter size and 12-day weight in mice and their relationship with postweaning growth. *Anim. Prod.*, 19: 13.

Harvey W.R. (1960). Least-squares analysis of data with unequal subclass numbers. Washington, D.C., U.S. Agricultural Research Service. ARS 20–8.

Hazel, L.N. and Lush, J.L. (1942). The efficiency of three methods of selection. *J. Hered.*, 33: 393.

Henderson C.R. (1972). Sire evaluation and genetics trends. Proceedings of the Animal Breeding and Genetic Symposium, July 1972, p. 10. American Society of Animal Science and American Dairy Science Association.

Henderson C.R. (1975). Best linear unbiased estimation and prediction under a selection model. *Biometrics*, 31: 423.

Hill W.G. (1971). Investment appraisal for national breeding programmes. *Anim. Prod.*, 13: 37.

Hill W.G. (1974). Prediction and evaluation of response to selection with overlapping generations. *Anim. Prod.*, 18: 117.

IUCN/UNEP/WWF. (1991). Caring for the Earth: A Strategy for Sustainable Living. Gland, Switzerland. World Conservation Union.

Jaenisch R. and Mintz, B. (1974). Simian virus 40 DNA sequences in DNA of healthy adult mice derived from preimplantation blastocysts injected with viral DNA. *Proc. Nat. Acad. Sci.* USA, 71: 1250-1254.

Jaenisch R. (1974). Infection of mouse blastocysts with SV 40 DNA: normal development of infected embryos and persistence SV 40-specific DNA sequences in the adult animals. *Cold Spring Harbor Symp. Quant. Biol.*, 39: 375380.

Jaenisch R. (1976). Germ line integration and Mendelian transmission of the exogenous Moloney leukemia virus. *Proc. Nat. Acad. Sci.* USA, 73: 1260.

Jimmy Borah, M. Firoz Ahmed and Pranjit Kumar Sarma, (2010). Brahmaputra River islands as potential corridors for dispersing Tigers: A case study from Assam, India. *International Journal of Biodiversity and Conservation*. Vol. - 2(11): 350-358.

Kennedy P.G.E. (2006). Human African trypanosomiasis - neurological aspects. *J Neurol* Volume 253 p.411-416

Kieffer N.M., Cartwright, T.C. and Sheek, J.E. (1972). Characterization of the double muscled syndrome: I. Genetics. College Station, Texas Agricultural Experiment Station. *Consolidated (Publ.)* PR-311-3131.

Koch R.M. Gregory, K.E. and Cundiff, L.V. (1974b). Selection in beef cattle. II. Selection response. *J. Anim. Sci.,* 39: 459.

Koch R.M., Gregory, K.E. and Cundiff, L.V. (1974a). Selection in beef cattle. I. Selection applied and generation interval. *J. Anim. Sci.,* 39: 449.

Krackhardt David, and Jeffrey R. Hanson. (1993). Informal Networks: The Company Behind the Chart. Harvard Business Review, 71(4):104-111.

Kräusslich H. and Brem, G. (1986). Economically important trait loci. Expert Consultation on Biotechnology for Livestock Production and Health. Rome, FAO. October 1986.

Laster, D.B. (1974). Factors affecting pelvic size and dystocia in beef cattle. *J. Anim. Sci.,* 38: 496.

Lathe R., Clark, A.J., Archibald, A.L., Bishop, L.O., Simons, P. and Wilmut, I. (1987). Novel products from livestock. Exploiting new technologies in animal breeding, p. 91-101. Oxford, Oxford University Press.

Lavitrano M., Camaioni, A., Fazio, V.M., Dolci, S., Farace, M.G. and Spadafora, C. (1989). Sperm cells as vectors for introducing foreign DNA into eggs: genetic transformation of mice. *Cell,* 57: 717-723.

Leggat P. A., Melrose, W., & Durrheim, D. N. (2004). Could it be lymphatic filariasis? *Journal of Travel Medicine,* 11 (1), 56-60.

Lerner I.M. and Donald, H.P. (1966). Modern development in animal breeding. London, Academic Press.

Lohse J.K., Robl, J.M. and First, N.L. (1985). Progress towards transgenic cattle. *Theriogenology* 23: 205.

Long C.R., Cartwright, T.C. and Fitzhugh, H.A. Jr. (1975). Systems analysis of sources of genetic and environmental variation in efficiency of beef production: cow size and herd management. *J. Anim. Sci.,* 40: 409.

Loskutoff N.M., Coren, B.R., Barrios, D.R., Bessoudo, E., Bowen, M.J., Stone, G. and Kraemer, D.C. (1986). Gene microinjection in bovine embryos facilitated by centrifugation. *Theriogenology,* 25: 168.

Lowrie R.C. Jr. (1983). Cryopreservation of the microfilariae of Brugia malayi, Dirofilaria corynodes and Wuchereria bancrofti. *The American Journal of Tropical Medicine and Hygiene,* 32 (1), 138-145.

Manguin, S., Bangs, M.J., Pothikasikorn, J., Chareonviriyaphap, T. (2010). Review on global co-transmission of human Plasmodium species and Wuchereria bancrofti by Anopheles mosquitoes. Infection, Genetics and Evolution: *Journal of Molecular Epidemiology and Evolutionary Genetics in Infectious Diseases,* 10(2):159-177.

Mann R., Mulligan, R.C. and Baltimore, D. (1983). Construction of a retrovirus packaging mutant and its use to produce helper-free defective retrovirus. *Cell*, 33: 153-159.

McCarthy J. (2000). Diagnosis of lymphatic filarial infection. In T. B. Nutman (Ed.),Lymphatic Filariasis (pp. 127-141). London: Imperial College Press.

McEvoy T.G., Stack, M., Barry, T. and Keane, B. (1987). Direct gene transfer by microinjection. Theriogenology, 27: 258.

McNeely J.A. (1988). Values and Benefits of Biological Diversity. In J. A. McNeely (ed.), Economics and Biological Diversity. Gland, Switzerland. International Union for the Conservation of Nature and Natural Resources. pp. 9-36.

Meganck R.A., and R.E. Saunier. (1983). What Trinidad and Tobago Must Know about Managing Our Natural Resources. *The Naturalist*, vol. 4, no. 8.

Melrose W.D. (2002). Lymphatic filariasis: new insights into an old disease. *International Journal for Parasitology*, 32 (8), 947-960.

Mercier J.C. (1987). Genetic engineering applied to milk-producing animals: some expectations. Exploiting new technologies in animal breeding, p. 122-131 Oxford, Oxford University Press.

Meyer H.H. and Bradford, G.E. (1974). Estrus, ovulation rate and body composition in selected strains of mice on ad libitum and restricted feed intake. *J. Anim. Sci.*, 38: 271.

Mintz B. (1977). Teratocarcinoma cells as vehicles for mutant and foreign genes. Genetic interaction and gene transfer. Brookhaven Symposia in Biology, 29: 82 Upton, NY, Brookhaven National Laboratories.

Morris C.A., Stewart, H.S. and Wilton, J.W. (1975). Choices among models of animal production systems. *J. Anim. Sci.*, 41: 253.

Myers Norman. (1993). The Question of Linkages in Environment and Development: We Can No Longer Afford to Split the World into Disciplinary Components.BioScience, vol. 43, no. 5. pp. 302-310.

Nancarrow, C., Marshall, J., Murray, J., Hazelton, I. and Ward, K. (1987). Production of a sheep transgenic with the ovine growth hormone gene. *Theriogenology*, 27: 263.

Nikolskala O. Lima, A. Kim, Y. Lonsdale-Eccles, J. Fukuma, T. Scharfstein, J. Grab, D. (2006). Blood-brain barrier traversal by African trypanosomes requires calcium signaling induced by parasite cysteine protease *The Journal of Clinical Investigation*. Volume 116 No. 10 p.2739-2747

Nordskog A.W., Tolman, H.S., Casey, D.W. and Lin, C.Y. (1974). Selection in small populations of chickens. *Poult. Sci.*, 53: 1188.

OAS. (1978). Environmental Quality and River Basin Development: A Model for Integrated Analysis and Planning. Washington, D.C. General Secretariat, Organization of American States.

OAS. (1984). Integrated Development Planning: Guidelines and Case Studies from OAS Experience. Washington, D.C. General Secretariat, Organization of American States.

OAS. (1987). Minimum Conflict: Guidelines for Planning the Development of American Humid Tropical Environments. Washington, D.C. General Secretariat, Organization of American States.

Olliver L. (1974). Optimum replacement rates in animal breeding. *Anim. Prod.,* 19: 257.

Oren, David C. (1988). Uma Reserva Biológica para o Marañhao. Ciencia Hoje, vol. 8, no. 44. pp. 37-45.

Orozco F. and Bell, A.E. (1974). Reciprocal recurrent selection compared to within-strain selection for increasing rate of egg lay of Tribolium under optimal and stress conditions. Genetics, 77: 143.

Palmiter R.D., Brinster, R.L., Hammer, R.E., Trumbauer, M.E., Rosenfeld, M.G., Birnberg, N.D. and Evans, R.M. (1982). Dramatic growth of mice that develop from eggs microinjected with metallothionein-growth hormone fusion genes. *Nature,* 300: 611 - 615.

Palmiter R.D., Norstedt, G., Gelinas, R.E., Hammer, R.E. and Brinster, R.L. (1983). Metallothionein-human GH fusion genes stimulate growth of mice. Sci., 222: 809-814.

Pays E. (2005). Regulation of antigen gene expression in *Trypanosoma brucei. Trends in Parasitology.* Volume 21 Number 11. 517-520

Pearson R.E. and Freeman, A.E. (1973). Effect of female culling and age distribution of the dairy herd on profitability. *J. Dairy. Sci.,* 56: 1459.

Pfarr K.M., Debrah, A.Y., Specht, S., Hoerauf, A. (2009). Filariasis and lymphoedema. *Parasite Immunology,* 31 (11), 664-672. doi:10.1111/j.1365-3024.2009.01133.x

Piedrahita J.A., Anderson, G.B., Martin, G.R., Bondurant, R.H. and Pashen, R.L. (1988). Isolation of embryonic stem cell-like colonies from porcine embryos. *Theriogenology,* 29: 286.

Powell R.L., Norman, H.D. and Dickinson, F.N. (1975). Analysis of the USDA-DHIA preliminary sire summary. *J. Dairy. Sci.,* 58: 551.

Price D.A. and Ercanbrack, S.K. (1975). Lamb production of Finnsheep crossbred ewe lambs. *J. Anim. Sci.,* 41: 255.

Public Health Agency of Canada. (2004). In Best M., Graham M. L., Leitner R., Ouellette M. and Ugwu K. (Eds.), Laboratory Biosafety Guidelines (3rd ed.). Canada: Public Health Agency of Canada.

Pumfrey R.A., Cunningham, P.J. and Zimmerman, D.R. (1975). Heritabilities of swine reproductive and performance traits. *J. Anim. Sci.,* 41: 256.

Rankin B.J. and Okidi, M.D. (1975). Twinning in a closed Hereford herd. *J. Anim. Sci.,* 41: 256.

Reed, M.L., Roessner, C.A., Womack, J.E., Dorn, C.G. and Kraemer, D.C. (1988). Microinjection of liposome-encapsulated DNA into murine and bovine blastocysts.*Theriogenology*, 29:293.

Rexroad Jr., C.E. and Wall, R.J. (1987). Development of one-cell fertilized sheep ova following microinjection into pronuclei. *Theriogenology*, 27: 611-619.

Riklefs R.E., Z. Naveh and R.E. Turner. (1984). Conservation of Ecological Processes. Gland, Switzerland. International Union for the Conservation of Nature and Natural Resources. (Commission on Ecology Paper 8)

Robertson E.J. (1986). Pluripotential stem cell lines as a route into the mouse germ line. Trends in Genetics, 2: 9-13.

Roditi I. Lehane, M.J. (2008). Interactions between trypanosomes and tsetse flies. *Current Opinion in Microbiology Volume 11.* p. 345-351

Roschlau, K., Rommel, P., Gazaryan, K.G., Andreewa, L., Roschlau, D., Hühn, R., Zackel, B., Strauss, M. and Schwerin, M. (1988). Microinjection of various vectors into pronuclei of bovine zygotes. Eleventh Int. Cong. on Animal Reproduction and Artificial Insemination, Dublin. June 1988.

Ross K., Brenig, B., Meyer, J. and Brem, G. (1988). Attempts to produce transgenic rabbits carrying MTI-HGH recombinant gene. In A.C. Beynen and H.A. Solleveld, eds.New developments in biosciences: their implications for laboratory animal science. Dordrecht, Martinus Nijhoff Publishers.

Rottmann, O.J., Stratowa, C., Hornstein, M. and Hughes, J. (1985). Tissue-specific expression of hepatitis B surface antigen in mice following hiposome-medicated gene transfer into blastocysts. *Zbl. Vot. Med.*, A 32: 676-682.

Rubenstein, J.L.R., Nicolas, J.F. and Jacob, B.F. (1986). Introduction of genes into preimplantation mouse embryos by use of a detective recombinant retrovirus. *Proc. Nat. Acad. Sci. USA*, 83: 330-368.

Ryan K.J., Ray C.G. (Eds.). (2004). Sherris Medical Microbiology An Introduction to Infectious Diseases (4th ed.). United States of America: McGraw-Hill.

Rylands A.B. (1991). The Status of Conservation Areas in the Brazilian Amazon. Washington, D.C. World Wildlife Fund.

Salter D.W., Smith, E.J., Hughes, S.H., Wright, S.E. and Crittenden, L.B. (1986). Retroviruses as vectors for germ line insertion in the chicken. Proc. 3rd World Congr. Genetics Appl. Livestock Prod. Lincoln, Nebraska, July 1986.

Sanders J.O., Cartwright, T.C. and Long, C.R. (1975). Casual components of maternally influenced characters. *J. Anim. Sci.*, 41: 257.

Sanyal P., (1999). Sundarbans- The largest mangrove diversity on Globe. *In:* D.N. Guha Bhakshi, P. Sanyal and K.R. Naskar (eds.). Sundarbans Mangal. Naya prakash, Calcutta: pp. 199-204.

Saunier Richard E. (1983). A Future Together? Development Forum, Vol. XI, no. 8, Nov-Dec.

Saunier Richard E. (1984). Regional Approaches Utilized in Development Planning. Natural Resource Technical Bulletin, no. 5. (AID-NPS Natural Resources Project).

Saunier Richard E. (1993). The Place of Tourism in Island Ecosystems. Paper presented to the Regional Conference on Health and Sustainable Tourism Development (Nassau, Bahamas, 9-11 Nov. 1993).

Schipper J., Chansson, J.S., Chiozza, F., Cox, N.A., Hoffmann, M., Katariya, V. (2008). The status of the world s land and marine mammals: diversity, threat and knowledge. *Science,* 322: 225-230.

Seidensticker J. and M.A. Hai, (1983). The Sundarbans Wildlife Management Plan. Conservation in the Bangladesh Coastal Zone, IUCN, Gland. : 120Burley F. William. (1988). Monitoring Biological Diversity for Setting Priorities in Conservation. In: E.O. Wilson (ed.), Biodiversity. Washington, D.C. National Academy Press, pp. 227-230.

Shaffer M.L. (1981). Minimum Population Sizes for Species Conservation. *BioScience*, vol. 31, no. 30. pp. 131-134.

Shenoy R.K. (2008). Clinical and pathological aspects of filarial lymphedema and its management. *The Korean Journal of Parasitology,* 46 (3), 119-125.

Simons, J.P., McClenaghan, M. and Clark, A.J. (1987). Alteration of the quality of milk by expression of sheep B-lactoglobulin in transgenic mice. *Nature,* 328: 530-532.

Skjervold H. (1966). Selection schemes in relation to artificial insemination. Report of proceedings, 9th International Congress of Animal Production, Edinburgh. p. 250.

Smith C., Meuwissen, T.H.E. and Gibson, J.P. (1987). On the use of transgenes in livestock improvement. *Anim. Breed.* Abstr., 55: 1-10.

Soriano P., Cone, R.D., Mulligan, C. and Jaenisch, R. (1986). Tissue-specific and ectopic expression of genes introduced into transgenic mice by retroviruses. *Sci.*234: 1409-1913.

Soulé Michael E. (1986). Conservation Biology: The Science of Scarcity and Diversity. Sunderland, Mass. Sinauer Assoc.

Staeheli P., Haller, O., Boll, W., Lindenmann, J. and Weissman, C. (1986). Mx protein: constitutive expression in 3T3 cells transformed with cloned Mx cDNA confers selective resistance to influenza virus. *Cell,* 44: 147-158.

Stewart C.L., Schuetze, S., Vanek, M. and Wagner, E.F. (1987). Expression of retroviral vectors in transgenic mice obtained by embryo infection. *EMBO-J.,* 6: 383-388.

Stewart C.L., Vanek, M. and Wagner, E.F. (1985). Expression of foreign genes from retroviral vectors in mouse teratocarcinoma chimeras. *EMBO-J.,* 4: 3701-3709.

Stuhlmann, H., Jähner, D. and Jaenisch, R. (1981). Infectivity and methylation of retroviral genomes is correlated with expression in the animal. *Cell,* 26: 221-232.

U.S. Meat Animal Research Center. (1975). Germ plasm evaluation program. Progress Report 2.

Udvardy M.D.F. (1975). A Classification of the Biogeographical Provinces of the World. Morges, Switzerland. International Union for the Conservation of Nature. (IUCN Occasional Paper No. 18)

US Department of Health and Human Services. (1999). Biosafety in Microbiological and Biomedical Laboratories. In J. Y. Richmond, R. W. McKinney (Eds.), (4th ed., pp. 118). Washington, D.C.: U.S. Government Printing Office.

Van der Putten, H., Botteri, F.M., Miller, A.D., Rosenfeld, M.G., Fan, H., Evans, R. and Verma, M. (1985). Efficient insertion of genes to the mouse germ line via retroviral vectors. *Proc. Nat. Acad. Sci.* USA, 82: 6148-6152.

Vassella E. Oberle, M. Urwyler,S. Renggli, C.K. Studer, E. Hemphill, A. Fragoso, C. Butikofer, P. Brun, R. Roditi,I. (2009). Major Surface Glycoproteins of Insect Forms of Trypanosoma brucei Are Not Essential for Cyclical Transmission by Tsetse, PLoS Volume 4 Issue 2 e4493.

Vize P.D., Michalska, A., Ashman, R., Seamark, R.F. and Wells, J.R.E. (1987). Improving growth in transgenic farm animals. EMBO Workshop Germline Manipulation of Animals, Nethybridge, Scotland, UK. 1987.

Wagner, E.F., Covarrubias, L., Stewart, T.A. and Mintz, B. (1983). Prenatal lethalities in mice homozygous for human growth hormone gene sequences integrated in the germ line. *Cell*, 35: 647-655

Wall R.J., Pursel, V.G., Hammer, R.W. and Brinster, R.L. (1985). Development of porcine ova that were centrifuged to permit visualization of pronuclei and nuclei. *Biol. of Reprod.*, 32: 645-651

Ward K.A., Franklin, I.R., Murray, J.D., Nancarrow, C.D., Raphael, K.A., Rigby, N.W., Byrne, C.R., Wilson, B.W. and Hunt, C.L. (1986). The direct transfer of DNA by embryo microinjection. Proc. 3rd World Congr. *Genetics Appl.* Livestock Prod. Lincoln, Nebraska. June 1986.

Ward K.A., Murray, J.D. and Nancarrow, D.D. (1986). The insertion of foreign DNA into animal cells. Expert Consultation on Biotechnology for Livestock Production and Health. Rome, FAO. July 1986.

Westman Walter E. (1985). Ecology, Impact Assessment, and Environmental Planning. New York. John Wiley and Sons.

Wilson E.O. (1984). Biophilia. Cambridge, Mass. Harvard University Press.

World Health Organization. (1993). Laboratory Biosafety Manual (2nd ed.)

WRI/UNEP/UNDP. (1992). World Resources 1992-93. New York. Oxford University Press.

Zimmerman D.R. and Chnningham P.J. (1975). Selection for ovulation rate in swine: population procedures and ovulation response. *J. Anim. Sci.*, 40: 61.

Appendices

Appendix-1

Scheduled Mammals
Schedule- I (Wild Life Protection Act)

S.No.	Schedule- I Mammals	Scientific Name
1.	Black Buck- Buck Black	*Antelope cervicapra*
2.	White Buck-Buck White	*Antilope cervicapra*
3.	Leopard Cat -Cat Jungle	*Felis bengalensis*
4.	Chinkara - Chinkara- Indian Gazella	*Gazella bennetti*
5.	Chowsingha	*Tetraceros quadricornis*
6.	Deer Brow- Antlered	*Cervus eldi eldi*
7.	Swamp Deer -Swamp Deer (Barasingha)	*Cervus duvauceli*
8.	Asiatic Elephant-Elephant Indian	*Elephas maximus*
9.	Hoolock Gibbon-Gibbon Hoolock	*Hylobates hoolock*
10.	Leopard/Panther	*Panthera pardus*
11.	Asiatic Lion-Lion Indian	*Panthera leo persica*
12.	Lion - Tailed Macaque—Macaque-Lion- Tailed	*Macaca silensus*
13.	Horned Rhinoceros-Rhinoceros Indian	*Rhinoceros unicornis*
14.	Royal Bengal Tiger	*Panthera tigris tigris*
15.	Wolf	*Canis lupus pallipes*
16.	Gaur	*Bos gaurus*

Appendix-1 Contd...

Scheduled Mammals

Schedule- I (Wild Life Protection Act)

S.No.	Schedule- I Mammals	Scientific Name
17.	Himalayan Black Bear- Bear Himalayan Black	*Selenarctos thibetanus*
18.	Sloth Bear—Bearsloth	*Melursus ursinus*
19.	Small Indian Civet—Civet Small Indian	*Viverricula indica*
20.	Common Palm Civet Or Toddy Cat— Civet Common Palm Toddy Cat	*Paradoxurus hermaphroditus*
21.	Jackal	*Canis aureus*
22.	Common Langur—Langur Common	*Presbytis entellus*
23.	Bonnet Macaque—Macaque Bonnet	*Macaca radiata*
24.	Rhesus Macaque —Macaque Rhesus	*Macaca mulatta*
25.	Stump Tailed Macaque—Macaque Stump Tailed	*Macaca speciosa*
26.	Indian Porcupine—Porcupine Indian	*Hystrix indica* (*Vulpes bengalensis*)
27.	Fox Common	*Vulpes bengalensis*

Appendix-2

Scheduled Birds

Schedule- I (Wild life Protection Act)

S.No.	Birds in captivity	Scientific name
1.	Hornbill Indian Great	*Buceros bicornis*
2.	Hornbill Grey	*Ocyceros birostris*
3.	Peafowl (White)	*Pavo cristatus*
4.	Spoonbill White	*Platalea leucorodia*

Scheduled Birds

Schedule- I (Wild life Protection Act)

Some Indian Common Bird species and their scientific Name

S.No.	Birds in captivity	Scientific name
1.	Eagle Crested Serpent	*Spilornis cheela*
2.	Yellow throated Sparrow	*Petronia xanthocollis*
3.	Egret Little	*Egretta garzetta*
4.	Ibis White	*Threskiornis melanocephala*
5.	Fowl Jungle Red	*Gallus gallus*
6.	Heron Grey	*Ardea cinerea*
7.	Kite	*Milvus migrans*
8.	Munia Black Headed	*Lonchura malacca*
9.	Munia Green	*Estrilda formosa*
10.	Munia Spotted	*Lonchura punctulata*
11.	Myna Hill	*Gracula religiosa*
12.	Owl Barn	*Tyto alba*
13.	Owl Screech	*Megascops*
14.	Owl Great Horned	*Bubo bubo*
15.	Parakeet Large Indian	*Psittacula eupatria*
16.	Parakeet Rose Ringed	*Psittacula krameri*
17.	Parakeet Red Breasted	*Psittacula krameri*
18.	Parakeet Blossom Headed	*Psittacula cyanocephala*
19.	Partridge Grey	*Francolinus pondicerianus*
20.	Pelican Rosy / White	*Pelecanus onocrotalus*
21.	Pheasant Kalij Indian	*Lophura leucomelana*
22.	Shikra	*Accipiter badius*
23.	Stork Black Necked	*Xenorhynchus asiaticus*
24.	Stork Lesser Adjutant	*Leptoptilos javanicus*
25.	Stork Painted	*Ibis leucocephalus*
26.	Vulture White	*Neophron percnopterus*

Append.ix-3

WILDLIFE INSTITUTE OF INDIA

Wildlife Institute of India was established in 1982 as an attached office of the Ministry of Environment and Forests. Subsequently, it was granted autonomous status in 1986. The institute is mandated by Government of India to carry out research on various aspects on Wild Life conservation, conduct training programmes for capacity building of Wild Life managers, build up repository of knowledge of Wild Life and provide technical and advisory services to the State and Central Governments in the country.

States/UTs	No of NPs	Area km²	No. of WLS	Area km²	No. of Cons Res Res.	Area km²	No. of Comm. Res Res.	Area km²	No. of PAs	Area km²
Andhra Pradesh	6	1388.39	21	11618.12					27	13006.5
Arunachal Pradesh	2	2290.82	11	7487.75					13	9778.57
Assam	5	1977.79	18	1932.01					23	3909.8
Bihar	1	335.65	12	2851.67					13	3187.32
Chhattisgarh	3	2899.08	11	3583.19					14	6482.27
Goa	1	107	6	647.91					7	754.91
Gujarat	4	479.67	23	16619.81	1	227			28	17326.5
Haryana	2	48.25	8	233.21	2	48.72			12	330.18
Himachal Pradesh	5	2271.38	32	7745.48					37	10016.9
Jammu & Kashmir	4	3925	15	10243.11	34	829.75			53	14997.9
Jharkhand	1	226.33	11	1955.82					12	2182.15
Karnataka	5	2472.18	22	4003.42	2	3.8	1	3.12	30	6482.52
Kerala	6	558.16	16	1822.86			1	1.5	23	2382.52
Madhya Pradesh	9	3656.36	25	7158.41					34	10814.8

Contd...

Appendix-3: Contd..

States/UTs	No ofNPs	Areakm²	No. of WLS	Area km²	No. of Cons Res Res.	Area km²	No. of Comm. Res.	Area km²	No. of PAs	Area km²
Maharashtra	6	1273.6	35	14152.7	1	3.49			42	15429.8
Manipur	1	40	1	184.4					2	224.4
Meghalaya	2	267.48	3	34.2					5	301.68
Mizoram	2	150	8	1090.75					10	1240.75
Nagaland	1	202.02	3	20.34					4	222.36
Orissa	2	990.7	18	6969.15					20	7959.85
Punjab	0	0	13	330.86	1	4.95		16.07	16	351.88
Rajasthan	5	3947.07	25	5379.26	3	222.27	2		33	9548.6
Sikkim	1	1784	7	399.1					8	2183.1
Tamil Nadu	5	307.85	21	3521.95	1	0.03			27	3829.83
Tripura	2	36.71	4	566.93					6	603.64
Uttar Pradesh	1	490	23	5221.88					24	5711.88
Uttarakhand	6	4915.44	7	2688.56	2	42.27			15	7646.27
West Bengal	5	1693.25	15	1203.28					20	2896.53
Andaman & Nicobar	9	1153.94	96	389.39					105	1543.33
Chandigarh	0	0	2	26.01					2	26.01
Dadra & Nagar Haveli	0	0	0	1	92.16				1	92.16
Daman & Diu	0	0	1	2.19					1	2.19

Contd...

Appendix-3: Contd..

Appendix-3: Contd...

States/UTs	No ofNPs	Area km²	No. of WLS	Area km²	No. of Cons Res Res.	Area km²	No. of Comm. Res.	Area km²	No. of PAs	Area km²
Delhi	0	0	1	27.82					1	27.82
Lakshadweep	0	0	1	0.01					1	0.01
Pondicherry	0	0	1	3.9					1	3.9
India	102	39888.12	517	120207.6	47	1382.28	4	20.69	670	161499

Appendix-4

Base line Data Collection for Ecology and Bio-diversity

Sampling Locations

Randomly selected quadrates in the proposed study area/project site and the other habitats within study area.

Terrestrial Environment

a. Sampling

(a) The part of the terrestrial environment within the study area will be surveyed by using site specific methodology for its flora and fauna. For present study of schedule of flora and/or faunal species, wild life protection act 1972 and amended time to time will be referred.

(b) Most of the villages in the study area and the sites of floristic and faunal importance likes, lakes, ravines, hills, hillocks and forest, if any present in the study area will be surveyed to document its floral and faunal diversity.

(c) For floristic survey, point quarter plot less/point centred quadrate sampling method will be followed.

(d) Vegetation measurements will be determined from points rather than being determined in an area with boundaries.

(e) For documentation of faunal diversity, opportunistic observation / Species list method / Direct sighting / Intensive Search / bird calls/ Micro-habitat search/ pugmarks and footprint observation / debarking observation and indirect sighting etc. will be followed.

(f) The Quantitative Assessment, like, frequency, abundance, diversity indices etc. will be followed of standard method.

(g) The sampling conducted only once during the study period/season.

(h) Secondary data collection from authenticated sources like BSI, ZSI, MoEF, EIC, FSI etc.

b. Parameters

1. Flora in the study area
   - Trees
   - Shrubs
   - Herbs
   - Climbers
2. Cultivated plants in the study area.
3. Floristic composition of the study area

4. Medicinal plants of the study area

5. Status of the forest, their category in the study area

7. Rare and endangered flora in the study area

8. Endemic plants in the study area

9. Fauna in the study area

- Reptiles

- Amphibians

- Birds

- Mammals

- Butterflies

10. Rare and Endangered fauna in the study area

11. Endemic fauna in the study area

12. Wild life and their conservation importance in the study area.

c. Evaluation of Ecological sensitivity

Ecological sensitivity of study area will be analyzed based on the following criteria-

(a) Wild life importance

(b) Floral Endemicity

(c) Faunal Endemicity

(d) State of Terrestrial vegetation

(e) State of wet land vegetation

(f) Mangrove vegetation

(g) Conservation importance

(h) Legal status (National park, Wild life sanctuary, Reserve forest, Wetlands, Agricultural lands)

(i) Lakes /reservoirs/dam

(j) Natural lakes and Swamps

(k) Breeding ground of Migratory and Residential birds

Aquatic Environment

The representative samples from the aquatic environment collected by Depth Sampler from the large inland water bodies (Lakes, dams, reservoir, large village ponds), if any in the study area, filtered in Plankton net (20 μm mesh size) using 1L capacity Polypropylene bottle having double stopper capacity. The sampling method followed of APHA 1995 and amended. The filtered samples will be concentrated by using the centrifuge. By using Lackey's drops method and light microscope the quantitative analysis will be carried out for phytoplankton and zooplankton. The standard flora and other literature will be followed for the qualitative evaluation of Plankton.

Parameters

a. Phytoplankton

- Cell count units/m^3
- Total genera
- Major genera

b. Zooplankton

- Population count units/m^3
- Total genera
- Major genera

Sources of Secondary Information for Ecology and Biodiversity

S.No.	Purpose	Source
1.	List of Plants(Floral Diversity)	Botanical Survey of India (BSI), Kolkata and regional officesRegional Forest DepartmentEnvironmental Information System (ENVIS), IndiaGovernment of India Directory
2.	List of Animals(Faunal Diversity)	Zoological Survey of India (ZSI), Kolkata and regional officesChief Wildlife Warden Environmental Information System (ENVIS), IndiaGovernment of India Directory
3.	Taxonomic studies	International Association for Plant Taxonomy (IAPT)International Plant Name Index (IPNI)Royal Botanic Garden, Kew, UK Zoological Survey of India (ZSI), KolkataBotanical Survey of India (BSI), Kolkata
4.	Forest and its type(Forest Diversity)	Forest Survey of India (FSI), DehradunIndian Council of Forestry Research & Education (ICFRE), DehradunFrench Institute PondicheryIndian Institute of Remote Sensing (IIRS), DehradunNational Remote Sensing Centre (NRSC)Ministry of Environment and Forests (MoEF), New Delhi
5.	Diversity of Western/Eastern Ghat	Salim Ali Institute of Ornithology and Natural History CoimbatoreTropical Botanical garden & research Institute CoimbatoreKerla Forest Research Institute Peechi, KerlaIndian Institute of Science BangaloreCentre for Ecological Science Bangalore
6.	Mountain Diversity/ Himalayan Diversity/North Eastern Diversity	G.B. Pant Institute of Himalayan Environment & Development Regional centers of ZSI DehradunWild Life Institute of India DehradunInstitute of Bioresource Shillong

Contd...

Appendix-4 :Contd...

S.No.	Purpose	Source
7.	Desert Biodiversity	Central Arid Zone Research Institute JodhpurBombay Natural History Society (BHNS), MumbaiSalim Ali Institute of Ornithology and Natural History CoimbatoreWild Life Institute of India DehradunWorld Wildlife Fund IndiaZoological Survey of India (ZSI),
8.	Wild Animals	Wildlife Institute of India (WII), DehradunEnvironmental Information System (ENVIS), India Ministry of Environment and Forests (MoEF), New Delhi
9.	List of Mangroves	Conservation and Management of Mangroves (CMM), New Delhi.Global Environment Facility (GEF)Ministry of Environment and Forests (MoEF), New Delhi
10.	List of Avifauna	Bombay Natural History Society (BHNS), MumbaiEnvironmental Information System (ENVIS), IndiaSalim Ali Centre for Ornithology and Natural History, CoimbatoreNature Club Surat (Gujarat)Bird Life International (UK) and its Regional Offices (www.birdlife.org)
11.	List of Medicinal Plants	Central Institute of Medical and Aromatic Plants (CIMAP), LucknowEnvironmental Information System (ENVIS), India
12.	Coastal and Marina diversity	Central Marine Fisheries Research Institute (CMFRI), New DelhiNational instate of Ocenography Goa.Botanical Survey of India Portblair.M.S. Swaminathan Reseach Foundation ChennaiMadras Science Foundation ChennaiCoastal Zone Management Authority (CZMA), New DelhiEnvironmental Information System (ENVIS), India Ministry of Environment and Forests (MoEF), New DelhiCentral Board of Irrigation and Power (CBIP)
13.	Wetland Diversity	Bombay Natural History Society (BHNS), MumbaiSalim Ali Institute of Ornithology and Natural History CoimbatoreWild Life Institute of India DehradunWorld Wild life Fund Zoological Survey of India (ZSI),KolkataWetland of India (MoEF) new Delhi.Environmental Information System (ENVIS), IndiaMinistry of Environment and Forests (MoEF), New Delhi
14.	Agricultural information	Indian Agricultural Research Institute (IARI), New DelhiMinistry of Environment and Forests (MoEF), New Delhi
15.	EndemicityRareEndangered	International Union for Conservation of Nature (IUCN)Wildlife Institute of India (WII), DehradunWorld Conservation Monitoring Centre (WCMC), UKNational Biodiversity Authority (NBA)*National Biodiversity Data Bank (NBDB)*

Contd...

Appendix-4 :Contd...

S.No.	Purpose	Source
16	Conservation plan	International Union for Conservation of Nature (IUCN)World Conservation Monitoring Centre (WCMC), UKWildlife Institute of India (WII), DehradunNational Bureau of Plant Genetic Resources (NBPGR), New DelhiNational Tiger Conservation Authority (NTCA)National Botanic Research Institute (NBRI), LucknowNational Dairy Research Institute (NDRI), Haryana
17	Offences/Crimes	Tiger and Other Endangered Species Crime Control Bureau (TOESCCB).Wildlife Crime Control Bureau (WCCB).
18	Heritage	National Museum of Natural History (NMNH), New DelhiNatural History Museum, London, UK
19	Island Diversity	Zoological Survey of India (ZSI),National Instate of Oceanography, GoaCentral Marine Fisheries Research Institute (CMRI), New Delhi
20	Effect of pollutants on biodiversity	Central Pollution Control Board (CPCB), New DelhiState Pollution Control Board (SPCB), StatesAmerican Public Health Association (APHA).

Appendix- 5

Helminth Diseases

Diseases	Infectious Agent	Discovery and	Disease Control Development and Implementation Research
Lympathic filariasis (Elephantiasis)	*Wuchereria bancrofti, Brugia timori nematode worms*	Drugs (adult worm), drug resistance, animal models, vaccine	Robust, easy and affordable easy and affordable diagnostics, improved vector control
Schistosomiasis (Bilharzia)	*Schistosoma flatworms*	Vaccines, drug resistance	Diagnostics, vector control
Ascariasis	*Ascaris lumbricoides*	Vaccines, drug efficacy	Easy and affordable diagnostics, improved vector control
Trichuriasis	*Trichuris trichiura* (whipworm).	Vaccines	Easy and affordable diagnostics, improved vector control
Hookworm	*Ancylostoma duodenale* and *Necator americanus*	Drugs and drug targets; drug resistance, vaccines	Easy and affordable diagnostics, improved vector control

Appedix-6

Protozoan Disease, Tests and Therapy

Name	Mode of Transmission	Symptoms
Flagellates		
G lamblia	Contaminated water, fecal-oral	Nausea, bloating, gas, diarrhea, anorexia
Dientamoeba	Fecal-oral, associated with *Enterobius*	Previously thought commensal; may *fragilis* cause diarrhea, abdominal, pain, nausea
Amoebas		
Entamoeba histolytica	Contaminated water, fecal-oral, contaminated food	Colitis, dysentery, diarrhea, liver abscess, other extraintestinal disease
Spore-forming (Coccidia)		
Cryptosporidium	Contaminated water, swimming pools, fecal-oral	Immunocompetent patients: Self-limited diarrhea Immunosuppressed patients: Severe and interminable diarrhea
Isospora belli	Fecal-oral	Same as in *Cryptosporidium*
Cyclospora cayetanensis	Fecal-oral, contaminated water and food	Same as in *Cryptosporidium*
Microsporidia (Septata intestinalis, Enterocytozoon bieneusi)	Fecal-oral, contaminated water	Same as in *Cryptosporidium*
Ciliates		
Balantidium coli	Fecal-oral (frequently associated with pigs)	Colitis, diarrhea
Other		
Blastocystis hominis	Fecal-oral	May cause mild diarrhea

Recommended Test

Organism	Size (mm)	Stain Used	Other Tests
E. histolytica	Trophozoite: 10-60 Cyst: 10-20	Wet mount,* trichrome, periodic Schiff	Enzyme-linked immunosorbent assay (ELISA)
G. lamblia	Trophozoite: 9-21 Cyst: 7-12	Wet mount,*trichrome, hematoxylin, Lugol	ELISA*
C. parvum	2-5	Modified acid-fast,* auramine-rhodamine, Sheafer method	ELISA*
I. belli	30x12	Wet mount,* modified acid-fast*	None
C. cayetanensis	8-10	Modified acid-fast,* wet mount	Electron microscopy
Microsporidia	1-2	Modified trichrome*	Electron microscopy, fluorescence methods, small intestine biopsy
D. fragilis	7-12	Iron hematoxylin,* trichrome*	None
B. coli	50-200	Wet mount,* concentration techniques	None
B. hominis	5-30	Trichrome,* iron * hematoxylin	None

Specific Therapy for Intestinal Protozoal Infections

Organism	Drugs, Pediatric Dose, and Treatment Duration
E. histolytica **(Luminal disease or** **colonization)**	Iodoquinol: 40 mg/kg/d PO divided tid for 20 d; not to exceed 2 g/d Paromomycin: 25-30 mg/kg/d PO divided tid for 7 d
E. histolytica **(Moderate colitis)**	Metronidazole: 50 mg/kg/d PO divided tid for 10 d Tinidazole: 50 mg/kg/d PO for 3 d; not to exceed 2 g/d
E. histolytica (Severe **colitis or liver abscess)**	Metronidazole: 50 mg/kg/d PO divided tid for 10 d Dehydroemetine*: 1-1.5 mg/kg/d divided bid PO for 5 d Tinidazole†: 50 mg/kg/d PO for 3-5 d; not to exceed 2 g/d
G. lamblia	Metronidazole: 15-20 mg/kg/d PO divided tid for 5 Tinidazole: 50 mg/kg/d PO once; not to exceed 2 g/dose Quinacrine‡: 6 mg/kg/d PO divided tid for 5 d; not to exceed 300 mg/d Furazolidone: 6 mg/kg/d PO divided qid for 7-10 d Paromomycin: 40 mg/kg/d PO divided tid for 7 d Nitazoxanide: 200-400 mg/d PO divided bid for 3 d
D. fragilis	Iodoquinol: 50 mg/kg/d PO divided tid for 20 d; not to exceed 2 g/d Paromomycin: 30 mg/kg/d PO divided tid for 7 d Tetracycline: 40 mg/kg/d PO divided qid for 10 d; not to exceed 2 g/d

Contd.

Contd...

Organism	Drugs, Pediatric Dose, and Treatment Duration
C. parvum	Paromomycin*: 30 mg/kg/d PO divided tid (duration unknown)
	Nitazoxanide: 200-400 mg/d PO divided bid for 3 d
I. belli	Trimethoprim/sulfamethoxazole (TMP/SMZ): 20/100 mg/kg/d PO divided
	bid for 10 d, followed by 10/50 mg/kg/d PO divided bid for 21 d
C cayetanensis	TMP/SMZ: 10/50 mg/kg/d PO divided bid for 3 d
Microsporidia	Albendazole* (adult dose): 800 mg/d PO divided bid
S. intestinalis	
Microsporidia	No treatment recommended; albendazole may decrease the number of
E bieneusi	organisms
B. coli	Tetracycline: 40 mg/kg/d PO divided qid for 10 d; not to exceed 2 g/d
	Metronidazole: 35-50 mg/kg/d PO divided tid for 5 d
	Iodoquinol: 40 mg/kg/d PO divided tid for 20 d
B. hominis	Metronidazole: 35-50 mg/kg/d PO divided tid for 10 d
	Iodoquinol: 40 mg/kg/d PO divided tid for 20 d
	Nitazoxanide: 500 mg/d PO divided bid for 3 d

'Efficacy is unknown.

§Recommended regimens are indicated only in patients who are immunosuppressed. A recent meta-analysis has not shown evidence for a reduction in the duration or frequency of diarrhea by nitazoxanide or paromomycin when compared with placebo in immunosuppressed patients, nevertheless, oocyst clearance was significantly reduced.

Appendix -7

Only Six Northern White Rhinos left in the World

The southern white rhino having common names White rhinoceros, square-lipped rhinoceros; Rhinocéros blanc (Fr); Rinoceronte. Scieitific name is Ceratotherium simum. Together with the greater one-horned rhino, the white rhino is the largest of all rhino species. Its name comes from the Dutch weit (wide), in reference to the animal's wide muzzle. It is also known as the square-lipped rhinoceros due to its squared (not pointed) upper lip. Compared to black rhinos, white rhinos have a longer skull, a less sharply defined forehead and a more pronounced shoulder hump. They have almost no hair and two horns. The front horn averages 60 cm, but occasionally reaches 150 cm in length. Size varies 150-185 cm in height, females weigh 1,400-1,700 kg, males weigh 2,000-3,600 kg. White rhinos appear to require thick bush cover, relatively flat terrain, water for drinking and wallowing, and short grass for grazing. They primarily inhabit grassy savanna and woodlands interspersed with grassy clearings. The ainmals tend to avoid the heat during the day, when they rest in the shade. They are usually active in the early morning, late afternoon and evening. During very hot periods, the cool and rid themselves of ectoparasites (external parasites) by bathing in mud in shallow pools. Adult males can spend almost their entire life in these areas, unless water is unavailable, in which case they follow a narrow corridor to a drinking site every 3-4 days. Females reach sexual maturity at 4-5 years of age but do not reproduce until they reach 6-7 years. In contrast, males tend not to mate until they are 10-12 years old. They can live up to 40 years. Breeding pairs may stay together for up to 20 days. Mating occurs throughout the year although peaks have been observed from October to December in South Africa and from February to June in East Africa. The gestation period is approximately 16 months with a period of 2-3 years between calves. Suni, a 37-year-old northern white rhino and only the second male of his kind left in the world, died recently of natural causes in the Ol Pejeta Conservancy reserve in Kenya. After his death merely six other specimens are now alive that still carries the legacy of this subspecies. Conservation efforts were heavily direct towards Suni, but now that the rhino is dead, all hope for the species lies with only one male and, of course, frozen sperm samples. All of the northern white rhino left in the world can only be finding in captivity; the last wild specimen died long ago. Suni was the first northern white rhino ever to be born in captivity, the conservancy said in a statement. He was one of four northern whites transferred from the Dvur Králové Zoo in the Czech Republic to Ol Pejeta in 2009 as part of the Last Chance to Survive project.

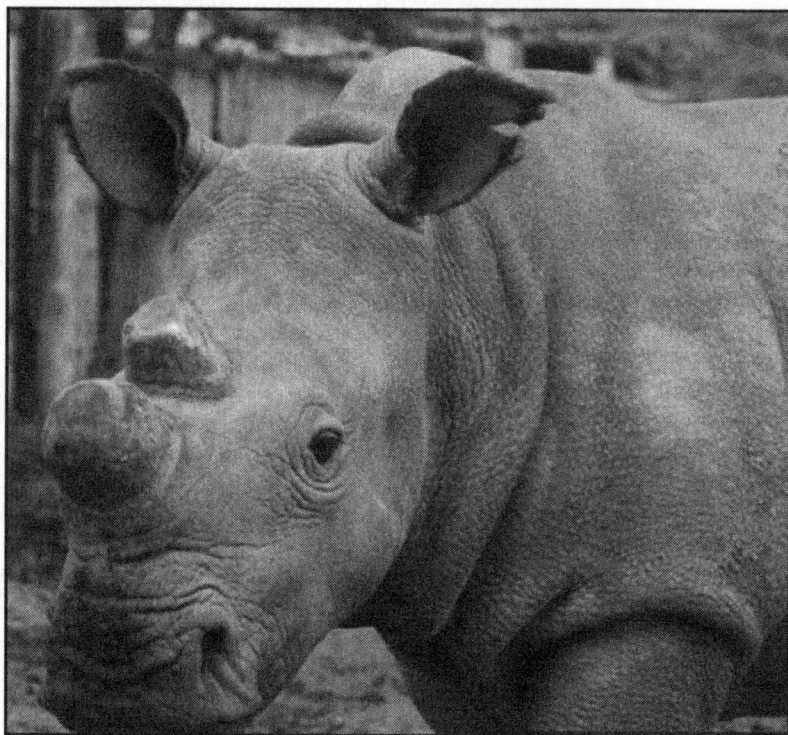

Rhino Suni at the Ol Pejeta Conservancy in Kenya

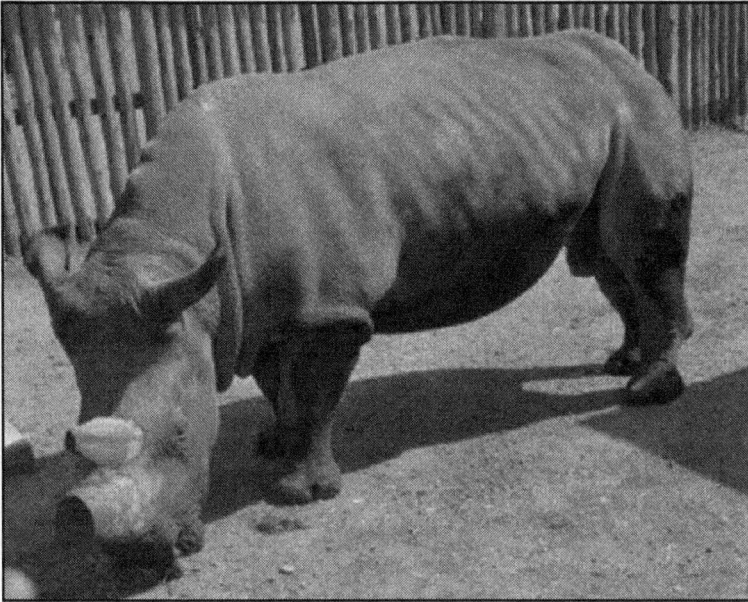

Rhino Suni after arriving at Ol Pejeta in 2009

The northern white rhino is one of two subspecies of the white rhino. The other subspecies, the southern white rhino, is estimated to number at about 20,000, according to the World Wildlife Fund. The northern white rhino seems to follow the same path at the hand of a common enemy, poachers. In fact, all African rhinos are under major threat from poachers, with some studies citing that wild rhinos could become extinct by 2020. It's not the meat or the skin the poachers are after; their trophy is the rhino's horn. Actually, this is what personally makes me the angriest. As it was not enough poachers are killing threatened species without any breach of conscious, they're doing it to supply a black market based on a whole load of mombo-jambo. All of the horns get shipped to south-east Asia where they're grounded into a powder that's thought to cure diseases such as cancer. The horn, made of a substance similar to human hair known as keratin, is more valuable by weight than gold ($65,000/kg). Of course, there isn't a published study that remotely links rhino powder with anti-cancer activity. Three northern white rhinos, Najin, Fatu and Sudan, remain at the Ol Pejeta Conservancy. One northern white rhino remains at the Dvur Králové Zoo and two remain at the San Diego Zoo.

Main Threats

Hunting and Poaching: Uncontrolled hunting in the colonial era was historically the major factor in the decline of white rhinos, and poaching for their horn continues to be the main threat. The white rhino is particularly vulnerable to hunting, because it is relatively unaggressive and occurs in herds. Efforts to protect the few remaining northern rhino have been severely disrupted because of the ongoing civil war in the

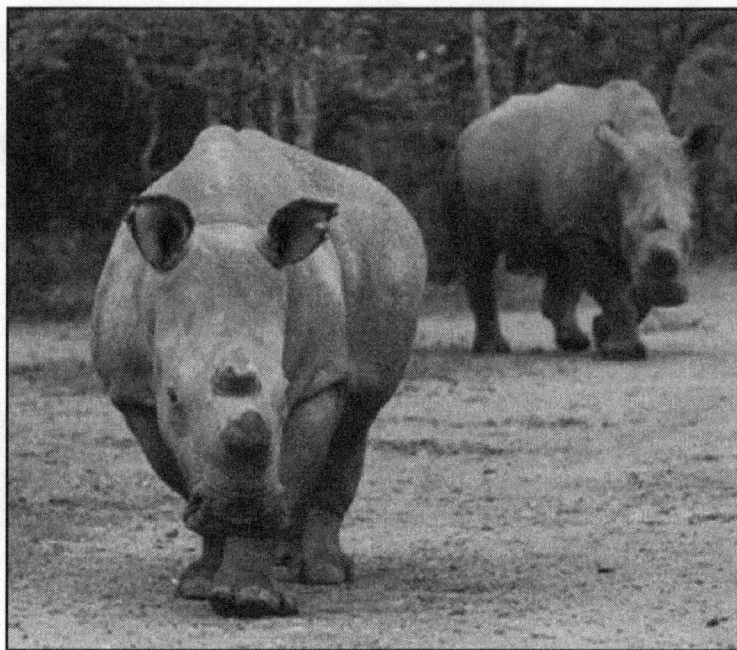

Sudan and Najin, two of the remaining northern white rhinos, at the Ol Pejeta Conservancy in Kenya

Democratic Republic of Congo and incursions by poachers coming mainly from Sudan. Thanks to the dedication of park staff through years of armed conflict in the region, this Critically Endangered subspecies still survives, but for how much longer?

Habitat Loss: Loss of habitat to agriculture and human settlement poses a secondary threat.

Appendix -8

Unique Bull (Murrah Buffalo- *Bubalus bubalis*)

A Unique Bull (Murrah Buffalo) in Haryana is worth Rs. 7 Crores. This bull by name Yuvraj is a celebrity in Haryana. The bull is owned by Karamvir Singh of Sunario, Kurukshetra and has the good fortune of sleeping in an air-conditioned room. It stood 1st in Meerut Cattle show on Oct 2014. At five years, he is 14-feet in length and is 5.7 feet tall. Now, its height is 5'.10", its weighs 1400 kgs, it is 14 feet wide. It is Water buffalo breed (*Bubalus bubalis*) and is considered as the foremost milking buffalo. Karamveer Dairy Farm has a fairly spacious, well designed and lush green area used as a multipurpose farm.

The owner is Karam Veer Singh who is bringing it up as his own son. Total 4 workers take of this bull. It has a special shed with a fan and security. He drinks 20 liters milk every day besides a bottle of country liquor. Its food is 15 kg grass and 5 kg

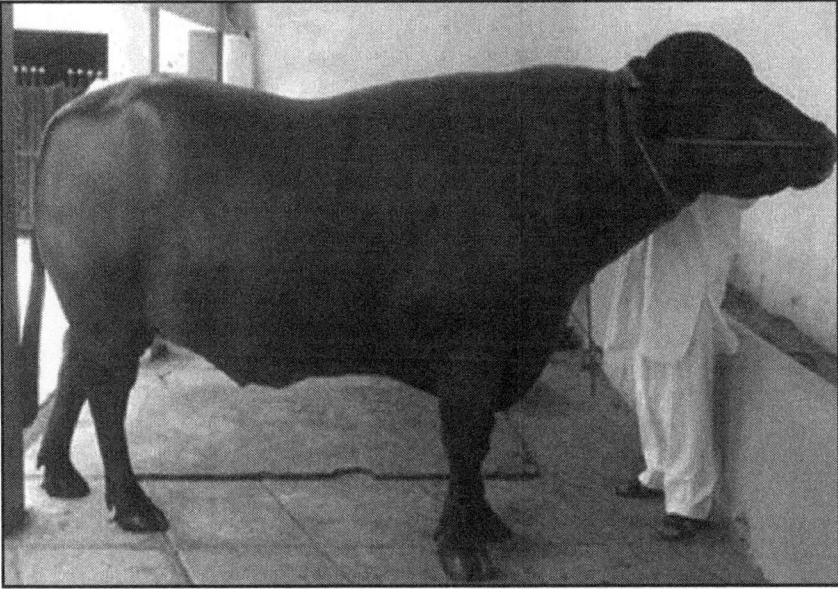

apples daily. It gives milk worth 30,000 per day. Apart from that 50 Lakhs per year earning is done through other sources. Chandigarh businessmen offered 7 crores to buy. But, still Karam Veer Singh rejected the offer. Karamvir Singh earn close to Rs 50 lakh a year from Yuvraj. Murrah is originally from Punjab and Haryana states of India and Punjab province of Pakistan, but has been used to improve the milk production of dairy buffalo in other countries, such as Italy and Egypt.

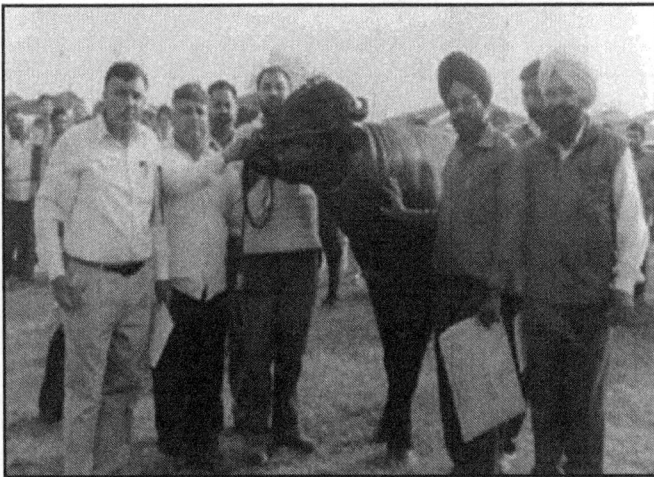

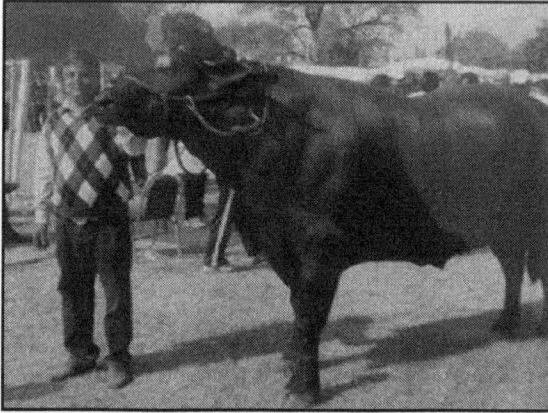

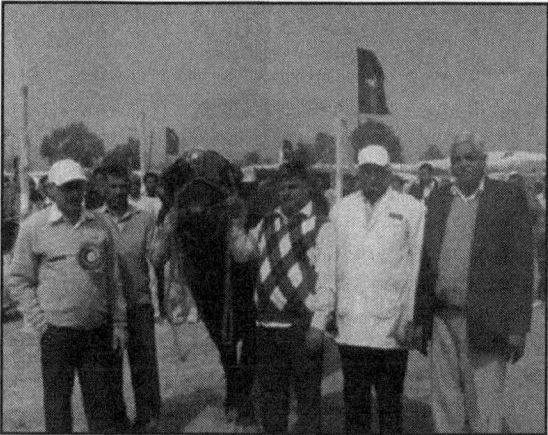

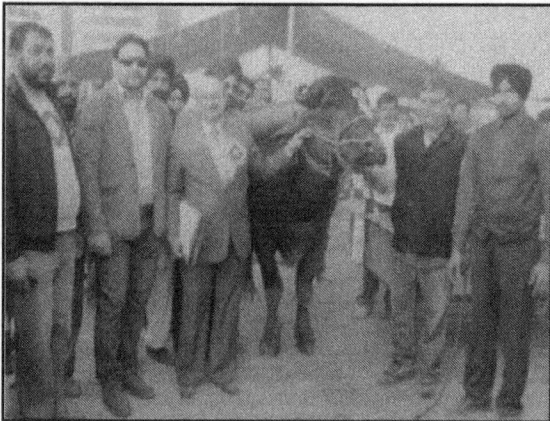